Fundamentals of Cancer Epidemiology

Philip C. Nasca, PhD
Professor of Epidemiology and Chair
Department of Biostatistics and Epidemiology
School of Public Health and Health Sciences
University of Massachusetts at Amherst
Amherst, Massachusetts

Harris Pastides, PhD, MPH
Professor of Epidemiology
Dean
Norman J. Arnold School of Public Health
University of South Carolina
Columbia, South Carolina

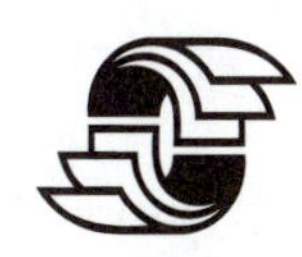

AN ASPEN PUBLICATION®
Aspen Publishers, Inc.
Gaithersburg, Maryland
2001

Library of Congress Cataloging-in-Publication Data

Fundamentals of cancer epidemiology/[edited by] Philip C. Nasca, Harris Pastides.
p. ; cm.
Includes bibliographical references and index.
ISBN 0-8342-1776-7
1. Cancer—Epidemiology. I. Nasca, Philip C. II. Pastides, Harris.
[DNLM: 1. Neoplasms—epidemiology. 2. Epidemiologic Methods.
3. Neoplasms—etiology. QZ 200 F9823 2001]
RA645.C3 F86 2001
614.5'9994—dc21
2001016068

Orders: (800) 638-8437
Customer Service: (800) 234-1660

Editorial Services: Joan Sesma
Library of Congress Catalog Card Number: 2001016068
ISBN: 0-8342-1776-7

Printed in the United States of America

1 2 3 4 5

With sincere appreciation to
my wife and best friend, Bonnie,
for her support and understanding;
to my children, Andrea, Christopher, Anthony, and Jason,
for their support and their ability to let me see the humorous side of life;
to the many students I have taught cancer epidemiology to over the years—
they have made teaching a delight.

PCN
Amherst, Massachusetts

With extreme gratitude to
my life partners, Patricia, Katharine, Andrew,
and Barbara—the best is yet to come!
to the students who I have had the honor of teaching over the past two decades—
they have made the hard work worthwhile;
to Robert Gilligan, MD, for providing so many experiences that led to insight,
understanding, and growth;
to Norman and Gerry Sue Arnold, who have taught me about cancer in ways
that books never could.

HP
Columbia, South Carolina

Contents

Contributors

Lisa Chasan-Taber, ScD
Assistant Professor of Epidemiology
Department of Biostatistics and Epidemiology
University of Massachusetts
Amherst, Massachusetts

James J. McSharry, PhD
Professor
Center for Immunology and Microbial Disease
Albany Medical College
Albany, New York

Wei Zheng, MD, PhD
Professor
Department of Medicine
Vanderbilt University School of Medicine
Nashville, Tennessee

Foreword

In order to address the diverse features of the cancer epidemic, scientists have advanced theories, developed research methods, and acquired knowledge directed toward the creation of effective intervention programs. As a result, a plethora of publications has emerged, aimed at equipping researchers and practitioners with the skills needed to study the complex causes of this widely feared disease and discover worthwhile treatments.

There are several books that address the morbidity, mortality, and risk factors of various cancers as well as the effectiveness of current treatments. *Fundamentals of Cancer Epidemiology* has some unique features that set it apart from others. It is primarily designed to be used by students in introductory survey courses on cancer epidemiology and by professionals administering cancer prevention and control programs. As a consequence, the book offers a succinct account of risk factors, methods of investigation, and approaches to intervention.

The book is intentionally not organized according to site-specific cancers. Rather, it first covers the biology of the cell, the use of biomarkers, and the role of genetic factors in cancer research. It then reviews the cancer risk factors that are found in the environment or are related to lifestyle. The reader, especially if new to this area of inquiry, can appreciate the magnitude of the cancer problem, the nuances of its genesis, and the means to lessen its burden by combating its risk factors.

The cancer researchers of the future and those who will be in a position to devise policies for the control and prevention of cancer must gain a broad understanding of and critical insight into the study of the putative causes of cancer and the application of intervention methods. They will find their needs met by this book.

Michel A. Ibrahim, MD, PhD
Professor of Epidemiology and Social Medicine
University of North Carolina at Chapel Hill

Preface

As long-time teachers of cancer epidemiology courses in graduate schools of public health, we often face the difficulty of selecting a course textbook. Although there are numerous books that cover aspects of cancer biology or present the epidemiology of cancer from a site-specific perspective, we felt that no single book offered a treatment of cancer epidemiology at a level appropriate for first-time students. In *Fundamentals of Cancer Epidemiology,* we offer students and others wishing to learn more about cancer an introduction to the current understanding of what cancer is, how it develops biologically and genetically, the "who, when, and where" of cancer (its descriptive epidemiology), and the determinants of cancer. Although this book is not a methods text per se, we have included discussions of pertinent methodological issues in order to provide students with an epidemiological framework for evaluating hypotheses concerning the etiologic role of various risk factors as well as for developing rational preventive measures.

The book is divided into two parts. The objective of the first part is to provide an overview of

- the magnitude and distribution of various cancers in the population (Chapter 1)
- the classification of human cancers (Chapter 2)
- the biology of the normal cell and the cancerous cell (Chapters 3 and 4)
- the role of experimental data in determining the etiology of various cancers (Chapter 5)
- the expanding role of biomarkers in epidemiologic research (Chapter 6)
- the epidemiologic study of genetic factors in cancer (Chapter 7)

The second part is devoted to cancer risk factors that, based on current evidence, have the potential to affect the incidence of various human cancers to a substantial degree. These risk factors include

- occupational exposures (Chapter 8)
- tobacco (Chapter 9)
- alcohol (Chapter 10)
- ionizing, nonionizing, and solar radiation (Chapter 11)
- viruses (Chapter 12); immunodeficiency (Chapter 13)
- endogenous hormones (Chapter 14)

- exogenous hormones (Chapter 15)
- nutritional factors (Chapter 16)

To add separate chapters on each major cancer site would have made the text too long for a standard introductory course. In any case, site-specific information is widely accessible in monographs and via the Internet (note that Appendix A contains a list of cancer-related informational web sites).

Fundamentals of Cancer Epidemiology is intended for use in cancer epidemiology courses in schools of public health as well as in schools of medicine, dentistry, and nursing and allied health programs. It is also directed toward individuals who work in cancer prevention and control programs in local, state, and federal agencies and who need a handy overview of the field. We assume that readers will have completed an introductory course in epidemiology. If they have not, we suggest that a good introductory epidemiology text be used in conjunction with this book. Although our overall goal was to create a text suitable for a typical 15-week graduate course, in developing it we assumed that it would be supplemented by instructor-prepared course notes and selected readings from the literature. In any case, whether the readers are graduate students or workers in the field of cancer prevention, our hope is that *Fundamentals of Cancer Epidemiology* will provide them with a basic understanding of cancer epidemiology and stimulate some to pursue their interest in this field as they continue their education or professional development.

Finally, we would like to acknowledge the help we received in bringing this book to completion. We offer sincere appreciation to Susan Hall, Jeannie McBride, and Rona Serhan for their assistance with important organizational tasks, including creating original artwork, obtaining permissions for the use of materials from other sources, and other activities too numerous to mention. They also read and critiqued the text from a student's point of view—an invaluable service. Thanks also to Sam Harper for his able research assistance and to Pam Pope for extensive editorial assistance in the "late stages." And special thanks to Ann Latrobe for supplying valuable information included in several of the chapters. Lastly, we are indebted to Christian Milord for his careful copyediting of the manuscript. Everyone involved with this project has made the book better; it was truly a team effort.

Philip C. Nasca
Harris Pastides

Chapter 1

The Descriptive Epidemiology of Cancer

Harris Pastides

Before epidemiologists or other health scientists can design studies to analyze the causes of a particular cancer, they must attain a thorough understanding of the distribution of new cases of the disease throughout communities or larger populations. Where is it found in greater frequency? Does it appear to cluster, and, if so, is there something unusual about the environment where it is most common? Are males or females affected more commonly? What about its distribution among racial, ethnic, and economic groups? Answers to these questions can provide critical leads about causation but the information will not be sufficient for determining the cause. Nevertheless, the design of an epidemiological study will benefit from such information.

Information about the distribution of cancer within the United States and internationally is facilitated by population-based cancer registries that record and summarize data on new cases of cancer in a population. Information, usually derived from registries, is available in publications from the American Cancer Society, the National Cancer Institute, the International Agency for Research on Cancer, and other organizations. Cancer incidence and mortality vary considerably throughout the United States by state and also by gender. Across the world, there is even greater variation in the frequency of cancer. Some of the variation is due to differing diagnostic standards and access to medical care, although some is undoubtedly due to an underlying difference in exposure to risk factors by the populations being compared. Migrant studies compare cancer incidence or mortality rates for ethnic populations that have relocated with the rates that prevail in the country of origin as well as the country of adoption. These studies can shed light on the relative importance of genetic and environmental factors in the etiology of cancer.

Cancer epidemiologists have justifiably achieved a prominent place alongside other scientists engaged in the search for the causes of and cures for cancer. Much of the esteem they have won is a result of high-profile studies linking cancer with tobacco, radiation, nutritional factors, and other risk factors. Less celebrated are the countless reports describing the frequency of occurrence of cancer, the time trends in cancer rates, and the national and international geographic patterns of cancer incidence and mortality. The statistics derived from these "descriptive epidemiology" studies nonetheless continue to serve as the foundations of analytic studies. This is because etiologic hypotheses are often generated after careful observation of where and when specific cancers seem to be occurring at a higher rate than the background or expected rate. Of course, an etiologic hypothesis thus generated may be verified or may be discredited by subsequent epidemiological or other scientific research.

Descriptive studies are typically less useful when designed to address etiologic questions. Sometimes community concerns about apparent clusters of cancer have led to the use of descriptive epidemiological studies to confirm or allay suspicions of environmental cancer hazards. For example, it has been suggested that women who live in areas in which nuclear energy reactors are situated suffer high rates of breast cancer mortality and that the high rates are due to radiation "fallout."[1] A comprehensive descriptive epidemiology study done by the National Cancer Institute (NCI) did not support this hypothesis,[2] in part because different boundaries dividing "exposed" and comparison populations were used, and additional descriptive studies would be unlikely to help in determining the validity of the hypothesis. Properly designed cohort or case-control studies would be far better able to address the issue of causality because they could estimate the lifetime radiation exposures of women, with and without breast cancer, and also adjust for potential confounding factors that might influence descriptive studies.

Regardless of whether the motivation for conducting descriptive studies is to generate or test hypotheses, they must be designed, conducted, and analyzed with no less care than studies intended to examine risk factor associations with cancer. If proper care is not taken, descriptive studies will divert scientific resources, especially public health department resources, away from more productive activities.

Descriptive epidemiology studies can also be used to evaluate cancer control activities. The US Food and Drug Administration and the numerous equivalent national agencies worldwide serve as arbiters of proposed new drugs, devices, and medical procedures. Descriptive studies can be used to monitor compliance and medical outcomes once new treatments are approved for practice. Additionally, these studies can help evaluate the effectiveness of educational, health promotional, screening, and other interventions aimed at reducing cancer risk among healthy persons and mitigating adverse outcomes among cancer patients.

SOURCES OF INFORMATION

There is a wealth of information available to students and others interested in learning about the incidence and mortality rates of cancer and related trends in the United States and worldwide. Some of the best sources, such as the National Cancer Institute, the American Cancer Society, and the World Health Organization's International Agency for Research on Cancer (IARC), offer documents published in print and electronically. The three organizations mentioned can be accessed through the World Wide Web and may provide expert information in response to specific questions, depending on their nature.

Incidence rates and five-year survival rates are published regularly by the SEER (Surveillance, Epidemiology, and End Results) Program of NCI.[3] This program periodically reports cancer statistics from regions encompassing about 10% of US inhabitants. Additionally, recent decades have seen an impressive increase in the number of states that operate populations-based cancer registries. These are excellent sources of up-to-date information and usually can provide detailed statistics on cancer rates at the level of special interest for a particular group of researchers (eg, the town or county level).

Table 1–1 provides a variety of World Wide Web addresses, including those for the American Cancer Society, the US National Cancer Institute, and the World Health Orga-

Table 1–1 Major Cancer Resources on the World Wide Web

Organization Name	*Address*
National Cancer Institute	http://cancernet.nci.nih.gov
American Cancer Society	http://www.cancer.org
World Health Organization	http://www.who.int/
SEER Cancer Statistics	http://www-seer.ims.nci.nih.gov
International Agency for Research on Cancer	http://www.iarc.fr/
Oncolink	http://cancer.med.upenn.edu

nization. The Web sites of these organizations can be extremely useful for students, cancer patients and their families, and others interested in statistical and related information (see also Appendix A).

THE MAGNITUDE OF CANCER

Cancer Incidence and Prevalence

Projecting the number of new cases of cancer in the United States is an important task given that we have no national cancer registration system. By applying a statistical forecasting model to annual age-specific cancer incidence rates and age-specific population projections from the US Census, researchers predicted that in 2000 about 1,220,100 Americans received a diagnosis of cancer exclusive of basal and squamous cell skin cancers and in situ carcinoma for all sites except the urinary bladder, with another 1.3 million Americans diagnosed with generally noninvasive skin cancers.[4]

Over the course of a lifetime, about one of every two males and one of every three females in the United States will develop an invasive cancer. This estimate should dispel the belief held by some that cancer is a rare condition. The prevalence of cancer obviously represents an enormous burden of physical pain, psychological distress (for the patients themselves and their families and friends), and financial cost (for under- and uninsured patients and for the society at large).

Figure 1–1 presents the estimated percent distribution of new cancer cases, by sex, in the United States in 2000 exclusive of in situ cancers and basal and squamous cell skin cancers. Among men, the prostate is the predominant site affected by cancer. In fact, about 3 of every 10 men who develop cancer in the United States will develop prostate cancer. Lung cancer, which has a much higher case-fatality rate, has been decreasing in men over the past decade owing to a reduction in smoking among men during the last several decades. Still, lung cancer is the second most common type of cancer in men, and many opportunities exist for reducing its incidence even further. Cancers of the colon and rectum in combination rank third in frequency among males in the United States (these cancers are often grouped together in statistical presentations because of the difficulty of specifying the site of origin exactly).

Among women, breast cancer is the most commonly diagnosed cancer; it is responsible for nearly one-third of all new cancer diagnoses in women in the United States.

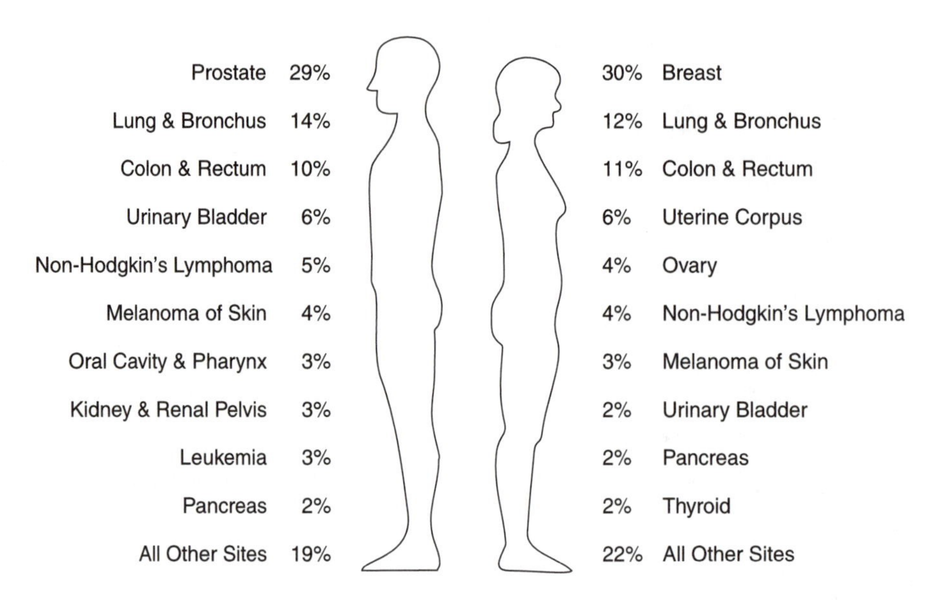

Figure 1–1 Estimated new cancer cases, 10 leading sites by sex, United States, 2000. *Note:* Data for all sites except the urinary bladder exclude basal and squamous cell skin cancers and in situ carcinomas. Also, percentages may not total 100% due to rounding. *Source:* Reprinted with permission from R.T. Greenlee, et al., Cancer Statistics 2000, *CA - A Cancer Journal for Clinicians*, Vol. 50, pp. 7–33, © 2000, Lippincott Williams & Wilkins.

Disappointingly, lung cancer is on the rise among American women and has surpassed colon and rectal cancers as the second most commonly diagnosed cancer. The upward trend in smoking among women, especially teenagers and younger women, ranks as one of the major public health failures of the recent past. Breast, lung, and colon and rectum cancers together account for over half of all the new cancers detected in women in the United States each year.

Cancer among children is much less common than among adults, yet it is the second leading cause of death among children aged 1–14 in the United States. It is estimated that between 8,000 and 9,000 new cases of cancer of all types are diagnosed in children each year. Three-quarters are cases of leukemia or brain and other central nervous system cancers.[5] Fortunately, five-year relative survival rates for childhood cancers at all sites combined improved from 56% in 1974–1976 to 75% in 1989–1995.

Since the early 1970s, the cancer incidence rate among children below age 15 has been rising. Relatively rapid increases in incidence have been observed for acute lymphoblastic leukemia, brain cancer (glioma), osteogenic sarcoma, and Wilms' tumor. The increases, because of their size, are unlikely to be due to statistical variability, improvement in diagnostic capabilities, or better reporting. The reasons for the rising incidence of these childhood cancers remain largely unknown, although numerous hypotheses about environmental causes, including residential proximity to electromagnetic fields and hazardous waste sites, have been put forth.

Cancer Mortality

In recent years, the American Cancer Society has reported an unprecedented reduction in the cancer death rate in the population of the United States.[5] Although a gradual decline in cancer mortality had been suspected since 1994, the first documented reversal in the upward trend occurred in 1998. On the surface, this turnaround would seem to be a cause for celebration. Yet some researchers see larger opportunities for influencing cancer mortality in the fields of primary and secondary prevention and view the vast sums of money spent on cancer treatment (part of the "war on cancer") as having had a disappointing payoff.

Bailar and Gornick,[6] for instance, conducted a comprehensive analysis of site-specific cancer mortality data collected by the National Center for Health Statistics and the National Cancer Institute and demonstrated that death rates had actually been rising slowly but steadily until recently. They suggest that the important recent declines in cancers of the cervix, endometrium, colon, rectum, stomach, and lung cancer in men are mainly the result of decreasing incidence or earlier detection rather than improved treatment and that the small increases in mortality from melanoma, cancer of the brain, prostate cancer, and breast cancer (in older women) reflect increasing disease incidence at these sites. These and other scientists have argued for a shift in funding priorities by the government and other sponsors to take advantage of the large cancer prevention opportunities that exist.

Researchers at the American Cancer Society have used similar data to estimate the number of cancer deaths that were expected in 2000.[5] In this year, about 552,000 Americans will die of cancer, or about 1,500 persons per day. That means cancer will be responsible for between one out of four and one out of five deaths, making it the second leading cause of death in the United States after heart disease. As epidemiology and preventive medicine have continued to achieve great success in elucidating the primary causes of heart disease and implemented effective primary and secondary prevention programs, death rates for this leading cause of death have declined markedly. Advances in clinical therapeutics and emergency medical services have, of course, also been significant. One consequence of this success, coupled with the slightly increasing trend in total cancer incidence, is that the relative proportion of total deaths due to cancer has been increasing.

Evidence that cancer mortality rates are declining in the United States was provided in a recent review of age-adjusted mortality rates from Vital Statistics of the United States reports and from the SEER Program. Data indicate that between 1990 and 1995 the reduction in total cancer mortality was 3.1%.[7] Major reductions were observed for lung cancer (3.9%) and for other smoking-related cancers (2%). Continued vigilance with respect to smoking, continued improvement in the design of cancer prevention programs, improvements in cancer treatment, and greater access to effective cancer treatment are expected to help sustain this decline in future years.

Figure 1–2 shows the sex-specific cancer death rates that were projected for the year 2000. As can be seen, these do not mimic the incidence rates shown in Figure 1–1. Although prostate cancer is the most common cancer among men and breast cancer is the most common cancer among women, lung cancer is the leading cause of cancer death

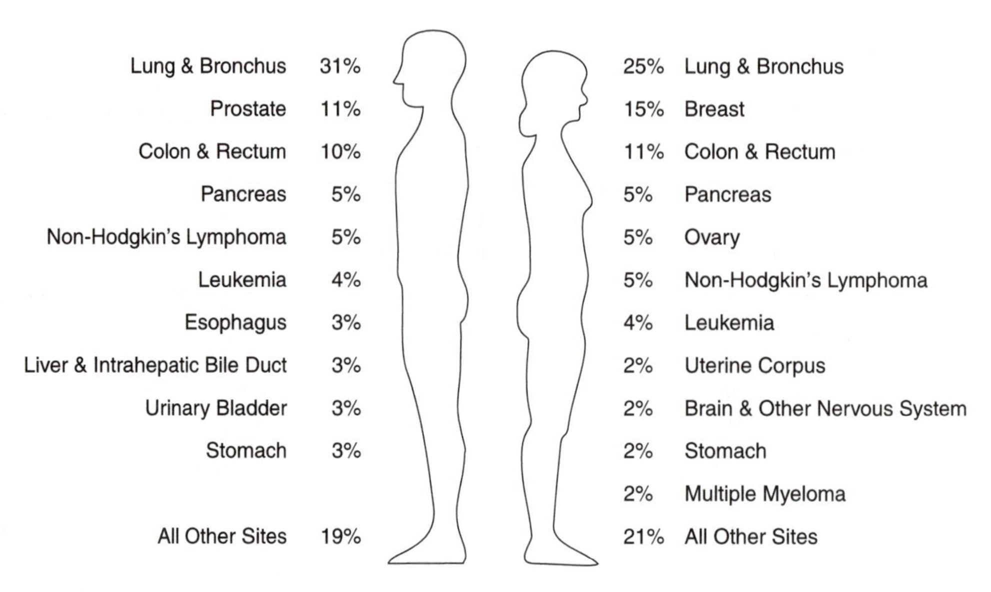

Figure 1–2 Estimated cancer deaths, 10 leading sites by sex, United States, 2000. *Note:* Data for all sites except the urinary bladder exclude in situ carcinomas. Also, percentages may not total 100% due to rounding. *Source:* Reprinted with permission from R.T. Greenlee, et al., Cancer Statistics 2000, *CA - A Cancer Journal for Clinicians*, Vol. 50, pp. 7–33, © 2000, Lippincott Williams & Wilkins.

among men and women in the United States. This is true despite the fact that lung cancer remains one of the most preventable cancers, and in fact prostate, breast, and colon and rectal cancers (other leading causes of cancer death in the United States) are also amenable to primary or secondary prevention techniques.

Cancer is the second leading cause of death among children aged 1–14 in the United States (following accidents) and is the leading fatal disease. About 1,500 deaths per year are attributable to cancer in this age group. In 1997, the cancer death rate, which has been falling for the past two decades, was 2.7 per 100,000 children aged 1–14, or 10.8% of total deaths.[5]

Given recent progress in the early identification of cancer and in cancer treatment, it is predictable that the prevalence of cancer will increase because patients will survive longer. In the United States, an estimated 10 million people currently have cancer. If that estimate is close to accurate, the prevalence of cancer is roughly 3.75% (based on a population estimate of approximately 267 million). Although the life expectancy of people with cancer who survive for at least five years is about the same as for people without cancer, the majority of the former will die of complications related to their cancer diagnosis.

Survival Rates

Cancer survival rates have improved immensely during this century. In the 1930s, fewer than 20% of patients diagnosed with cancer survived for five years. Today about

60% can expect five years of survival, and the five-year survival rate for children under age 15 is about 75%. Undoubtedly, the rapid improvement in survival rates is attributable to several factors, including advances in clinical diagnostics and therapeutic interventions and more effective public health strategies (these have jointly resulted in earlier diagnosis of cancer). The promotion of public awareness of early warning signs of cancer and the introduction of mass screening programs aimed at uncovering latent or "subclinical" cancer have created an environment in which cancer is being identified at earlier stages than ever before. Yet work is needed in this area to extend the opportunities for enhanced survival to the economically disadvantaged segments of the US population, which have not realized the same increases in survival as the rest of the population.

Temporal Trends

As described above, total cancer incidence and mortality in the United States has been rising slightly until recently, when both indicators saw a slight decline. Between 1930 and 1992, the age-adjusted rate of total cancer mortality rose by 17%, from 143 per 100,000 population to 192 per 100,000. The major contributor to this rise was the increase in lung cancer deaths among both males and females. Figures 1–3 and 1–4 show that, during the same period in which the lung cancer mortality rate was increasing, mortality rates for most of the other leading causes of cancer death either decreased (eg, stomach cancer in males and females and uterine cancer in females) or remained fairly constant. In fact, if the lung cancer death rate is omitted, the total age-adjusted death rate for cancer declined 15% between 1950 and 1991.[8] Unfortunately, the lung cancer death rate is continuing to rise among women.

The percentage change in cancer mortality, on a site-specific basis, over the past 30 years is presented in Table 1–2. Site-specific declines in mortality rates may be attributed to declining incidence, earlier diagnosis, advances in treatment and care in general, or any combination thereof. As can be seen, declines have occurred for over half of the cancer sites listed for both males and females.

In examining cancer incidence and mortality trends, it is usually preferable to compare rates on a site-specific or histology-specific basis. Total cancer incidence and mortality rates are each a weighted average of the site-specific rates, and therefore a large increase or decrease in one type of cancer over time may obscure a smaller opposite trend among other cancer types. Also, improvements in diagnostic accuracy could lead to the misperception that a specific cell or histologic type of cancer has been increasing.

GEOGRAPHIC VARIATION OF CANCER

A careful examination of the geographic variation in cancer rates and in cancer risk factors is an excellent starting point for generating hypotheses about the etiologic factors that are responsible for cancer. Indeed, descriptive studies should precede case-control and cohort studies, for, among other things, they can help epidemiologists find the best populations for recruiting subjects. Assisted by information from geographic cancer surveys, which may include maps where incidence or mortality patterns are "geocoded," investigators may decide to select subjects in areas where the occurrence of a particular cancer is high in order to test etiologic hypotheses regarding risk factors for that cancer.

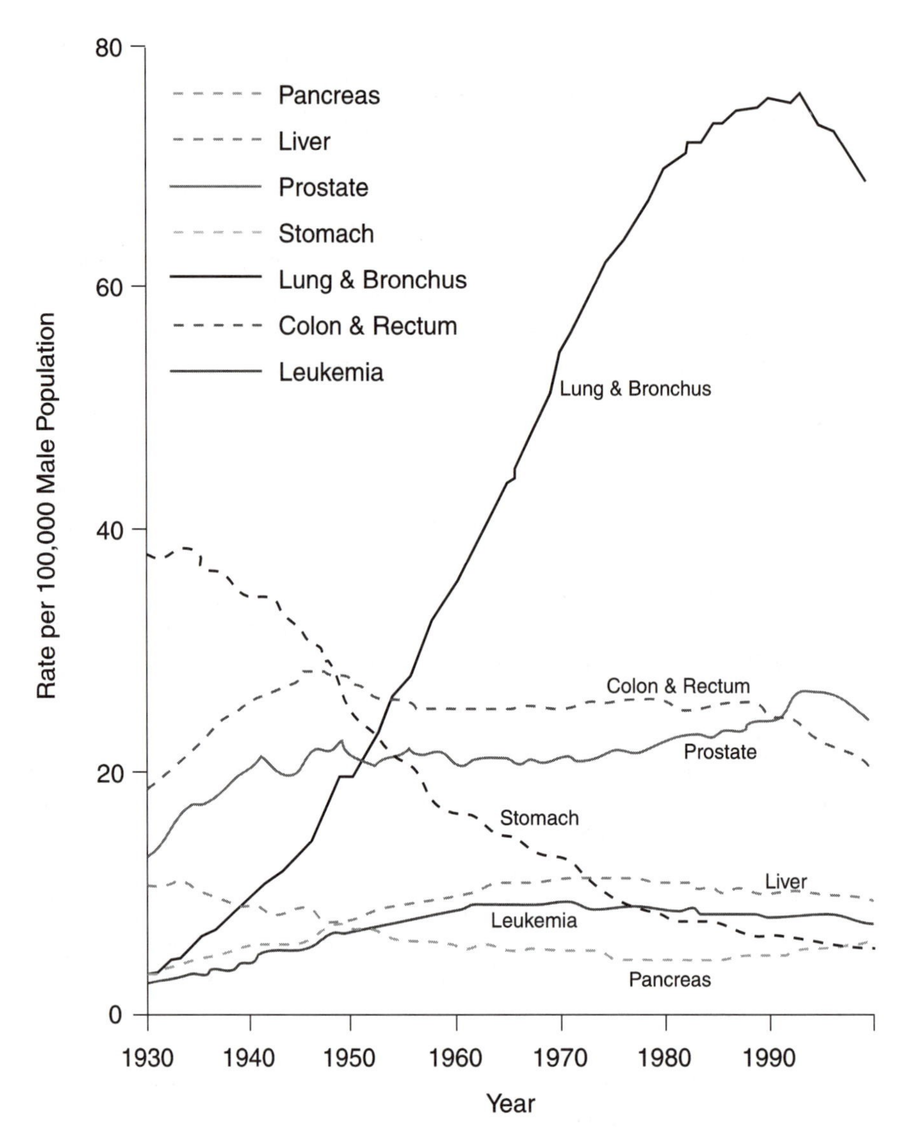

Figure 1–3 Age-adjusted cancer death rates, males by site, United States, 1930–1996. *Note:* Rates are per 100,000 and are age-adjusted to the 1970 US standard population. Also, due to changes in ICD coding, numerator information has changed over time. Rates for cancers of the liver, lung and bronchus, and colon and rectum are affected by these coding changes. *Source:* Reprinted with permission from R.T. Greenlee, et al., Cancer Statistics 2000, *CA - A Cancer Journal for Clinicians*, Vol. 50, pp. 7–33, © 2000, Lippincott Williams & Wilkins.

In China, for example, epidemiologists noted that there was a very high incidence of cancer of the esophagus in Linxian, a small city in the northeast, and in towns located in concentric rings around it. Descriptive studies showed that one in four residents were dying from it and that the rate of the disease declined with increasing distance from Linxian. The discovery of the high esophageal cancer rate in this locale was followed by speculation about environmental and dietary habits that could be causing the apparent

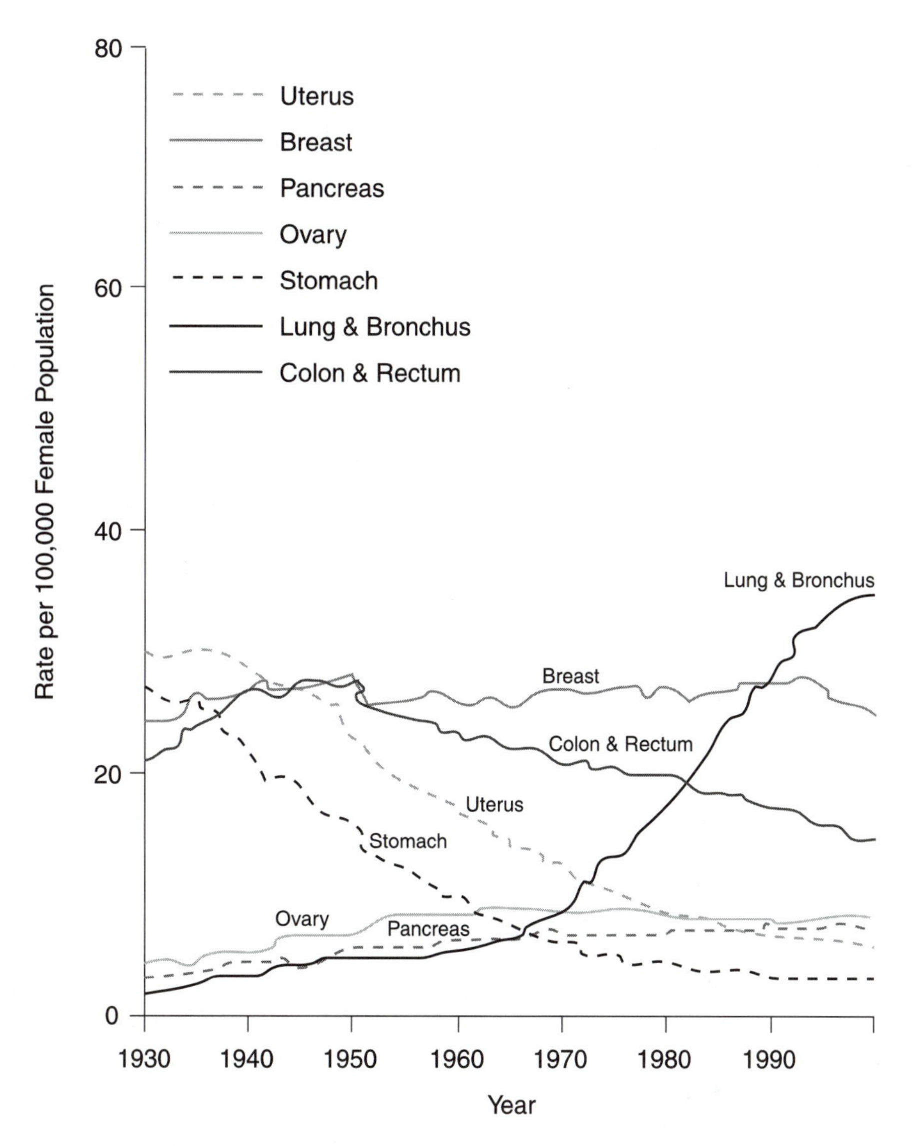

Figure 1–4 Age-adjusted cancer death rates, females by site, United States, 1930–1996. *Note:* Rates are per 100,000 and are age-adjusted to the 1970 US standard population. Due to changes in ICD coding, numerator information has changed over time. Rates for cancers of the uterus, ovary, lung and bronchus, and colon and rectum are affected by these coding changes. Uterine cancer death rates are for uterine cervix and uterine corpus combined. *Source:* Reprinted with permission from R.T. Greenlee, et al., Cancer Statistics 2000, *CA - A Cancer Journal for Clinicians*, Vol. 50, pp. 7–33, © 2000, Lippincott Williams & Wilkins.

---

epidemic. Theories cited as possibilities the temperature of the food (too hot), the scraping of the esophagus through the practice of eating dried corn husks, the eating of moldy bread, and a deficiency of molybdenum in the soil. After much focused analytic investigation, the purported link between the epidemic and dietary factors gained plausibility, although a newer case-control study noted a serologic association between papillomavirus 16 infection and the risk of esophageal cancer in a province of China.[9]

Table 1–2 Thirty-Year Trends in Cancer Death Rates per 100,000 Population, 1960–1962 and 1990–1992

Sites	*Sex*	*Rates in 1960–62*	*Rates in 1990–92*	*Percent Change*
All Sites	Male	185.3	220.0	19%
	Female	135.4	141.9	5%
Oral	Male	6.0	4.5	–25%
	Female	1.6	1.6	0%
Esophagus	Male	4.8	6.1	27%
	Female	1.2	1.5	25%
Stomach	Male	16.2	6.7	–59%
	Female	8.2	3.0	–63%
Colon & Rectum	Male	25.2	23.0	–9%
	Female	22.4	15.5	–31%
Colon	Male	17.3	19.1	10%
	Female	17.3	13.2	–24%
Rectum	Male	7.9	3.8	–52%
	Female	5.1	2.3	–55%
Liver	Male	6.3	5.5	–13%
	Female	6.0	3.3	–45%
Pancreas	Male	10.6	10.1	–5%
	Female	6.4	7.2	12%
Larynx	Male	2.7	2.5	–7%
	Female	0.3	0.5	67%
Lung	Male	40.2	74.4	85%
	Female	6.0	32.3	438%
Melanoma	Male	1.5	3.1	107%
of skin	Female	1.1	1.5	36%
Other skin	Male	1.6	1.3	–19%
	Female	0.7	0.3	–57%
Breast	Male	0.3	0.2	–33%
	Female	25.9	26.9	4%
Cervix uteri	Female	8.9	2.9	–67%
Other uterus	Female	6.3	3.4	–46%
Ovary	Female	8.7	8.0	–8%
Prostate	Male	20.7	26.7	29%
Bladder	Male	7.2	5.7	–21%
	Female	2.7	1.7	–37%
Kidney	Male	3.9	5.3	36%
	Female	2.0	2.5	25%
Brain	Male	4.3	5.2	21%
	Female	2.8	3.5	25%

continues

Table 1–2 continued

Sites	*Sex*	*Rates in 1960–62*	*Rates in 1990–92*	*Percent Change*
Non-Hodgkin's Lymphoma	Male	5.0	8.1	62%
	Female	3.3	5.2	58%
Hodgkin's disease	Male	2.3	0.7	–70%
	Female	1.3	0.4	–69%
Multiple myeloma	Male	2.1	3.8	81%
	Female	1.5	2.5	67%
Leukemia	Male	9.1	8.3	–9%
	Female	5.7	4.9	–14%

Source: Reprinted by permission of the American Cancer Society, Inc.

Unfortunately, descriptive epidemiology studies are too frequently overlooked in favor of analytic studies, either because they seem methodologically unsophisticated or because they do not provide direct evidence about causation. Yet the execution and interpretation of descriptive epidemiology studies of cancer is quite complex owing to the migratory patterns of modern populations as well as the lack of universally available, high-quality data on cancer incidence and mortality in defined populations. Furthermore, descriptive studies have historically provided a large number of productive leads about environmental, nutritional, lifestyle, and other types of risk factors. The often-cited estimate that approximately 80% of the worldwide cancer burden is related to environmental (nongenetic) factors is derived from the results of descriptive studies.[10]

Cancer incidence, the rate of newly diagnosed cancers in a defined population, is the preferred measure for uncovering differences in the geographic occurrence of cancer. Unfortunately, in many countries, especially developing nations, there are insufficient resources for providing reliable data on incidence. The problems include unequal distribution of health care resources, difficulty in gaining access to information about persons residing in remote areas, and the unavailability of the advanced technical tools required for diagnosing cancer. Also, even when diagnostic technology is available, there is often no reliable registration system for recording and tabulating cancer incidence rates in a defined population. In these cases, cancer mortality rates may provide somewhat better information about the underlying cancer risks in a population, since registration of the fact and cause of death, accompanied by basic descriptive characteristics of the decedent, is practiced everywhere.

Mortality rates are recorded in a relatively standardized manner throughout the world, in part due to the World Health Organization's International Classification of Diseases (ICD). The ICD provides uniform nomenclature for disease classification and a recommended format for death certificates.[11] As is well known, however, substantial errors in recording the cause of death can occur as a result of numerous factors, including lack of intensive medical investigation into the cause of death, poor access to health services, and the increasingly low autopsy rates in many countries. The problem of recording errors is likely to be exacerbated when cancer is the underlying cause of death because the patient is likely to have undergone a complex clinical course in the period leading to his or her demise.[12] Careful and intensive clinical and laboratory investigations are usually required to make an accurate identification of the primary site of cancer in an individual.

Note also that, because cancer is predominately a disease of older persons, nations with an older population profile would be expected to have higher cancer death rates. Therefore, international comparisons of cancer death rates must be age-adjusted. Often the World Health Organization's "standard world population" is used for this purpose.[13]

For cancers with a relatively low survival rate, such as those of the lung, liver, and stomach, differences in mortality rates should serve as reasonable approximations of differences in incidence rates. For cancers with more favorable survival rates, such as those of the breast and prostate, the use of mortality rates could result in a biased interpretation. For example, the recorded death rates for prostate cancer may be similar in a developed and a developing country, yet the developed country might in fact have a higher incidence rate but also a higher survival rate (due to advanced screening and treatment modalities). Therefore, when survival rates are substantially different between geographic regions, comparing mortality rates to arrive at an understanding of the underlying risk of cancer is not recommended.

Geographic and Ethnic Variation within the United States

In the most recent tabulations that compare the number of estimated new cancers and cancer deaths in the United States, by state, the range is dramatically wide. States like California, Florida, and New York have many more cancers recorded than do smaller states. Obviously, more populous states will have more cancers diagnosed. However, even if we calculate cancer incidence and mortality rates per 100,000 population, we shouldn't take the rates as evidence of environmental risks until we adjust them in light of the age distributions of the states. States like Florida and Arizona have much "older" populations because of the large retirement communities that abound there. Consequently, cancer rates in these states will appear higher than in the "younger" states from which people tend to migrate upon retirement. Table 1–3 lists age-adjusted cancer mortality rates for all 50 states and the District of Columbia for the period 1989–1994. Once age has been taken into account, any apparent excess cancer risk in states like Florida and Arizona disappears. Note, however, that there is still variability. For example, the District of Columbia, New Jersey, and Maryland have cancer death rates that are 25–50% higher than states like Utah, New Mexico, and Hawaii. Such differences in rates may be used to generate hypotheses about environmental, lifestyle, and ethnic or racial determinants of cancer. They may also indicate differences in the proportion of these populations that have access to health insurance or health services in general.

In the United States, as in most countries, there is a clear divide in morbidity and mortality rates along racial and ethnic lines; this situation is no different for cancer. By carefully describing the risk differentials and interpreting them in light of multifactorial etiologic theories, scientists can take the first steps toward effective cancer control.

In the case of all diseases, the number of deaths among certain minority groups, including Asians, Hispanics, Native Americans, and Pacific Islanders, is underestimated

Table 1–3 Cancer Mortality by State, 2000.

State	*Reported Death Rate per 100,000*	*State*	*Reported Death Rate per 100,000*
Alabama	179	Montana	159
Alaska	167	Nebraska	155
Arizona	155	Nevada	184
Arkansas	181	New Hampshire	181
California	156	New Jersey	179
Colorado	142	New Mexico	146
Connecticut	163	New York	169
Delaware	195	North Carolina	175
Dist. of Col.	212	North Dakota	155
Florida	166	Ohio	180
Georgia	175	Oklahoma	170
Hawaii	133	Oregon	166
Idaho	148	Pennsylvania	177
Illinois	178	Rhode Island	178
Indiana	178	South Carolina	178
Iowa	160	South Dakota	155
Kansas	159	Tennessee	181
Kentucky	192	Texas	168
Louisiana	193	Utah	122
Maine	185	Vermont	172
Maryland	184	Virginia	177
Massachusetts	178	Washington	162
Michigan	173	West Virginia	184
Minnesota	156	Wisconsin	163
Mississippi	182	Wyoming	157
Missouri	176	United States	170

Note: Average annual mortality rate for 1992–1996, age-adjusted to the 1970 US standard population.
Source: Reprinted with permission from R.T. Greenlee, et al., Cancer Statistics 2000, *CA - A Cancer Journal for Clinicians*, Vol. 50, pp. 7–33, © 2000, Lippincott Williams & Wilkins.

because these groups are underreported on death certificates.[14] Nevertheless, it is widely appreciated that cancer incidence and age-adjusted mortality rates vary by ethnic and racial status. For example, cancer death rates are higher in African Americans than in Caucasians for most sites. For the period 1990–1996, the difference in cancer incidence was 9% and the difference in mortality was 25% for all sites combined.[5] Although cancer accounts for a smaller proportion of total deaths among African Americans than among all races combined, the age-adjusted rates for African Americans are still higher.

In the 1950s and 1960s, cancer death rates were much more similar for African Americans and Caucasians than currently. However, in the last three decades death rates have climbed more precipitously among African American men and women than among Caucasians.[15] Currently, African Americans have a marked excess risk of cancers of the gastrointestinal system (including the esophagus, larynx, stomach, and liver); the excess is also notable for prostate cancer and cervical cancer. The likely reasons for the observed excess cancer risk in African Americans are partially known. A higher proportion of African American men are exposed to several behavioral risk factors for cancer, including tobacco use and adverse dietary constituents. Also, in comparison with Caucasians, African American men and women have higher case-fatality rates because they are diagnosed at a later stage of cancer.[16] The increased cancer risk experienced by African Americans represent a multitude of economic and sociocultural factors that afford numerous opportunities for public health interventions, including health education and screening.

Other minority groups exhibit a complex pattern of cancer incidence and mortality, with nearly all having some higher site-specific cancer rates and some lower rates than Caucasians. For example, Native Americans have generally higher prostate cancer mortality rates and lower colon and rectum cancer mortality rates than other groups. Asian Americans and Pacific Islanders (mainly the indigenous residents of Hawaii) experience a relatively high rate of death from cancer of the liver and stomach and a relatively low rate of death from leukemia and oral cavity cancers. The same group also has a lower rate of urogenital cancers, including bladder, kidney, cervix, endometrium, ovary, and prostate cancers, than whites.[17] The description of cancer rates and risk factors among Hispanic Americans is especially challenging given the heterogeneous populations that make up this group. Table 1–4 shows the ten leading causes of cancer deaths and the percentage of total cancer deaths by racial or ethnic group in the United States in 1993. The table does not contain rates and therefore does not allow a comparison of cancer mortality between the ethnic groups, but it does indicate the relative ranking of cancer mortality, by site, within the groups.

Five-year survival rates are lower for African Americans than Caucasians, as seen in Table 1–5. Taking all cancer sites together, 48% of African Americans and 61% of Caucasians survived five years or more. For a cancer in which survival is known to be strongly related to the stage at diagnosis, like female breast cancer, the survival differences are pronounced (71% among African Americans and 86% among Caucasians). On the other hand, for a cancer that is difficult to diagnose and is usually detected at a later stage, like stomach cancer, the five-year survival rates are nearly identical (22% among African Americans and 19% among Caucasians). This suggests that the decreased survival time for African Americans is largely due to lack of early detection, at least in part, in which case the public health community faces the challenge of increasing the number of screening and other prevention activities in targeted communities to narrow the gap.

International Geographic Variation

Studies of international variation are not possible without a large body of data to facilitate the elucidation of geographic patterns of cancer.[18] One of the most useful sources of information about the international cancer rates is the monograph series "Cancer Incidence in Five Continents."[19] Data on worldwide cancer incidence are presented and are used to support theories regarding the vast differences in the rates of specific cancers as well as in the total cancer burden in populations worldwide. It should be pointed out that the available data suffer from important limitations, namely, the

Table 1–4 Reported Deaths for the 10 Leading Cancer Sites and Percentage of Total Cancer Deaths by Ethnic or Racial Group, United States, 1994

	Caucasian	*African American*	*Native American**†	*Asian American & Pacific Islander**	*Hispanic American*‡
	All Sites 465,797 (100%)	All Sites 59,939 (100%)	All Sites 1,507(100%)	All Sites 7,067 (100%)	All Sites 16,635 (100%)
1	Lung & Bronchus 131,763 (28%)	Lung & Bronchus 15,658 (26.1%)	Lung & Bronchus 418 (27.7%)	Lung & Bronchus 1,521 (21.5%)	Lung & Bronchus 2,969 (17.8%)
2	Colon & Rectum 50,310 (10.8%)	Colon & Rectum 6,222 (10.4%)	Colon & Rectum 148 (9.8%)	Colon & Rectum 727 (10.3%)	Colon & Rectum 1,646 (9.9%)
3	Female Breast 37,960 (8.1%)	Prostate 5,650 (9.4%)	Female Breast 107 (7.1%)	Liver 645 (9.1%)	Female Breast 1,368 (8.2%)
4	Prostate 28,912 (6.2%)	Female Breast 5,083 (8.5%)	Prostate 82 (5.4%)	Stomach 569 (8.1%)	Prostate 1,015 (6.1%)
5	Pancreas 23,104 (5%)	Pancreas 3,255 (5.4%)	Stomach 63 (4.2%)	Female Breast 494 (7.0%)	Pancreas 926 (5.6%)
6	Non-Hodgkin's Lymphoma 20,161 (4.3%)	Stomach 2,206 (3.7%)	Pancreas 62 (4.1%)	Pancreas 413 (5.8%)	Stomach 867 (5.2%)
7	Leukemia 17,852 (3.8%)	Esophagus 1,948 (3.2%)	Non-Hodgkin's Lymphoma 55 (3.6%)	Non-Hodgkin's Lymphoma 295 (4.2%)	Non-Hodgkin's Lymphoma 836 (5.0%)
8	Ovary 12,256 (2.6%)	Leukemia 1,653 (2.8%)	Kidney 53 (3.5%)	Leukemia 288 (4.1%)	Leukemia 806 (4.8%)
9	Brain 11,465 (2.5%)	Multiple Myeloma 1,639 (2.7%)	Liver 49 (3.3%)	Prostate 258 (3.7%)	Liver 733 (4.4%)
10	Stomach 10,732 (2.3%)	Non-Hodgkin's Lymphoma 1,297 (2.2%)	Leukemia 40 (2.7%)	Ovary 173 (2.4%)	Ovary 439 (2.6%)

Note: Because each column includes only the top 10 cancer sites, site-specific numbers and percentages do not add up to the totals for all sites. Also, data for all sites except the urinary bladder exclude basal and squamous cell skin cancers and in situ carcinomas.

*Numbers are likely to be underestimates because of underreporting of Asians and Native Americans.

†Includes American Indians, Eskimos, and Aleuts.

‡Persons classified as Hispanic may be of any race. Hispanic origin is reported for all states except New Hampshire and Oklahoma.

Source: Adapted with permission from S.H. Landis, Cancer Statistics 1998, *CA - A Cancer Journal for Clinicians*, Vol. 48, pp. 6–29, © 1998, Lippincott-Raven Publishers.

overrepresentation of population-based cancer registries in developed nations, differences in the quality and coverage of the registries, and differences in the cancer classification systems used or the way they are used. For example, code 158 of the ninth revision of the International Classification of Diseases (ICD-9) is for malignant neoplasm of retroperitoneum and peritoneum. Under this code, the Finnish cancer registry includes only mesotheliomas (ie, cancers of the peritoneum only), whereas registries in Fortaleza,

Table 1–5 Five-Year Relative Cancer Survival Rates by Race, United States, 1989–1995

Site	*Caucasian Relative 5-Year Survival Rate for 1989–1995 (%)*	*African American Relative 5-Year Survival Rate for 1989–1995 (%)*
All Sites	61	48
Brain & Other Nervous System	30	39
Breast (female)	86	71
Cervix (uterus)	71	59
Colon	62	52
Endometrium (uterus)	86	56
Esophagus	13	9
Hodgkin's Disease	83	76
Kidney & Renal Pelvis	61	58
Larynx	66	53
Leukemia	44	34
Liver and Intrahepatic Bile Duct	6	3
Lung & bronchus	14	11
Melanoma-Skin	88	68
Multiple Myeloma	28	31
Non-Hodgkin's Lymphoma	52	41
Oral cavity	56	34
Ovary	50	47
Pancreas	4	4
Prostate	93	84
Rectum	60	51
Stomach	19	22
Testis	96	88
Thyroid	95	89
Urinary bladder	82	62

Note: Data for all sites except the urinary bladder exclude basal and squamous cell skin cancers and in situ carcinomas.
Source: Adapted with permission from R.T. Greenlee, et al., Cancer Statistics 2000, *CA - A Cancer Journal for Clinicians*, Vol. 50, pp. 7–33, © 2000, Lippincott Williams & Wilkins.

Brazil, and Cali, Colombia, and several in Hungary exclude "mesothelioma, not otherwise specified, of the peritoneum." To complicate matters further, the cancer registry of South Australia also includes tumors of the retroperitoneum in this category. As another example, under code 180, cervical cancer, registries in Romania and certain states in Brazil include carcinoma-in-situ of the cervix. Investigators need to be aware of these and other reporting inconsistencies. Nevertheless, comparing and interpreting data provided by international registries can be done with reasonable confidence that the data are generally consistent.

CANCER IN DEVELOPING NATIONS

In 1994, IARC reported on a comprehensive survey of 10 countries and geographical regions, 5 of which are in the developing stage (Africa, China, Asia [excluding China and Japan], Melanesia/Polynesia, and Latin America). Data on oral cavity, larynx, lung, esophagus, stomach, liver, pancreas, bladder, and kidney cancer as well as lymphomas and leukemias were collected and reported as age-standardized, sex-specific rates.[20] The bias created by failing to compare age-standardized cancer rates is vitally important and has been recognized for decades. Owing to the strong correlation between risk of developing cancer and age and also owing to the younger age distribution of populations in developing areas, age-adjustment must be performed if the cancer rates of different regions, countries, and local areas are to be compared without bias.

Of the 7.6 million new cancer cases that are diagnosed worldwide annually, over half are estimated to be in developing nations, and the overall cancer incidence is 1.8 times higher for males and 1.3 times higher for females in developing nations than in developed nations. Rates are higher for all cancer sites except for cancers of the mouth and pharynx, the esophagus, and the liver. Rate ratios vary from 4.0 (kidney cancer) to 1.2 (stomach cancer). Rate ratios are, on average, lower among females. Stomach cancer was the most common cancer among the 11 sites studied, but it was followed closely by lung cancer and then by oral cancer, which is especially prevalent in Asia. In Southeast Asia, oral cancer often involves the tongue and gum and is attributable to chewing tobacco. In China, cancer of the nasopharynx (the part of the pharynx most proximal to the nasal cavity) is the most common cancer. Its high incidence there has been attributed to viruses, nutritional factors, and occupational exposures.

Table 1–6 shows the age-adjusted mortality rates by sex for three common sites and for all sites combined in eight countries.

Table 1–6 Age-adjusted Death Rates per 100,000 Population for Selected Sites for Eight Countries, 1994–1997

	All Sites		*Breast*	*Lung and Bronchus*		*Oral*	
Country	*Male*	*Female*	*Female*	*Male*	*Female*	*Male*	*Female*
Australia*	156.7	98.2	19.9	38.8	13.6	4.1	1.2
China†‡	149.9	83.5	5.0	37.3	15.8	2.6	1.1
Finland*	142.3	85.0	16.8	41.2	6.9	2.2	1.0
Israel*	127.1	104.5	25.1	27.1	8.7	1.5	0.7
Mexico*	85.0	78.9	9.3	16.2	6.0	1.9	0.7
Poland	204.9	107.6	16.1	71.3	11.1	6.3	1.1
United Kingdom*	164.2	116.5	24.5	46.6	20.5	2.9	1.1
United States§	156.0	108.3	20.0	52.3	26.6	3.2	1.1

Note: Rates are age-adjusted to the World Health Organization world standard population.
*Data for 1994–1995.
†Data for 1994 only.
‡Oral cancer mortality rate includes nasopharynx only.
§Data for 1994–1997.
Source: Adapted with permission from R.T. Greenlee, et al., Cancer Statistics 2000, *CA - A Cancer Journal for Clinicians*, Vol. 50, pp. 7–33, © 2000, Lippincott Williams & Wilkins.

MIGRANT STUDIES

The substantial variation in the frequency of occurrence of cancer by geographic location offers important clues about cancer etiology. By studying groups who migrate from one country to another, evidence can be amassed to determine whether their cancer rates remain the same as those of the country of origin or become more like those of the new country of residence. In cases where a group of immigrants maintain in the new country their old rate for a particular cancer, it is reasonable to suspect the presence of genetic component causes. In cases where the cancer rate changes to approximate the rate for the original inhabitants of the new country, it is reasonable to suspect the presence of environmental or lifestyle component causes.

Of course, observations of cancer rate stability or change must be interpreted in light of specific theories about cancer causation. For example, causation for a particular cancer might be multifactorial, which means the cancer can be caused by various factors operating together within one "causal web" or "causal wheel." Etiologic factors that are present in every causal web are said to be "necessary causes" whereas factors required by one web but not another are referred to as "component causes." The minimum set of factors contained within one cancer web compose a "sufficient cause"[21] (the set could include a combination of genetic, environmental, and lifestyle factors). If a migrant group settles into a cancer rate intermediate between the rates of the country of origin and the adopted country, genetic and environmental component causes might both be in play. However, the migrant group's cancer rate could merely be in a period of transition and still be changing, and in such a case a cross-sectional "snapshot" estimate of the migrant cancer rate would be a misleading basis for causal inference by itself.

One landmark descriptive study done by IARC compared cancer rates between Africans residing in Ibadan, Nigeria; African Americans; and Caucasian Americans.[19] (Although perhaps of greater historical interest than currently relevant, the study is noteworthy because it helped pioneer the methodology of migrant studies.) Data retrieved from the population-based cancer registries in Nigeria and the United States in the 1960s are presented in Table 1–7. As pointed out by Doll and Peto,[10] the comparisons are to some degree limited, since the ancestors of African Americans were not chiefly from Nigeria; nevertheless, some inferences can be made. Most obvious is the general similarity between the cancer rates of African Americans and Caucasian Americans. The contrast between the cancer rates of Nigerians and African Americans is so great that it is not plausible to assume they result mainly from genetic dilution through interbreeding. Migrant studies of Japanese who migrated to Hawaii, Britons who went to Fiji, and Central Europeans who went to North America and Australia, among other studies, lead to similar inferences.[10]

SUMMARY

A comprehensive description of the distribution of cancer within a population according to geographic, temporal, and demographic characteristics is required before analytic studies can be designed to assess causal factors. The information generated from descriptive epidemiology studies often uncovers opportunities to reduce the incidence

Table 1–7 Comparison of Cancer Incidence Rates for Ibadan, Nigeria, and for Two Representative Populations of African Americans and Caucasians in the United States (Annual Incidence per Million People)*

Primary Site of Cancer	*Patients' Sex*†	*Ibadan, Nigeria 1960–1969*	*United States*‡ *African Americans*	*Whites*
Colon	M	34	349	294
			353	335
Rectum	M	34	159	217
			248	232
Liver	M	272	67	39
			86	32
Pancreas	M	55	200	126
			250	122
Larynx	M	37	236	141
			149	141
Lung	M	27	1,546	983
			1,517	979
Prostate	M	134	724	318
			577	232
Breast	F	337	1,268	1,828
			1,105	1,472
Cervix uteri	F	559	507	249
			631	302
Corpus uteri	F	42	235	695
			208	441
Lymphosarcoma§	M	133	10	4
at ages <15 yr	F		5	3

*Ages 35–64 years, standardized for age as in source text.

†For brevity, wherever possible only the male rates have been presented, and sites for which rates among US Caucasians resemble those in the country of origin of the non-Caucasian migrants have been omitted.

‡For each type of cancer, upper entry shows incidence in San Francisco Bay area, 1969–1973; lower entry shows incidence in Detroit, 1969–1971.

§Including Burkitt's lymphoma. The cited rates are the average of the age-specific rates at ages 0–4, 5–9, and 10–14 years.

Source: Reprinted with permission from *Cancer Incidence in Five Continents, Vol. III,* IARC Scientific Publications, © 1976, International Agency for Research on Cancer.

and mortality rates of cancer in the United States and worldwide. Students and researchers must not be too quick to look beyond descriptive statistics regarding "person, place, and time." The methodological competence that is required to manipulate, compare, and interpret descriptive data is taught in basic and intermediate epidemiology and biostatistics courses and should, therefore, be within reach of most persons using this text. Care is always needed in interpreting comparisons and trends, however, especially if the data have been derived from different sources or cover different time periods.

Statistics concerning the worldwide distribution of cancer highlight the contrasting risk profiles between persons who are of different races and ethnic backgrounds and who live in different physical, social, and economic environments. Careful interpretation of the statistics has led to many causal hypotheses and to some breakthroughs in the identification of etiologic agents. Recent cancer incidence and mortality data suggest that the slight, steady rise in the US cancer burden may have been reversed. Whether the trend is currently downward, substantial declines can be realized by using the information already in hand. There continue to be unmet opportunities for targeting prevention activities toward communities where cancer incidence or mortality remains high.

Discussion Questions

1. Of major concern to society is whether cancer is more common today than in the past. Discuss this issue from a US perspective and use incidence and mortality data to help address it. How does the issue of changing trends in cardiovascular incidence affect the way we interpret the importance of cancer in our society?
2. Comparing cancer incidence rates between geographic locations affords opportunities to determine the causal factors responsible for the variation. Provide several reasons why such comparisons must be made judiciously, especially when cancer rates are being compared internationally.
3. Migrant studies have been used to help determine the relative importance of genetic and environmental factors in the causation of cancer. From your own experience or travels, identify three communities or populations with a large immigrant component and indicate how descriptive studies might help uncover information about the causes of cancer that could be useful to epidemiologists.
4. It has been alleged that industrial pollution from a large manufacturing facility that opened in 1954 was responsible for an apparent excess in lung cancer in the part of the county where the facility was located. How might you use available cancer statistics to provide a fuller basis for evaluating this allegation? Assume that the county is in a state in which there has been reasonable access to health care and that cancer registration has been conducted since the 1940s.

References

1. Gould J. *The Enemy Within.* New York: Four Walls Eight Windows; 1996.
2. Jablon MA, Hrubec Z, Boice JD. Cancer in populations living near nuclear facilities. *JAMA.* 1991;265: 1403–1408.
3. National Cancer Institute. *SEER Cancer Statistics Review, 1973–1992.* Bethesda, MD: National Institutes of Health; 1995.
4. American Cancer Society. *Cancer Facts and Figures, 1998.* Atlanta, GA: American Cancer Society; 1998.
5. Greenlee RT, Murray T, Bolden S, Wingo PA. Cancer statistics, 2000. *CA Cancer J Clin.* 2000;50:7–33.
6. Bailar JC III, Gornick HL. Cancer undefeated. *N Engl J Med.* 1997;336:1569–1574.
7. Cole P, Rodu B. Declining cancer mortality in the United States. *Cancer.* 1996;78:2045–2048.
8. Parker SL, Tong T, Bolden S, Wingo PA. Cancer statistics, 1996. *CA Cancer J Clin.* 1996;65:5–27.
9. Han C, Qiao G, Hubbert NL, et al. Serologic association between human papillomavirus type 16 infection and esophageal cancer in Shaanxi Province, China. *J Natl Cancer Inst.* 1996;88:1467–1471.
10. Doll R, Peto R. *The Causes of Cancer.* Oxford: Oxford University Press; 1981.
11. US Department of Health and Human Services. *The International Classification of Diseases, 9th Revision.* 3rd ed. Bethesda, MD: US Department of Health and Human Services; 1989.

12. Percy C, Stanek E, Gloeckler L. Accuracy of cancer death certificates and its effects on cancer mortality statistics. *Am J Public Health.* 1981;71:242–250.
13. World Health Organization. *World Health Statistics Annuals 1987–1993*. Geneva, Switzerland: World Health Organization; 1993.
14. Kochanek KD, Hudson B. Advance report of final mortality statistics 1992. *Monthly Vital Statistics Report* (National Center for Health Statistics). 1995; 43(suppl):6.
15. Boring CC, Squires TS, Heath CW Jr. Cancer statistics for African Americans. *CA Cancer J Clin.* 1992;42:125.
16. Bal DG. Cancer in African Americans. *CA Cancer J Clin* 1992;42:5–6. Editorial.
17. Goodman, MT. Cancer incidence among Asian-Americans. In: Jones LA, ed. *Minorities and Cancer.* New York: Springer-Verlag; 1989.
18. Cook-Mozaffari, J. The geography of cancer. In: Vessey MP, Gray M, eds. *Cancer Risks and Prevention.* Oxford: Oxford University Press; 1985.
19. International Agency for Research on Cancer. *Cancer Incidence in Five Continents.* Vol 3. Lyon, France: International Agency for Research on Cancer; 1976.
20. Pisani P. Burden of cancer in developing nations. In: Perch N, Matos E, Vainio H, et al. *Occupational Cancer in Developing Countries*. Lyon, Fr
21. Rothman KJ. *Modern Epidemiology.* Boston: Little, Brown and Co; 1986.

Chapter 2

Basic Terminology

Philip C. Nasca

The overall objective of this chapter is to provide an introduction to basic terminology that the first-time student may find useful when exploring articles and books related to cancer epidemiology. The chapter is designed to introduce the reader to a number of basic concepts that apply to benign and malignant neoplasms, tumor metastases, tumor staging, and grading classification schemes and to a number of approaches to standardizing the anatomic and morphological classification of cancers. It also defines basic terms used in cancer diagnosis and management. Finally, it briefly discusses ways in which diagnostic difficulties may affect epidemiological studies of various cancers.

Different terms are often used to describe the benign and malignant growths referred to in this volume. *Neoplasm* literally means "new growth," and a neoplasm can be defined as an abnormal mass of tissue that is uncoordinated with the normal tissues of the affected organ. A neoplasm may also persist even after the stimulus that produced the growth is removed.[1] This definition implies two important facts about neoplasms. First, neoplasms exhibit growth in excess of normal tissue regeneration, suggesting that they have somehow escaped the biologic restraints on growth that govern normal cellular replication and tissue growth. Second, the stimuli provoking neoplastic changes at the cellular level are often permanent and inherited by all cellular progeny. The occurrence of permanent and heritable changes at the cellular level that lead to uncontrolled cellular proliferation and tissue growth will be referred to throughout the text as *neoplastic transformation.* The term *tumor* is often commonly used interchangeably with the term *neoplasm.* (Note that a comprehensive glossary of terms used in the field of cancer epidemiology is provided in Appendix B.)

PATHOLOGIC FEATURES OF CANCER

The normal architecture of an organ involves standard relationships between specific groups of cells, whereas in neoplastic growth the relationships between cells are significantly altered, as shown in Figure 2–1. In normal epithelial tissues, the layers of epithelial cells are arranged in a regular and ordered manner, and cells replicate at the rate necessary to replace lost cells and to maintain the normal structure and functions of the tissues. The most common forms of cancer occur in the epithelial tissues. The epithelial tissues are separated from the underlying connective tissue, blood and lymphatic vessels, and nerves by a basement membrane. Neoplasms of epithelial origin tend to show structural differences when compared with the normal architecture of the tissue within which the tumor originated. In neoplastic growth, many more cells are produced

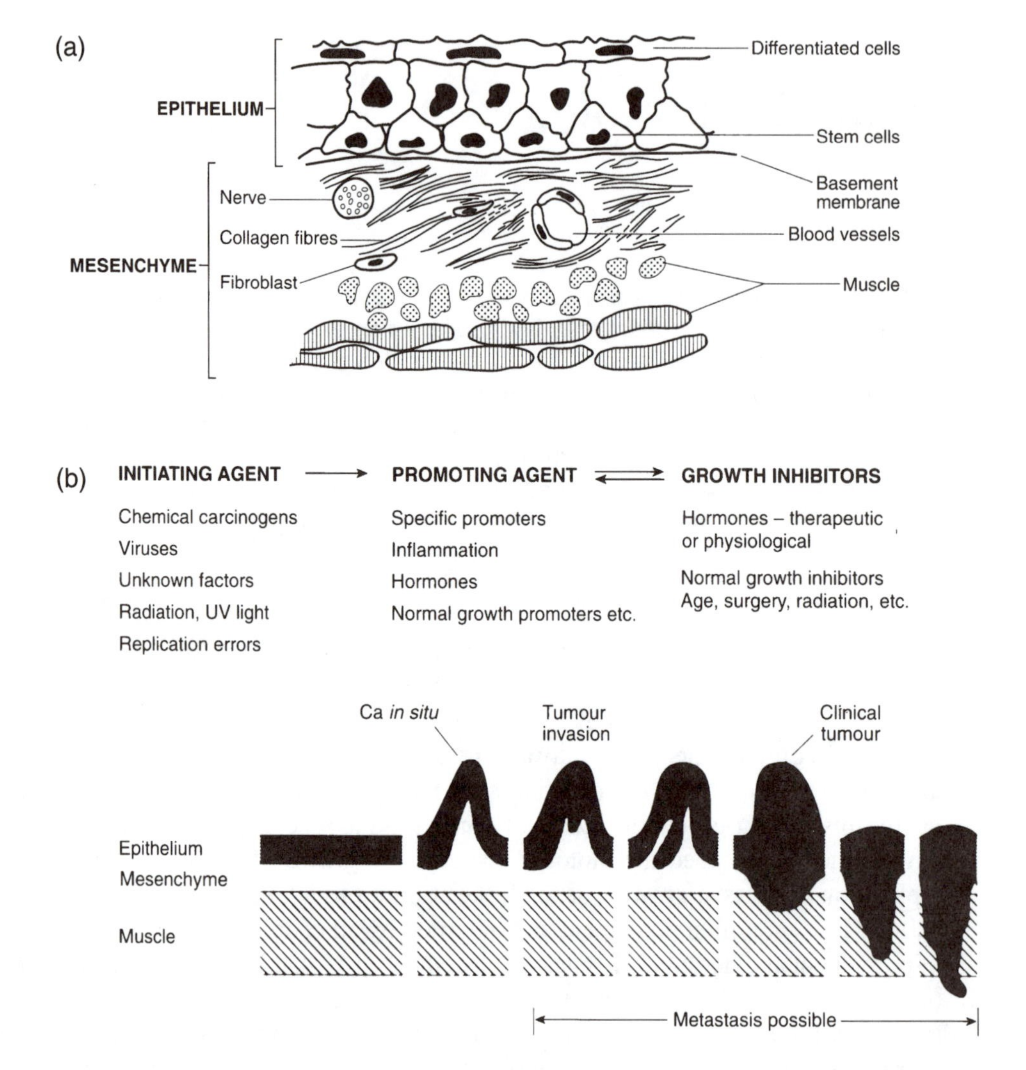

Figure 2–1 (a) A typical tissue showing epithelial and mesenchymal components and (b) factors influencing tumor development showing progression from a normal to an invasive tumor. *Source:* Reprinted from L.M. Franks and N.M. Teich, *Introduction to the Cellular and Molecular Biology of Cancer, 2nd Edition*, pp. 2 and 5, © 1991, by permission of Oxford University Press.

than are needed to replace lost cells. The architecture of neoplastic tissue is not orderly, and many layers of epithelial cells are arranged in irregular patterns.[2]

Neoplastic cells are distinguished from normal cells by a loss of cellular differentiation. The term *degree of differentiation* refers to the extent to which the neoplastic cells continue to resemble morphologically and functionally the normal cells of the tissue within which the neoplasm develops. Neoplasms defined as well differentiated have cells that are morphologically similar to cells normally found in the tissue of origin and that maintain many of the functions of normal cells. In poorly differentiated neoplasms, the neoplastic cells have a primitive appearance and suffer a loss of normal functioning. The reduction in differentiation is an important characteristic of malignant neoplasms, and it is referred to as *anaplasia.*

A number of morphologic and functional changes at the cellular level indicate the presence of anaplasia. The cells and their nuclei show variation in size and shape, which is referred to as *pleomorphism.* Neoplastic cells may be either much larger than normal cells in the same tissue or uncharacteristically smaller and more primitive in appearance than normal cells. The nuclei of neoplastic cells may show variability in their shapes, have large amounts of dark staining DNA, and take up an exceptionally large proportion of the total volume of the cell. While the ratio of nuclear to cytoplasmic material is on the order of 1:4 to 1:6 in normal cells, this ratio may approach 1:1 in neoplastic cells. These neoplastic cells may also show evidence of frequent cell divisions, indicating rapid cellular proliferation. Evidence for cellular proliferation might include the presence of large nucleoli and large numbers of mitoses.[3(p243)]

Microscopic studies of cancer cells also show gross changes in the cellular cytoskeleton. The cytoskeleton of normal cells is composed of actin fibers, which are arranged in an orderly cablelike fashion. These actin cables serve to provide structure to the cell and are connected to receptors on the cell surface, which in turn anchor the cell to the intracellular matrix. In cancer cells, these actin cables are either lost or become disorganized, and the cancer cells lose their adherence to the intracellular matrix.[4(pp39–42)]

BENIGN AND MALIGNANT NEOPLASMS

Neoplasms are classified as either benign or malignant based on a number of important characteristics, which are summarized in Table 2–1. Benign neoplasms are usually well differentiated, whereas malignant neoplasms range from well differentiated to poorly differentiated. Systems of tumor grading have been developed by pathologists to describe the degree of differentiation observed in a particular epithelial tumor. Tumor grade as a measure of differentiation is clinically important as a measure of tumor progression and as a prognostic factor often related to the tumor's response to treatment, disease recurrence rates, and patient survival.

Rate of growth is also a critical distinguishing feature of benign and malignant neoplasms. Benign neoplasms tend to grow at a relatively slow pace and may take years to develop into a significant mass. Malignant tumors generally tend to grow faster, with growth rates inversely correlated with the degree of differentiation. Doubling time, the amount of time needed for the tumor to double in mass, is used as a measure of tumor growth. Benign tumors usually have long doubling times, whereas the doubling time for malignancies with high case-fatality rates can be quite short.

Benign tumors, which are encapsulated by connective tissue, tend to remain confined within the tissue of origin. Malignant tumors may gain the ability to penetrate the basement membrane, a thin extracellular layer of mucopolysaccharides and proteins that separates the epithelial tissues from the underlying connective tissues, blood vessels, and lymphatics. This ability to penetrate the basement membrane leads to local invasion and destruction of adjacent tissues.

METASTASIS

Penetration of the basement membrane also provides the tumor with access to local blood and lymphatic vessels, thus providing a route for the tumor to spread to other organs of the body. The process of systemic spread, referred to as *metastasis,* is another important distinguishing feature of malignant neoplasms. Metastasis can occur through a

Table 2–1 Morphologic and Functional Differences between Benign and Malignant Tumors

Characteristic	*Benign Tumors*	*Malignant*
Structure	Structurally similar to tissue within which tumor originated	Architecture of tumor disorganized and not typical of tissue of origin
Differentiation	Well differentiated	Poorly differentiated (anaplastic)
Rate of growth	Slow rate of growth	Rapid rate of growth, with short doubling time
Mode of growth	Expansion (encapsulated)	Penetration and destruction of surrounding tissues
Metastases	No metastases	Metastases common through local tissue invasion and transport of malignant cells through the bloodstream or lymphatic system
Response to therapy	Rare for tumor to recur	Recurrent disease common after initial therapy
Prognosis	Usually excellent; inaccessible tumors can be fatal	More often fatal than benign tumors

number of mechanisms, including by direct extension of the tumor into various natural body cavities, such as the peritoneal cavity, and, most commonly, by penetration of the nearby lymph nodes and blood vessels for transport to other vital organs.

Research has shown that most cancers contain subpopulations of cells of varying biologic characteristics. Cells may vary with respect to rate of growth, karyotype, pigment production, receptor content, degree of immunogenicity, and susceptibility to cytotoxic drugs.[4] Subpopulations of cells probably exist at diagnosis, and these may have a greater potential to metastasize than other subpopulations of cells, possibly because they possess a greater ability to withstand exposure to chemotherapeutic agents. These metastatic cancer cells spread to other organs in the body via the circulatory and lymphatic systems by invading new blood vessels formed by tumor angiogenesis or by entering existing blood vessels or lymphatics. The metastatic cells enter and leave the circulatory system by excreting a number of substances that break down the vessel wall (Figure 2–2).[5] The process of metastatic spread is a highly complicated biological process. A more detailed description of how metastases occur can be found in the article by Fidler.[5]

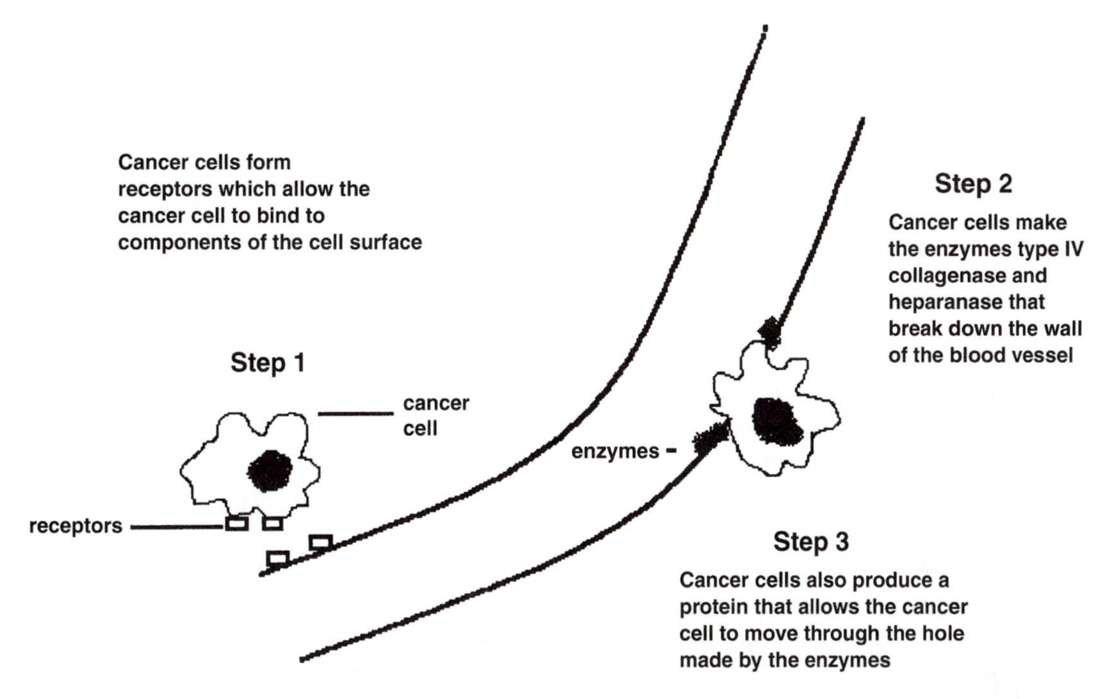

Figure 2–2 The migration of cancer cells through blood vessels.

CANCER DIAGNOSIS

A diagnosis of cancer is usually confirmed by obtaining a biopsy specimen or tumor sample by surgical excision, needle aspiration, or the collection of exfoliated cells from body fluids, among other methods. The specimen is then examined by a pathologist, who determines if the tissues are neoplastic, notes the behavior (benign or malignant) of the neoplasm, and notes the cell type. The pathologist will also determine the tumor grade (as a measure of degree of differentiation) and will examine any lymph nodes submitted by the clinician for evidence of cancer. The exact histology (or cell type) and tumor grade will help the clinician plan the proper course of therapy and establish a probable prognosis. In the pathology laboratory, the tumor specimen is fixed, sectioned, and stained as part of the preparation of slides for examination by the pathologist. The fixation process is designed to help preserve and stabilize the tissues. The protein structure of the specimen is cross-linked with specific fixatives, such as formalin, or proteins are precipitated with alcohol-based chemicals, such as methacarn. The lipids and water are then removed from the tissue and the specimen is impregnated either with paraffin wax (for light microscopy) or resin (for ultrastructural studies).

If the specimen is to be viewed under a light microscope, a device called a *microtome* is used to cut thin sections of the tumor from the paraffin block. These thin sections are stained with acidic or basic dyes to highlight the nucleus, cytoplasm, and extracellular matrix, and they are then placed on slides for examination under the microscope. A device called a *cryostat* can be used to cut thin sections from a specimen that has been snap frozen with liquid nitrogen at –80°C. In addition to providing materials for initial diagnoses, paraffin blocks can be maintained for many years and have been used extensively in molecular-epidemiological studies. Recent innovations in gene amplification methods have led to studies of gene-environmental interactions that utilize DNA and RNA extracted from paraffin blocks.[6]

MOLECULAR PATHOLOGY

A number of useful molecular pathology techniques have emerged in recent years to aid the clinician in cancer diagnosis and management. For a detailed account of these techniques, the reader is referred to the excellent review article by Sklar and Costa.[7] Some of the techniques are in the field of immunohistochemistry, some involve the measurement of total DNA content, and some are in the field of diagnostic molecular genetics.[7]

Immunohistochemical techniques include a number of complicated laboratory techniques, including one in which antibodies are tagged with fluorescent molecules to bind with antigens expressed by various tumor cells. Innovations in immunohistochemistry have led to the development of more refined classification systems for tumors and a significant reduction in the proportion of tumors that are unclassified. Immunohistochemical techniques can also help sort out different cell types in tumors with mixed cellularity, help identify metastatic tumor cells in secondary sites, and occasionally help distinguish benign from malignant tumors. More recently, immunohistochemical classification of tumors has been used to develop markers to help establish prognoses. For example, recent studies have shown the multidrug resistance of tumors that overexpress p53 antigen, and the overexpression is thought to reflect a point mutation in the tumor suppressor gene, a mutation that leads to inactivation of p53 protein.[7]

Predictions of the course of a cancer can also be based on measurements of the DNA content within cancer cells. A commonly used prognostic marker is the number of chromosomes present in the cells. Cancer cells frequently show abnormal numbers of chromosomes, or ploidy. The presence of ploidy indicates a poorly differentiated tumor and suggests a poor prognosis for the patient. In addition, cancer cells can be examined for the proportion of cells that have doubled their DNA in preparation for cell division. This measure, called the *S-phase fraction,* has been shown to correlate with increased tumor aggressiveness. Finally, a number of molecular techniques developed over the past 20 years can be used to examine cells obtained from the fluids or tissues of cancer patients for specific nucleotide sequences that indicate the presence of specific genes known to be associated with specific forms of cancer.[7] (See Chapter 7 for a discussion of these techniques and their use in epidemiological research.)

A growing number of circulating tumor markers have been shown to be useful in establishing the initial diagnosis of the cancer and in helping to predict a patient's prognosis. These markers are also useful for monitoring the course of the patient's disease or the tumor's response to therapy.[7] Blood tests can be used to obtain baseline measures of certain biomarkers at the time of diagnosis and following treatment for the purpose of monitoring the patient for any recurrence of cancer. A significant increase in the value of one of these markers over the baseline value taken after initial treatment may signal the return of the disease. Table 2–2 contains a brief description of some of the biomarkers currently used by physicians to help manage the patient's disease in the optimal fashion.

Some tests are performed at the time of initial diagnosis to help plan future treatments in the event that the cancer recurs. It is now standard practice for physicians to send a portion of the breast cancer biopsy specimen to a laboratory so that estrogen and

Table 2–2 Selected Antigens Analyzed by Immunohistochemistry in the Diagnosis and Characterization of Tumors

Antigen	*Comments on Tissue and Tumor Specificities*
Actin	Isoform specific for smooth muscle and myofibroblasts Sarcomeric isoform specific for striated muscle
α-Fetoprotein	Liver, visceral endoderm; yolk sac tumors, hepatocellular carcinoma
α-Lactalbumin	Breast epithelium, ductal and lobular carcinoma of the breast; hidradenoma papilliferum
CA 19.9	Monosialo Lewis A antigen; pancreatobiliary carcinoma, transitional cell tumors
CA 125	Mucinous epithelial tumors of the ovary, cervix, endometrium, gastrointestinal tract, breast
Cadherin	Carcinoma; expression inversely correlated to differentiation
Carcinoembryonic antigen (CEA)	Adenocarcinoma of the gastrointestinal tract, etc.
CD31	Endothelial cells
CD34	Endothelial cells, bone marrow stem cells
Chromogranins	Neuroendocrine tumors
Cytokeratins	Epithelial tumors, less commonly other types
Desmin	Striated and parenchymal smooth muscle
Epithelial membrane antigen	Adenocarcinomas, mesothelioma, meningioma
Factor VIII	Megakaryocytes, platelets, mast cells, endothelium, endothelial tumors
Factor XIII	Megakaryocytes, fibroblasts, macrophages, dermal fibrous histiocytomas
GFAP	Glial cells, astrocytomas, oligodendrogliomas, ependymomas, schwannomas
GCDFP-15	Apocrine differentiation in breast and skin; some breast carcinomas
HMB-45	Melanoma, angiomyolipoma, some neural crest tumors
Hormone receptors	Estrogen: carcinoma of the breast, desmoid tumor Progesterone: carcinoma of the breast
HCG-β	Syncytiotrophoblast; germ cell tumors, ectopic production in lung and other carcinomas
Human placental lactogen	Trophoblast, germ cell tumors, gastric and lung carcinomas
Immunoglobulins	Lymphoid and plasma cell tumors
Integrins	Expressed in tumors according to cell lineage
Ki-67	Proliferation antigen in cycling cells, all tumor types
Laminin	Basement membrane component, epithelial; smooth muscle and endothelial tumors
Leukocyte common antigen	Panlymphocytic; negative in other cell types
LeuM-1	Hodgkin's disease, adenocarcinoma
Leu-7	Neural and neuroendocrine tumors, prostatic carcinoma
MyoD-1	Skeletal muscle tumors, alveolar soft part sarcoma

continues

Table 2–2 continued

Antigen	*Comments on Tissue and Tumor Specificities*
Myoglobin	Skeletal and myocardial muscle
Myosin	Isoforms specific for smooth and striated muscle
Neurospecific enolase	γ/γ and γ/α predominantly in neural and neuroendocrine tumors; present in many other tumor types
Notch	Present in some stem cells; stains epithelial tumors and lymphomas
p53	Prolonged half-life in many tumor types
P-glycoprotein	Normal colon, endothelial, and adrenal cells; associated with multidrug resistance
Placenta-like alkaline phosphatase	Present in gonadal and extragonadal germ cell tumors; marker of in situ germ cell neoplasia
Prostate-specific antigen	Present in normal, hyperplastic, and neoplastic prostate; specific for that organ
Prostatic acid phosphatase	Carcinoma of the prostate, transitional cell carcinoma, carcinoids and other tumors
S-100	Peripheral nerve sheath tumors, central gliomas, cartilaginous and adipose tumors; marks myoepithelial cells
Surfactant apoprotein	Primary pulmonary adenocarcinoma
Synaptophysin	Neuroectodermal and neuroendocrine tumors
Thyroglobulin	Thyroid tumors of follicular cell origin
Vimentin	Mesenchymal tumors; high-grade epithelial tumors
Numerous antigens for stages of B- and T-lymphocytic lineage and activation	Hematolymphoid tumors

Source: Reprinted with permission from J.L. Sklar and J.C. Costa, *Cancer: Principles and Practice of Oncology, 5th Edition*, V.T. DeVita, Jr., S. Hellman, and S.A. Rosenberg, eds., © 1997, Lippincott Williams & Wilkins.

progesterone receptor assays can be done. These assays determine if the patient's breast cancer grows in response to the hormones estrogen and progesterone. The results play an important role in determining a suitable management plan for recurrent disease. If the breast cancer is estrogen receptor positive, then the patient may be treated with an estrogen antagonist, such as the drug tamoxifen.[8] Estrogen and progesterone receptor status has also been used by epidemiologists to determine if breast cancers categorized as receptor positive or negative exhibit different epidemiological characteristics. (More is said about this approach in Chapter 10.)

Finally, it is also possible for a patient who is diagnosed with a cancer at one anatomic site to develop a second primary cancer at a different anatomic site many years later. Such multiple primary cancers sometimes involve paired organs, such as the ovary or breast. It is therefore necessary for the patient to undergo regular monitoring of the initially unaffected side. Women with breast cancer are usually given a mammographic and clinical examination of the initially unaffected breast at regular intervals to detect the development of new primary disease in the second breast or to detect metastatic spread from the original primary cancer.

CANCER STAGING

A powerful predictor of recurrent disease and length of survival is the extent to which the patient's disease has become locally invasive, has spread to other adjacent organs, or shows evidence of already having spread to distant organs, including bones, the liver, the lungs, and the central nervous system. The clinician will utilize the results of the clinical examination of the patient, observations obtained during surgical intervention, and the results of the pathologist's report to determine the extent of disease at the time of diagnosis. Determining the extent of disease is referred to as *cancer staging.* A number of special imaging tests may also be performed to discover if the cancer has spread into organs such as the liver and into a bone. The information gained is then used to categorize the patient's stage of disease at the time of diagnosis.

Tumor staging systems range from simple to sophisticated. The simpler systems include categories for in situ cancers (tumors limited to the first layer of epithelial cells), invasive cancers that are still restricted to the original primary site, invasive cancers that have spread to adjacent organs, and cancers that have already metastasized at the time of diagnosis. A more sophisticated and widely used system is the TNM system, where *T* stands for the size of the tumor, *N* stands for the extent of regional lymph node involvement, and *M* stands for evidence of metastases. The TNM system was developed jointly by the International Agency for Research on Cancer (IARC) and the American Joint Committee on Cancer (AJCC).[9] Data are extracted from the patient's record for each of the three variables and entered into an algorithm developed for each tumor type. The contributions of the three variables are combined to create a final stage for the tumor.

An example of the TNM staging process is presented in Exhibit 2–1, which shows the definitions that are applied to the individual staging components of tumor size, nodal involvement, and evidence of distant metastases for patients with primary cancers of the breast. The exhibit also shows how various combinations of these individual components are translated into a final stage at diagnosis. Exhibit 2–2 presents an example of how a breast cancer patient's medical history is converted into an appropriate TNM stage.

In addition to general systems, such as the TNM, specialized systems have been developed for certain tumors. These include the Dukes System for staging cancers of the colon and rectum,[10] the Columbia system for breast cancers,[11] and the International Federation of Gynecologists and Obstetricians (FIGO) system for staging tumors of the female reproductive organs.[12]

Tumors that are not locally invasive represent the most curable form of a malignancy and present ideal targets for early detection programs. A number of screening techniques for tumors have been developed, including cytological testing for early cancer of the uterine cervix and mammographic screening for early breast cancer. Early detection and prompt treatment of cancer of the uterine cervix is associated with a better than 90% five-year survival rate.[13(p139)] Conversely, lesions that are not discovered early continue to grow, invade local tissues, and sometimes metastasize, and patients with undetected lesions have significantly decreased survival rates.

Exhibit 2–1 TNM Staging Form for Breast Cancer

TNM Staging for Breast Carcinoma

Primary Tumor (T)

TX	Primary tumor cannot be assessed
TO	No evidence of primary tumor
Tis	Carcinoma *in situ*: Intraductal carcinoma, lobular carcinoma *in situ,* or Paget's disease of the nipple with no tumor
T1	Tumor 2 cm or less in greatest dimension
T1mic	Microinvasion 0.1 cm or less in greatest dimension
T1a	Tumor more than 0.1, but not more than 0.5 cm in greatest dimension
T1b	Tumor more than 0.5 cm, but not more than 1 cm in greatest dimension
T1c	Tumor more than 1 cm, but not more than 2 cm in greatest dimension
T2	Tumor more than 2 cm, but not more than 5 cm in greatest dimension
T3	Tumor more than 5 cm in greatest dimension
T4	Tumor of any size with direct extension to (a) chest wall or (b) skin, only as described below.
T4a	Extension to chest wall
T4b	Edema (including peau d'orange) or ulceration of the skin of breast or satellite skin nodules confined to same breast
T4c	Both (T4a and T4b)
T4d	Inflammatory carcinoma

Note: Paget's disease associated with a tumor is classified according to the size of the tumor.

Regional Lymph Nodes (N)

NX	Regional lymph nodes cannot be assessed (e.g., previously removed)
N0	No regional lymph node metastasis
N1	Metastasis to movable ipsilateral axillary lymph node(s)
N2	Metastasis to ipsilateral axillary lymph node(s) fixed to one another or to other structures
N3	Metastasis to ipsilateral internal mammary lymph node(s)

Pathologic Classification (pN)

pNX	Regional lymph nodes cannot be assessed (e.g., previously removed)
pN0	No regional lymph node metastasis
pN1	Metastasis to movable ipsilateral axillary lymph node(s)
pN1a	Only micrometastasis (none larger than 0.2 cm)
pN1b	Metastasis to lymph node(s), any larger than 0.2 cm
pN1bi	Metastasis in 1 to 3 lymph nodes, any more than 0.2 cm and all less than 2 cm in greatest dimension
pN1bii	Metastasis to 4 or more lymph nodes, any more than 0.2 cm and all less than 2 cm in greatest dimension
pN1biii	Extension of tumor beyond the capsule of a lymph node metastasis less than 2 cm in greatest dimension
pN1biv	Metastasis to a lymph node 2 cm or more in greatest dimension
pN2	Metastasis to ipsilateral axillary lymph node(s) fixed to one another or to other structures
pN3	Metastasis to ipsilateral internal mammary lymph node(s)

continues

Exhibit 2–1 continued

Distant Metastasis (M)

MX	Distant metastasis cannot be assessed
M0	No distant metastasis
M1	Distant metastasis (includes metastasis to ipsilateral supraclavicular lymph node[s])

Stage Grouping

Stage 0	Tis	N0	M0
Stage I	T1	N0	M0
Stage IIA	T0	N1	M0
	T1	N1	M0
	T2	N0	M0
Stage IIB	T2	N1	M0
	T3	N0	M0
Stage IIIA	T0	N2	M0
	T1	N2	M0
	T2	N2	M0
	T3	N1	M0
	T3	N2	M0
Stage IIIB	T4	Any N	M0
	Any T	N3	M0
Stage IV	Any T	Any N	M1

Source: Used with permission of the American Joint Committee on Cancer® (AJCC®), Chicago, Illinois. The original source for this material is the AJCC® Cancer Staging Manual, 5th edition (1997) published by Lippincott-Raven Publishers, Philadelphia, Pennsylvania.

CLASSIFICATION OF NEOPLASMS

Neoplasms are usually classified according to the type of tissue in which the tumor first develops and the anatomic site of the tumor within the body. Neoplasms that arise from the epithelial tissues are referred to as carcinomas, whereas neoplasms that arise from the connective tissues, such as bone, muscle, and fibrous tissues, are referred to as sarcomas. Tumors of epithelial origin constitute approximately 90% of all cancers, while sarcomas are relatively rare, representing only 2% of all cancers. In addition, approximately 8% of all cancers are classified as leukemias (malignancies of the hematopoietic system) or lymphomas (malignancies of the lymphatic system).[14(p17)]

Histological classification may further specify the type of epithelial or connective tissue in terms of either function or morphology. A tumor originating in glandular tissue would be classified as an adenocarcinoma, implying a tumor of epithelial origin whose cells normally perform an excretory function. Classification of a tumor as a papillary carcinoma implies an epithelial tumor that exhibits fingerlike projections when viewed

Exhibit 2–2 Example of How a Breast Cancer Patient's Medical History Is Converted into an Appropriate TNM Stage

Case History

A 52-year-old, postmenopausal, previously healthy woman visited her family physician after detecting a lump in her right breast. Upon questioning she stated she felt otherwise well. She denied having any pain or discharge from the nipple. On examination the physician noted a nontender, mobile, firm mass, approximately 3 cm in diameter, adjacent to the areola at "10 o'clock." In addition, two nontender and movable enlarged lymph nodes were palpated in the right axillary region. The left breast and axilla were normal on examination. Enlarged lymph nodes were not detected elsewhere, nor was the liver found to be enlarged. Physical examination was otherwise unremarkable and the patient appeared healthy.

Subsequent mammography revealed a singular mass, 2.5 cm in greatest diameter, with irregular borders and microcalcifications. No abnormalities were detected in the left breast. Fine-needle biopsy of the mass showed infiltrating intraductal carcinoma.

Nuclear bone scanning for metastases was negative, as was a CT scan of the chest and abdomen.

Modified radical mastectomy with axillary lymph node dissection was performed. Adjuvant chemotherapy and radiotherapy was initiated.

Histologic examination revealed moderately well differentiated, infiltrating papillary ductal carcinoma. Blood vessel and lymphatic invasion was noted. Surgical margins were free of tumor cells. Metastatic tumor growth was found in three axillary lymph nodes. Tests for cancer cell hormone receptors were positive.

Staging by TNM Classification

I. Clinical-Diagnostic Classification. The tumor was palpated as being more than 2 cm but less than 5 cm in greatest diameter and was mobile, indicating no fixation to the underlying pectoral fascia and/or muscle (T2). The enlarged lymph nodes were movable and nontender, suggesting tumor growth rather than inflammatory reaction (N1). Clinical workup did not detect any distant metastases (M0). Thus the overall clinical-diagnostic TNM classification is T2N1M0, which represents Stage IIB disease.

II. Postsurgical Treatment-Pathological Classification. At operation the tumor was found to be 2.5 cm in maximum diameter and was not fixated to the pectoralic fascia or muscle (T2). The enlarged axillary lymph nodes were not fixated to one another or to the surrounding structures but gross metastatic carcinoma was evident (N1). No evidence of distant metastases was found (M0). Surgical margins were free of tumor growth. The tumor was found to be moderately well-differentiated. Thus the overall pathological TNM classification is T2N1M0, representing Stage IIB disease.

under the microscope. A connective tissue tumor that originates in bone would be classified as an osteogenic sarcoma.

The term for a neoplasm that has the appearance of originating from embryonic tissues is given the suffix *-blastoma.* Examples include *neuroblastoma* (for neural tumors) and *retinoblastoma* (for ocular tumors). The term for a type of tumor might include the name of the scientist who first reported the cancer in the medical literature. Examples include *Hodgkin's disease,* which refers to a tumor of the lymphatic system; *Wilms' tumor,* which refers to a childhood cancer; and *Kaposi's sarcoma,* the name of a cancer that has reached epidemic proportions in AIDS patients within the past decade.[14]

For many years, leukemias have been classified as lymphatic, myelogenous, or monocytic based on the type of affected blood cell. These cancers have also been classified as acute or chronic based on their clinical behavior. More recent advances in medicine have led to further refinement of leukemia classification through immunological subtyping. For instance, acute leukemias involving the lymphocytes can be subtyped as originating from either T or B lymphocytes. Further subtyping of the T- and B-cell acute lymphocytic leukemias can be accomplished by special laboratory tests that measure cell surface antigens, enzymes, and gene arrangements.[6(pp266–268)]

Some cancers exhibit a mixture of different cell types within the same tumor. Cancers of the central nervous system include a spectrum of tumors that develop in the astrocytes (supporting cells of the central nervous system), the ependymal cells (which line the ventricles of the brain and spinal cord), and cells that make up the meninges (the covering of the brain).[15] Tumors of the brain and nervous system may be composed of a specific cell type or as a mixture of cells. Mixed cellularity also occurs in tumors of other anatomic sites, such as adenosquamous carcinomas of the vagina, which contain both glandular and squamous cell components.

Neoplasms are also classified according to the primary anatomic site within the body where the tumor first appeared. Combining the histological and anatomic terminology, a breast tumor of the glandular epithelium with fingerlike projections might be described as a *papillary adenocarcinoma of the breast.*

A number of disease coding systems have been utilized to incorporate various aspects of cancer classification. For several decades, cancer registries around the world have stored incidence data in computerized form using various versions of the International Classification of Disease (ICD) coding system.[16] The ICD provides a detailed coding system based on the first or primary anatomic site of the tumor. The organ within which the cancer first developed is assigned a three-digit code ranging from 140 through 208 for malignant neoplasms, 210 through 229 for the benign neoplasms, and 230 through 239 for in situ tumors and tumors of uncertain or unspecified behavior. A cancer of the large intestine, for instance, would be assigned the code number 153 for anatomic site. A fourth digit is available to provide further specification of the tumor's location within the organ. A cancer originating within the ascending colon would be assigned the four-digit code 153.6.

As new versions of the ICD have been developed, registries have developed transmutation tables to allow researchers to equate older and newer codes for particular sites and thus extract computerized data for cancers of a particular anatomic site over several decades. Because the ICD codes for many cancers have not changed substantially from the 7th through the 10th revision, it is possible to conduct epidemiological analyses of long-term time trends for these cancers. In addition, ICD codes are used for identifying cause of death, and therefore cancer mortality data can be easily extracted from vital records systems for analysis and comparison with incidence data.

IARC has developed an International Classification of Diseases for Oncology (ICD-O), which provides codes to indicate the anatomic site of origin, the histological classification of the tumor, and the tumor behavior (benign, uncertain or unknown behavior, in situ neoplasms, malignant neoplasms of primary origin, and malignant neoplasms of secondary origin).[17] As an example, the anatomic site codes for cancers of the colon are shown in Table 2–3. A malignant adenocarcinoma of the ascending colon would be coded as C18.2 by anatomic site (Table 2–3) and M-8140/3 for histology. The

Table 2–3 International Classification of Disease for Oncology, 2nd Revision, Codes for Cancers of the Colon

Anatomic Site	*Site Code*
Malignant neoplasm of the colon	C18
Cecum	C18.0
Appendix	C18.1
Ascending colon	C18.2
Hepatic flexure	C18.3
Transverse colon	C18.4
Splenic flexure	C18.5
Descending colon	C18.6
Sigmoid colon	C18.7
Overlapping lesions of the colon	C18.8
Colon, unspecified	C18.9

Source: Reprinted with permission from C. Percey, V. Van Holten, and C. Muir, eds., *International Classification of Diseases for Oncology (ICD-0), 2nd Edition,* © 1990, World Health Organization.

digit 3 after the slash indicates that the behavior of this tumor is considered to be malignant and primary in origin. Data are generally stored in population-based cancer registries using the ICD and ICD-O coding systems.

CASE IDENTIFICATION PROBLEMS AND EPIDEMIOLOGICAL RESEARCH

Epidemiological research studies that are designed to identify risk factors for a particular cancer need to aggregate data according to the primary site of the cancer rather than the secondary sites of metastases. Possible confusion between primary and secondary cancers varies according to anatomic site, and distinguishing true multiple primary cancers from metastatic cancers is often quite difficult. In North America and Europe, where primary liver cancers are rare but where the liver is a frequent site of metastases for other primary site cancers, separating the small number of primary liver cancers from those that represent metastatic spread is hard to do.

The degree of difficulty encountered when attempting to determine the primary anatomic site of a patient's cancer varies widely. Brain cancers, for example, can occur in physical locations in which any attempt to obtain a biopsy specimen is likely to cause harm to the patient. An epidemiologist who designs a case-control study of malignant central nervous system tumors might therefore elect to eliminate cases without histological confirmation. However, the decision to eliminate these cases, because their number is likely to be large, could result in selection bias. For example, extreme levels of a particular carcinogenic agent may be more strongly associated with advanced cancers than with early-stage cancers. These high levels of exposure may increase the chances of developing cancers of the central nervous system and may also lead to more rapid tumor growth in those who do develop such cancers. Consequently, excluding advanced cancers could lead to an underestimate of the strength of the association between the carcinogen and cancers of the central nervous system. An alternative approach would be to have an expert neurologist review the clinical and radiological evidence as a basis for placing these clinically diagnosed tumors into several categories, such as "probably malignant," "possibly malignant," and "probably benign." Separate analyses of standard risk factors could be conducted for the histologically confirmed cases and the various clinical groups defined above. Similarity of findings in these subgroups would provide some assurance that a combined analysis of histologically confirmed and clinically diagnosed cases was warranted.

Difficulties also arise when the clinical course of the cancer tends to be silent and local or distant metastases have occurred in a large percentage of cases. As regards ovarian cancer, 54% of women younger than age 50 and 77% of women aged 50 and older are diagnosed with tumors that have already spread beyond the original primary site into adjacent or distant organs.[13] In this instance, it is often difficult to determine the primary site of the cancer, and the epidemiologist may inadvertently include cases in which the primary cancer is not ovarian. A process similar to that used for central nervous system tumors can be utilized to manage this source of case heterogeneity.[18]

A related problem faces the epidemiologist who is interested in not only identifying risk factors for a specific primary site of cancer but also analyzing separately the histological subtypes that exist for that primary site. For a number of cancers, the determination of a specific cell type is relatively straightforward, and the investigator is probably justified in accepting the histological diagnoses reported by the individual hospital pathologists. However, there are other cancers, such as central nervous system tumors, ovarian cancers, and the lymphomas, in which histological classification is more problematic. For epidemiological case-control studies, the investigator usually selects potential cases from the tumor registry or hospital discharge lists based on the ICD or ICD-O codes. However, the histological subtype of these tumors may be difficult to determine, and there is often disagreement among pathologists concerning proper classification. It is not uncommon for the epidemiologists to obtain representative pathologic slides from the hospital in which the diagnosis occurred for each cancer case identified from the cancer registry or hospital discharge files. These slides are then reviewed by an expert pathologist or panel of pathologists, who classify the histological subtypes of the tumors using special classification systems developed for these cancers. This process helps to standardize the histological diagnoses within the case series and decreases the possibility of misclassification.

SUMMARY

Malignant and benign neoplasms are dissimilar in terms of degree of differentiation, rate of growth, mode of growth, ability to metastasize, response to therapy, and eventual prognosis. Local invasion and metastases involve many complicated biological adaptations by the cancer cells, including angiogenesis, clonal selection, and the production of specialized enzymes. Cancers are classified on the basis of the initial anatomic location of the primary tumor and the histological features of the tumor cells. Classifying cancers according to the degree of differentiation of the tumor cells and the initial stage of the cancer at diagnosis provides important indicators of the prognosis following treatment. Anatomical and histological classification systems for categorizing tumors also have an important impact on the use of routinely collected cancer data in epidemiological research.

Discussion Questions

1. Discuss the basic differences between benign and malignant neoplasms.
2. Discuss the pathologic features of malignant neoplasms in terms of various structural differences between normal cells and cancer cells.
3. Discuss the various components of the TNM tumor staging system and how these components are combined to create a summary cancer stage for each patient.
4. Discuss various ways in which tumor markers are used in cancer medicine.
5. Discuss the anatomic and histologic classification systems that are used to code benign and malignant neoplasms.
6. Discuss the process of spread of cancer through distant metastasis.

References

1. Wills RA. *The Spread of Tumors in the Human Body.* London: Butterworth & Co; 1952.
2. Franks, LM. What is cancer? In: Franks LM, Teich NM, eds. *Introduction to the Cellular and Molecular Biology of Cancer.* 3rd ed. New York: Oxford University Press; 1997:1–20.
3. Cotran RS, Kumar V, Robbins SL. *Robbins Pathologic Basis of Disease.* 5th ed. Philadelphia: WB Saunders Co; 1994.
4. Varmus H, Weinberg RA. *Genes and the Biology of Cancer.* New York: WH Freeman & Co; 1993:39–42.
5. Fidler IJ. Molecular biology of cancer: invasion and metastasis. In: DeVita VT, Jr, Hellman S, Rosenberg SA, eds. *Cancer: Principles and Practice of Oncology.* 5th ed. Philadelphia: JB Lippincott Co; 1997:135–152.
6. Lemoine NR, Stamp GWH. The molecular pathology of cancer. In: Franks LM, Teich NM, eds. *Introduction to the Cellular and Molecular Biology of Cancer.* 3rd ed. New York: Oxford University Press, 1997:343–352.
7. Sklar JL, Costa J. Principles of cancer management. In: DeVita VT, Jr, Hellman S, Rosenberg SA, eds. *Cancer: Principles and Practice of Oncology.* 5th ed. Philadelphia: JB Lippincott Co; 1997:259–284.
8. Nayfield SG, Karp JE, Ford LG, et al. Potential role of tamoxifen in prevention of breast cancer. *J Natl Cancer Inst.* 1991;83:1450–1459.
9. Sobin LH, Wittekind C, eds. *TNM Classification of Malignant Tumours.* 5th ed. New York: John Wiley & Sons; 1997.
10. Dukes CE. Discussion on major surgery on carcinoma of the rectum, with or without colostomy, excluding the anal canal and including the rectosigmoid. *Proc R Soc Med.* 1957;50:1031–1035.
11. Miller EB. Five-year review of carcinoma of the breast: analysis according to Columbia Classification. *Ann Surg.* 1966; 163:4:629–633.
12. International Federation of Gynecology and Obstetrics. Announcements: FIGO Stages—1988 revision. *Gynecol Oncol.* 1989;35:125–127.
13. Ries LAG, Miller BA, Kosary CL, Harras A, Edwards BK, eds. *SEER Cancer Statistics Review, 1973–1991: Tables and Graphs, National Cancer Institute.* Bethesda, MD: National Institutes of Health; 1994. Pub. No. 94-2789.
14. Cooper GM, *Elements of Human Cancer.* Boston: Jones & Bartlett Publishers; 1992.
15. Kleihues P, Burger PC, Scheithauer BW, in collaboration with LH Sobin and pathologists in 14 countries. *Histological Typing of Tumours of the Central Nervous System.* 2nd ed. Berlin: Springer-Verlag; 1993.
16. World Health Organization (WHO). *The International Classification of Diseases, 10th Revision.* Vol 1. Geneva: World Health Organization; 1992.
17. Percey C, Van Holten V, Muir C, eds. *International Classification of Diseases for Oncology (ICD-O).* 2nd ed. Geneva: World Health Organization; 1990.
18. Nasca PC, Greenwald P, Chorost S, et al. An epidemiologic case-control study of ovarian cancer and reproductive factors. *Am J Epidemiol.* 1984; 119:705–713.

Chapter 3

Biology of Normal Cells

James McSharry

This chapter describes the functions of eukaryotic cells at the molecular level. It begins with a description of the functional components of a eukaryotic gene and the mechanisms involved in gene activation, the transcription of a gene into messenger RNA, and the translation of a messenger RNA into a protein. This description is followed by a discussion of the regulation of gene expression. The remainder of the chapter describes the processes involved in DNA replication and cell division. An account of the cell cycle is followed by an account of the mechanisms involved in regulation of the cell cycle.

Normal cells follow set patterns for gene expression, cell division, cell differentiation, and cell death. Under ordinary circumstances, normal differentiated cells do not undergo cell division, and only certain genes are expressed to produce macromolecules that function to help maintain homeostasis. This chapter presents a brief overview of the mechanisms for the regulation of gene expression and for the regulation of DNA synthesis and cell division in normal eukaryotic cells. The reader is referred to several excellent textbooks for a more detailed description of these topics.[1–3]

THE EUKARYOTIC CELL

Figure 3–1 illustrates the structure of a eukaryotic cell (a cell containing a defined nucleus). The cell is surrounded by a plasma membrane composed of lipids and proteins. Some of the proteins contain carbohydrate side chains attached to certain amino acids. These are known as *glycoproteins.* A glycoprotein that extends from the exterior of the cell through the plasma membrane into the cytoplasm is called a *transmembrane glycoprotein.* The transmembrane portion anchors the glycoprotein into the plasma membrane of the cell.

Some transmembrane glycoproteins serve as receptors for chemicals present in the extracellular environment that regulate the activities of cells. The cytoplasmic tails of the transmembrane glycoproteins interact with a number of proteins that are located on the cytoplasmic side of the plasma membrane. These proteins pass signals from the cell surface to other cytoplasmic proteins, called *transcription factors,* that become activated and pass into the nucleus where they activate particular genes on chromosomes. The nucleus of each cell of human origin contains 22 pairs of chromosomes, plus one X and one Y chromosome in males and two X chromosomes in females. The chromosomes are composed of DNA and proteins. The DNA contains all of the information required for a cell to function. The nuclear material is contained within the nuclear envelope, which has pores for transport of materials in and out of the nucleus.

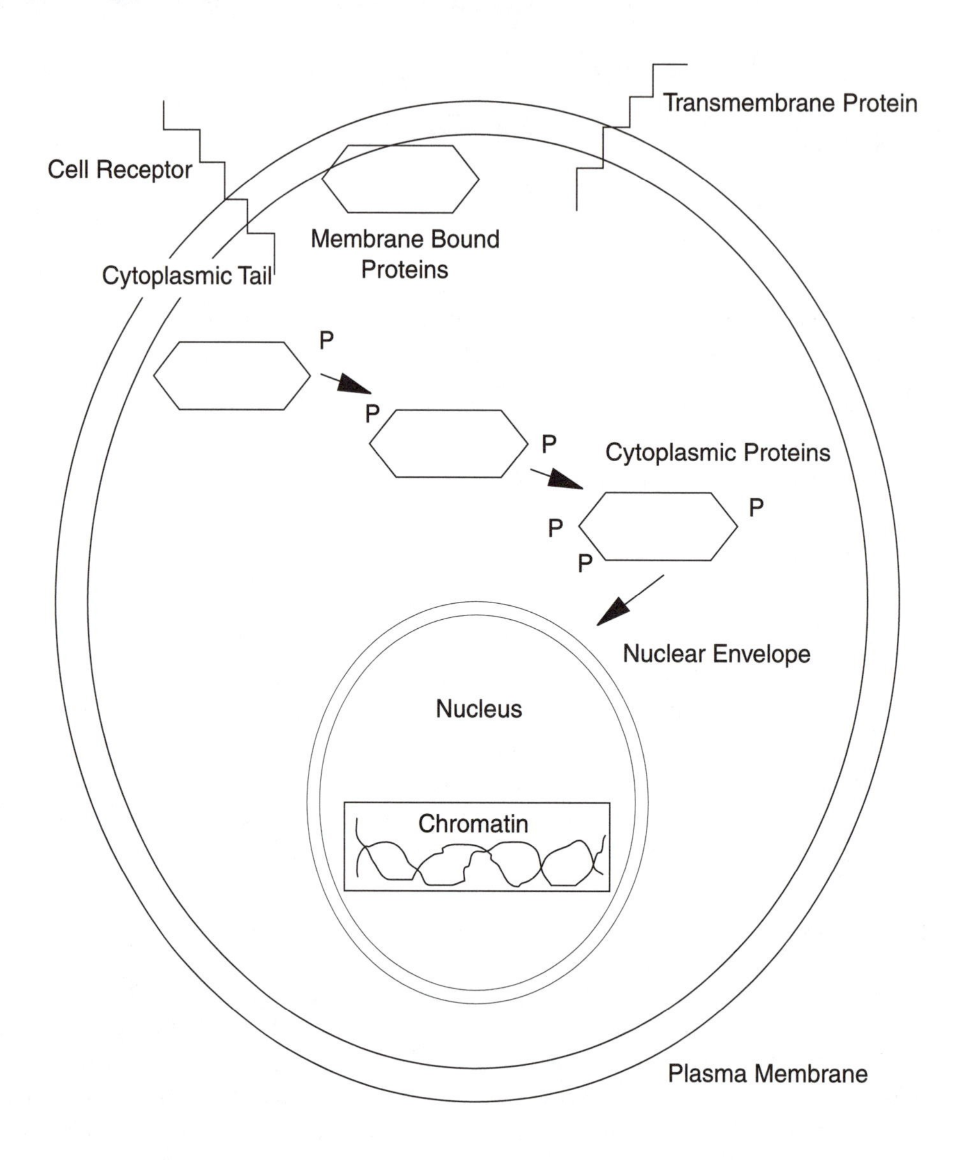

Figure 3–1 The eukaryotic cell. Shown are the locations of some of the important molecules involved in the regulation of gene expression and cell division. The exterior proteins are receptors for ligands that stimulate the cell to initiate an activity. In the figure, the cell receptor is a transmembrane protein that encompasses an exterior segment, a segment that passes through the plasma membrane, and a segment within the cytoplasm. The hexagons on the inner side of the plasma membrane represent membrane-bound molecules that receive signals from the transmembrane receptor and pass the signals to other proteins (hexagons) in the cytoplasm, which proteins then pass the signals to the nucleus. The nucleus contains the genetic material, which is composed of linear arrays of genes covered with proteins that form the chromosomes. The chromosomes in the nucleus together make up the chromatin. The arrows indicate the flow of information from the cell surface through the cytoplasm into the nucleus. The *P*s on some of the hexagons indicate phosphorylation of the cytoplasmic proteins.

GENE EXPRESSION IN NORMAL EUKARYOTIC CELLS

All cells in a human body arose from a single cell, the fertilized egg. In subsequent cell division, the full genetic content of that cell was copied and passed on to all progeny cells. Therefore, every cell in the human body has the genetic potential to code for the same proteins. However, most cells of the human body are differentiated cells that perform certain specialized functions by producing specific proteins. Therefore, the expression of genes in a eukaryotic cell is highly regulated. To understand the regulation of gene expression, we must first understand the structure of a eukaryotic gene.

The Functional Organization of the Eukaryotic Gene

Each eukaryotic gene is contained within chromosomes in the nucleus of the cell. The DNA in each chromosome is wound around a core of histone proteins, known as the *nucleosome,* which keeps the genes silent. Figure 3–2 shows the functional components of a eukaryotic gene. *Enhancer regions* are cis-acting transcriptional regulatory elements (nucleotide sequences on the DNA) that are located at some distance upstream (5') or downstream (3') from the *start site* of the gene. *Promoter sequences* are cis-acting transcriptional regulatory elements located between the 5' enhancer region and the 5' start site of the gene. The *TATA box* is so called because it is a stretch of AT rich nucleotides located very near the 5' start site of a gene. The start site is located at the beginning of the *open reading frame* (ORF), which consists of a sequence of nucleotides that have the potential to code for a protein. A *leader sequence* often occurs between the start site and the first nucleotide that is copied into precursor RNA. A signal for the formation of the *poly A tail* that is added to the 3' end of all messenger RNAs occurs near the 3' end of the gene. *Exons* are stretches of nucleotides in the DNA that will code for a protein. *Introns* are intervening sequences of nucleotides in the DNA that will not code for a protein because they are removed from the precursor RNA sequence after the DNA is copied (transcribed) into precursor RNA.

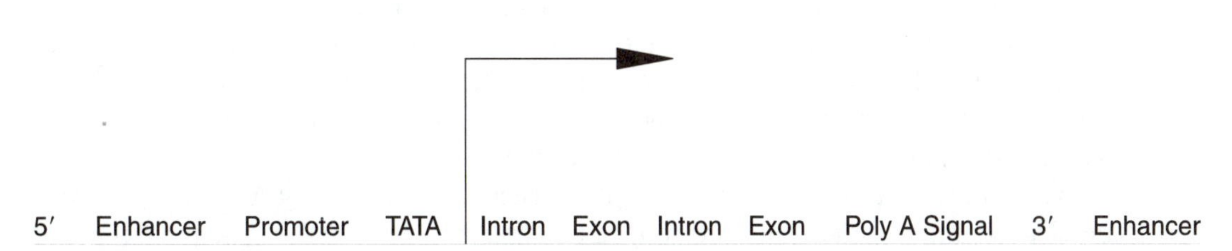

Figure 3–2 Structure of a eukaryotic gene. A eukaryotic gene is composed of cis-acting elements (nucleotide sequences on the DNA) called *enhancers, promoters,* and the *TATA box* (situated upstream of the start site, on the 5' side) and of coding sequences downstream of the start site, including introns (intervening sequences), exons (coding sequences), and a signal sequence for the addition of 50 to 250 adenosines to the 3' end of messenger RNAs. The start site is a codon where the DNA-dependent RNA polymerase begins to copy the DNA into precursor RNA. Enhancer regions can be at either end or both ends of the DNA sequence. Once they bind transcription factors, they can bend the DNA to initiate the copying of the DNA into RNA, a process known as transcription.

Activation of a Gene of the Chromosome

To activate a particular gene, a specific signal must be sent from the outside of the cell to the nucleus. There are a number of different signaling pathways used by different kinds of cells to pass information from the external environment through the cytoplasm and into the nucleus of the cell to activate a gene.[4–9] One type of a signaling pathway involves cell surface receptors that are tyrosine kinases. The binding of a specific chemical (ligand) to specific cell surface transmembrane glycoprotein receptors causes the receptors to dimerize and activate a kinase that is associated with their cytoplasmic portion. The kinase phosphorylates tyrosines on the cytoplasmic portion of each receptor in the dimer. This allows particular proteins present on the cytoplasmic side of the plasma membrane to bind to the cytoplasmic portion of the receptor. Formation of this complex of proteins on the cytoplasmic side of the plasma membrane initiates a cascade of phosphorylation and dephosphorylation events that activate a number of *transcription factors* (proteins that bind to specific regions on the DNA to initiate transcription) present in the cytoplasm. These activated transcription factors dimerize and enter the nucleus, where they push aside the histone proteins on the chromosome and activate particular genes that contain cis-acting sequences recognized by the transcription factors. Once the gene, along with its 5' and 3' enhancer regions, is exposed, other transcription factors bind to enhancer and promoter regions of the gene and begin to initiate transcription (the copying of the DNA into *precursor RNA).* Particular transcription factors bind to specific enhancer regions at the 3' end of the gene, causing the DNA to bend and activate other transcription factors that are bound to the promoter regions at the 5' end of the gene (near the start site). The TATA box–binding protein (TBP) binds to the TATA box and allows the binding of additional transcription factors to itself. In total, this transcription complex recruits approximately 50 proteins, including DNA-dependent RNA polymerase II, that are required to initiate transcription at the proper start site so that the gene will be copied into precursor RNA with the correct nucleotide sequence.

Transcription and Translation of the Messenger RNA

The flow of information from DNA to protein is illustrated in Figure 3–3. A particular gene is activated as described above and transcribed into a molecule of precursor RNA in the nucleus. Small nuclear RNAs and proteins bind to the precursor RNA and process the RNA into a functional molecule. The precursor RNA is processed by the addition of *7-methyl guanosine* to the 5' end of the RNA and by the addition of a chain of 50 to 250 *adenosines* to the 3' end of the RNA (which form the poly A tail). The introns are cleaved out, and the exons are spliced together into appropriate functional units of nucleotides called *messenger RNA* (mRNA). The processed mRNA associates with transport proteins in the nucleus to form a ribonucleoprotein complex that is transported out of the nucleus into the cytoplasm. Here the mRNA associates with ribosomes and is translated into a protein. The protein is further processed by the addition of fatty acids and sugars (acylation and glycosylation) and is folded, cleaved, and assembled into functional units of homopeptides or heteropeptides. The completed protein is transported either into the compartments of the cell where it performs its function or out of the cell to influence extracellular events.

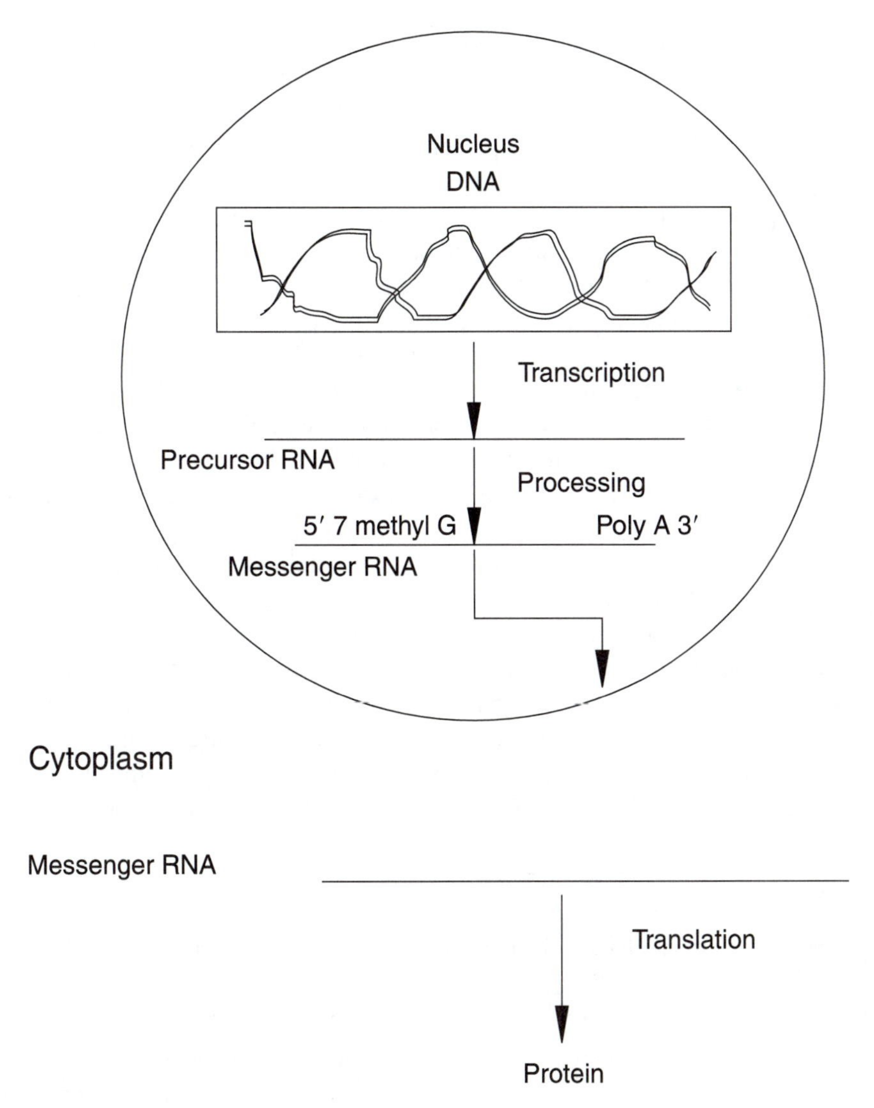

Figure 3–3 The flow of information. Information flows from the DNA in the nucleus into precursor RNA in the nucleus (transcription); the precursor RNA is processed into messenger RNA in the nucleus; and the messenger RNA is transported into the cytoplasm of the cell, where it is translated into proteins.

Regulation of Gene Expression

Since every cell in the body contains the same genetic material and normal differentiated cells only express a small amount of this genetic material, gene expression must be highly regulated. How does regulation of gene expression occur? In the normal cell, gene expression is controlled by the interaction of specific external signals (peptide hormones and steroid hormones) with specific cell surface or cytoplasmic receptors, followed by the passage of a signal from the cell surface or the cytoplasm into the nucleus of the cell. Specificity of gene expression is controlled in differentiated cells by the presence or absence of specific signals. For example, gene expression might be influenced by (1) the presence or absence of specific peptide hormones or steroid hormones in the extracellular environment, (2) the presence or absence of specific cell surface receptors for peptides or of cytoplasmic receptors for steroid hormones, (3) the presence or absence of specific cytoplasmic proteins (transcription factors), and (4) the availability of specific cis-acting factors (enhancer and promoter regions) on the genes contained on the chromosomes in the nucleus of the cell. Exhibit 3–1 lists some of the factors involved in the regulation of gene expression. Activation of specific genes is controlled to a large extent by phosphorylation and dephosphorylation of proteins on the cytoplasmic side of the plasma membrane, in the cytoplasm, and in the nucleus of the cell.[10]

The regulation of gene expression can be very complex (involving many proteins in the passing of a signal from the exterior of the cell to the nucleus) or it can be relatively simple (involving only a few proteins). An example of a simple pathway for regulation of gene expression is the induction of the antiviral state in cells in response to interferon α (illustrated in Figure 3–4).[11] Interferon α, a protein secreted by virus-infected cells, attaches to the external portion of the interferon α receptor on the surface of neighboring cells. Binding of interferon α to the receptor causes two receptors to dimerize and activate two kinases (TK), Tyk2 and Jak1, on the cytoplasmic side of the plasma membrane. These kinases phosphorylate several inactive proteins in the cytoplasm, Stat1α, Stat1β, and Stat2. Phosphorylation activates these proteins, allowing them to form a complex with a fourth protein, p48. This complex enters the nucleus and binds to the interferon-stimulated response element (ISRE) found on the promoter regions of a number of

Exhibit 3–1 Some Factors Involved in the Regulation of Gene Expression, DNA Synthesis, and Cell Division in Eukaryotic Cells

Polypeptide Growth Factors
- Insulin
- Platelet-derived growth factor (PDGF)
- Epidermal growth factor (EGF)

Polypeptide Growth Factors Receptors
- Insulin receptor
- Platelet-derived growth factor receptor (PDGFr)
- Epidermal growth factor receptor (EGFr)

Steroid Hormones
- Cortisone
- Glucocorticoids
- Vitamin D
- Thyroid hormone
- Retinoic acid

Cytoplasmic Factors
- GTP- and GDP-binding proteins (Ras)
- Tyrosine kinases (Src)

Transcription Factors
- Fos, Jun, and Myc

Tumor Suppressor Proteins
- pRB, p53

Cyclins and Cyclin-dependent Kinases
- Cyclins A, B, D, and E
- Cyclin-dependent kinases

Inhibitors of Cyclin-dependent Kinases
- p16, p21, p27

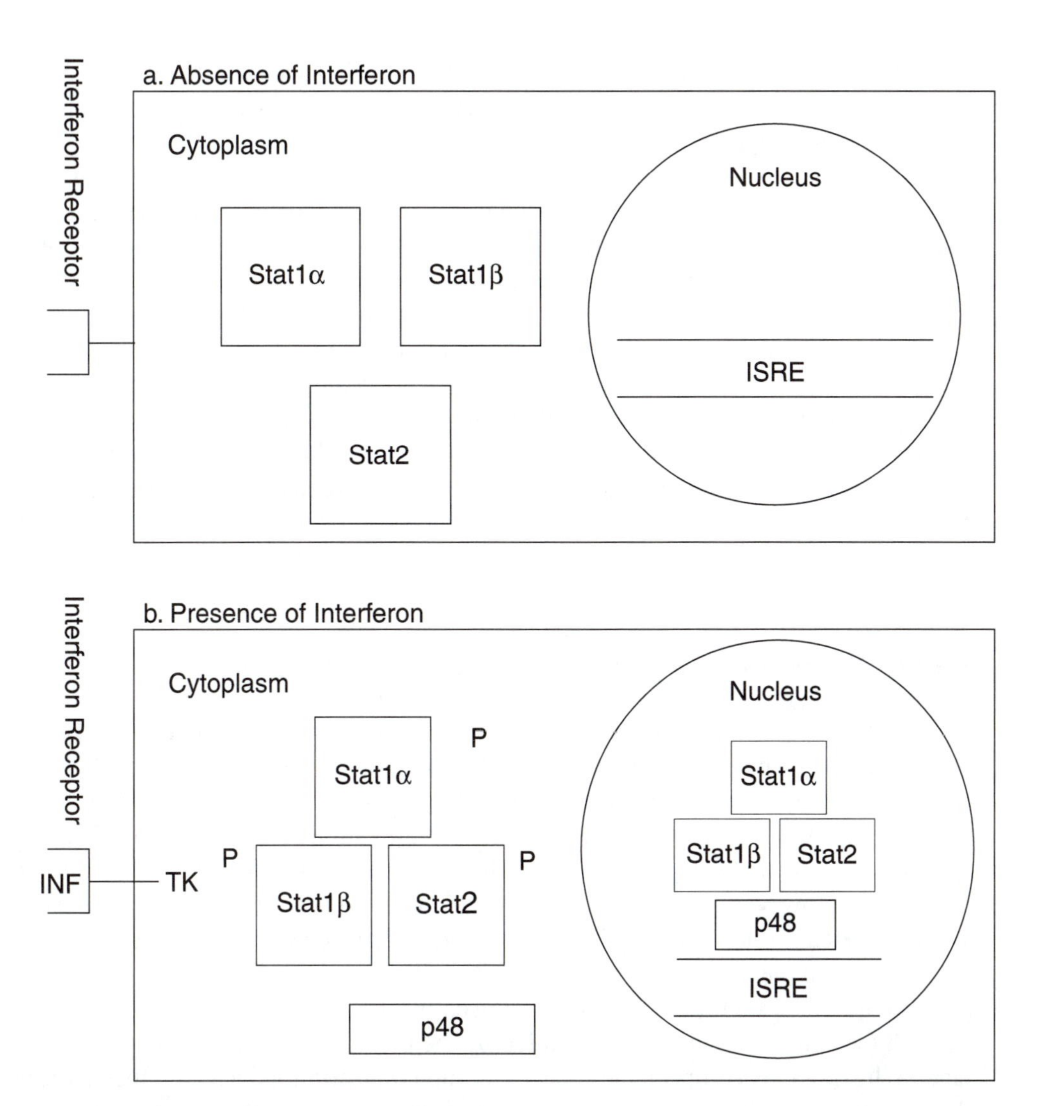

Figure 3–4 Regulation of gene expression. (A) In the absence of interferon, the cell has a number of inactive proteins sitting in the cytoplasm, and the nucleus contains DNA with a number of genes possessing interferon-sensitive response elements (ISRE). (B) The binding of interferon to the cell surface transmembrane receptor passes a signal from the outside of the cell to the cytoplasmic tail of the transmembrane protein. This causes activation of TK (tyrosine kinase, an enzyme that phosphorylates tyrosine residues on some proteins), which is situated on the inner surface of the plasma membrane. The activated TK then phosphorylates the inactive proteins in the cytoplasm, allowing them to form a complex that migrates into the nucleus and bind to the ISRE elements upstream (5') of some of the genes. Binding to the ISRE elements activates these genes, leading to the production of proteins that set up the antiviral state in the cell.

---

genes. Transcription of these genes leads to the formation of three proteins that protect the cell from virus infection.[12] When the signal is stopped by degradation of the short-lived interferon α, the interferon α receptor does not bind interferon α and pass a signal to activate the cytoplasmic proteins, and the specific genes for the antiviral state are not turned on, thereby ending the antiviral state in the cell. Therefore, the presence or absence of the signal (interferon α) allows for either positive or negative regulation of this system, respectively.

Thus, gene expression in differentiated eukaryotic cells is highly regulated. The factors involved in the regulation of gene expression include external factors, cell surface and cytoplasmic receptors, transcription factors, and cis-acting regions on the activated gene. Activation of gene expression depends on the availability of all of these factors. When the factors are not available, activation of a particular gene does not occur. (Cis-acting elements are present on all genes, but they are not always available, in particular, when activated transcription factors have not removed the histone proteins from that region of the chromosome. Therefore, all genes are not activated at the same time.) For activation to be regulated, the activating factors must be short-lived, there to initiate the events and gone within minutes to hours so that the gene is not always turned on. As explained in Chapter 4, one of the major problems in cancer cells is the formation of defective proteins that activate gene expression, DNA synthesis, and cell replication in an unregulated manner.

DNA REPLICATION AND CELL DIVISION IN NORMAL CELLS

Most normal differentiated cells do not replicate their DNA and divide but express certain genes that maintain homeostasis. What prevents normal differentiated cells from dividing or allows them to divide only when they are supposed to? A number of specific proteins prevent the cell from undergoing DNA replication and cell division. These proteins are called *tumor suppressor proteins* because they prevent normal cells from forming tumors. However, when a cell has to divide to form new cells, the negative signals are inactivated by the specific phosphorylation and/or dephosphorylation of particular amino acids on the tumor suppressor proteins, allowing the cell to enter a very specific program for DNA synthesis and cell division called the *cell cycle*. Entry into and passage through the cell cycle is highly controlled by the presence or absence of environmental factors (ligands), receptors on the cell surface, and transcription factors in the cytoplasm. When specific transcription factors become activated, they migrate into the nucleus and bind to specific genes required for the cell to enter the cell cycle, replicate its DNA, and divide. This section briefly describes the major players in DNA replication and cell division and its regulation in normal eukaryotic cells. The reader is referred to excellent texts and review articles for more detailed information.[1–3,13–17]

As illustrated in Figure 3–5, cell division follows an orderly process called the *cell cycle,* which is divided into four parts, G_1 (gap 1), S (synthesis), G_2 (gap 2), and M (mitosis). In the G_1 phase, the cell prepares to duplicate its DNA. The G_1 phase can be further divided into early G_1, during which the cell prepares to undergo DNA synthesis but remains uncommitted to DNA synthesis, and late G_1, during which the cell becomes committed to begin to replicate its DNA. The point that separates early G_1 from late G_1 is called the *restriction point*. In the S phase, the DNA is duplicated from a 2n content to a 4n content. In the G_2 phase, the duplicated DNA is condensed into chromosomes in preparation for separation into two progeny cells (which occurs in the M phase). During the M phase, the duplicated DNA is separated into 22 pairs of chromosomes plus the two

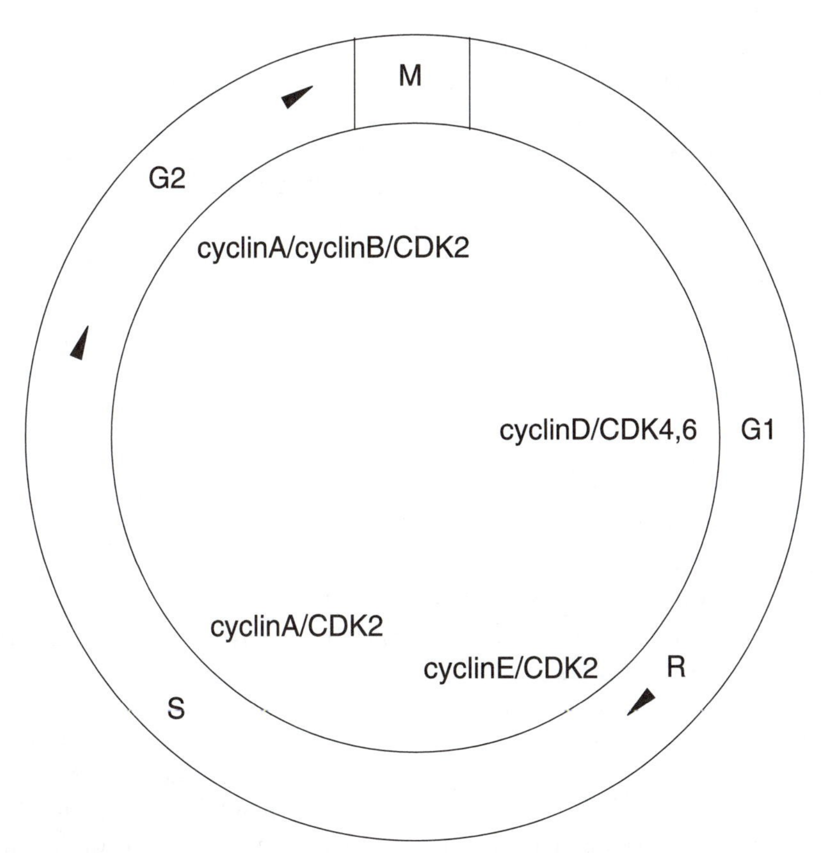

Figure 3–5 The cell cycle. Shown is the sequence of events that occur during DNA replication and cell division in eukaryotic cells. At the top of the figure, M represents mitosis, during which the duplicated DNA is separated into two sets of chromosomes and the cell divides into two daughter cells. G_0 is a resting state outside of the cell cycle. In this state, the cell expresses certain genes by copying them into messenger RNA and translating them into proteins in response to specific external signals. DNA repair can occur during G_0, but DNA replication does not occur during G_0. DNA replication is prevented during G_0 by the association of the tumor suppressor protein pRB with the universal transcription factor E2F, the interaction of tumor growth factor β with cell surface receptors, and the interaction of cyclin-dependent kinase inhibitors p15 and p27 with the cyclin-dependent kinases. G_1 is a gap in DNA synthesis in which the cell receives signals from the external environment for the cell to enter the S phase of the cell cycle. G_1 is separated into two parts, early G_1 and late G_1, that are separated by R (the restriction point). In the S phase, the DNA is duplicated. G_2 represents a gap in which the duplicated DNA is condensed into chromosomes before separation in the M phase. Cyclins and cyclin-dependent kinases drive progression through the cell cycle. Cyclin D/CDK 4,6 complex is active during the early G_1 phase of the cell cycle; cyclin E/CDK 2 complex is active during the late G_1-S transition. Cyclin D and E are degraded at the end of the G_1 phase of the cell cycle. Cyclin A is active during the S phase, and cyclins A and B are active during the G_2 phase of the cell cycle. At mitosis (M), cyclins A and B are degraded. In the presence of DNA damage, the gene for p53, the guardian of the genome, is expressed. p53 activates the gene for p21, which activates the genes for the proteins that perform DNA repair. p53 functions at the interfaces of the cell cycle phases (G_0-G_1, G_1-S, and S-G_2) by preventing passage from one phase of the cell cycle to the next. p53 functions to stop the cell cycle until DNA repair has been complete. If the DNA damage is too great, then p53 sets the cell into programmed cell death (apoptosis). In this manner, using both positive and negative signals, cell growth and division are regulated in the normal eukaryotic cell.

sex chromosome, and the cell divides into two cells (cytokinesis), each with a nucleus containing the proper number of chromosomes. After cell division, the two progeny cells can reenter the cell cycle or instead can enter a prolonged resting state, called G_0. In G_0, the cell continues to metabolize, activate, and express genes that produce proteins required for the proper function of the cell and to repair damaged DNA, but the cell does not replicate its DNA and does not divide. The signals that the cell receives from the external environment soon after mitosis will determine whether the cell enters G_0 or reenters the cell cycle (phase G_1).

Entry into the Cell Cycle

Cells that are going to reenter the cell cycle receive positive signals from the external environment in the form of growth factors such as epidermal growth factor (EGF; see Figure 3–6). EGF is a 52–amino acid peptide that stimulates DNA replication and cell division in epidermal tissues by binding its specific receptor, the epidermal growth factor receptor (EGFr), which is found on the surface of cells in epidermal tissues. The EGFr is a transmembrane glycoprotein cell surface receptor with a ligand-binding site external to the plasma membrane, a transmembrane portion, and a signaling portion on cytoplasmic side of the plasma membrane.

In a normal cell, the binding of EGF to the EGFr causes two receptors to dimerize. Dimerization activates a tyrosine kinase activity associated with the cytoplasmic tail of the receptor, and this activity phosphorylates tyrosine residues. The phosphorylated dimers attract and bind GRB, a connector protein. Then GRB binds with Sos (the guanine nucleotide exchange factor), and together they can interact with the inactive Ras-GDP complex. Thus, a complex consisting of activated EGFr dimers, GRB, Sos, and Ras-GDP is formed at the cytoplasmic side of the plasma membrane.

The interaction of Sos with Ras-GDP dissociates GDP from the complex and allows GTP, which is present in excess, to bind to Ras, causing its activation. The activated Ras-GTP complex initiates a phosphorylation cascade (Figure 3–7) that results in the phosphorylation of a number of cytoplasmic proteins, including Raf (a serine/threonine kinase), MEK (a dual-specificity kinase), and MAP kinase (another serine/threonine kinase). The phosphorylated MAP kinase phosphorylates various cytoplasmic and nuclear proteins to set up physiological effects.[18] The Ras-GTP complex is rapidly inactivated by the GTPase-activating protein (GAP), turning off the signal. Thus, through the interaction of extracellular ligands, growth factor receptors, proteins associated with the cytoplasmic membrane, and the Ras-GTP complex, signals are sent from the cell surface to the nucleus to activate specific genes to produce specific proteins.

Some of these proteins are involved in DNA replication and cell division, such as the immediate early proteins cyclin D, cyclin E, Jun, and Fos. These proteins are involved in the initiation of the G_1 phase of the cell cycle. The immediate early proteins are short-lived transcription factors. In the early, uncommitted portion of the G_1 phase of the cell cycle, pRB (the retinoblastoma protein) is bound to E2F, the general transcription factor, effectively preventing the cell from entering the late G_1 phase of the cell cycle.

When the cell has to enter the cell cycle and replicate its DNA, cyclin D and cyclin E interact with their cyclin-dependent kinases (CDKs)—CDK4/6 and CDK2, respec-

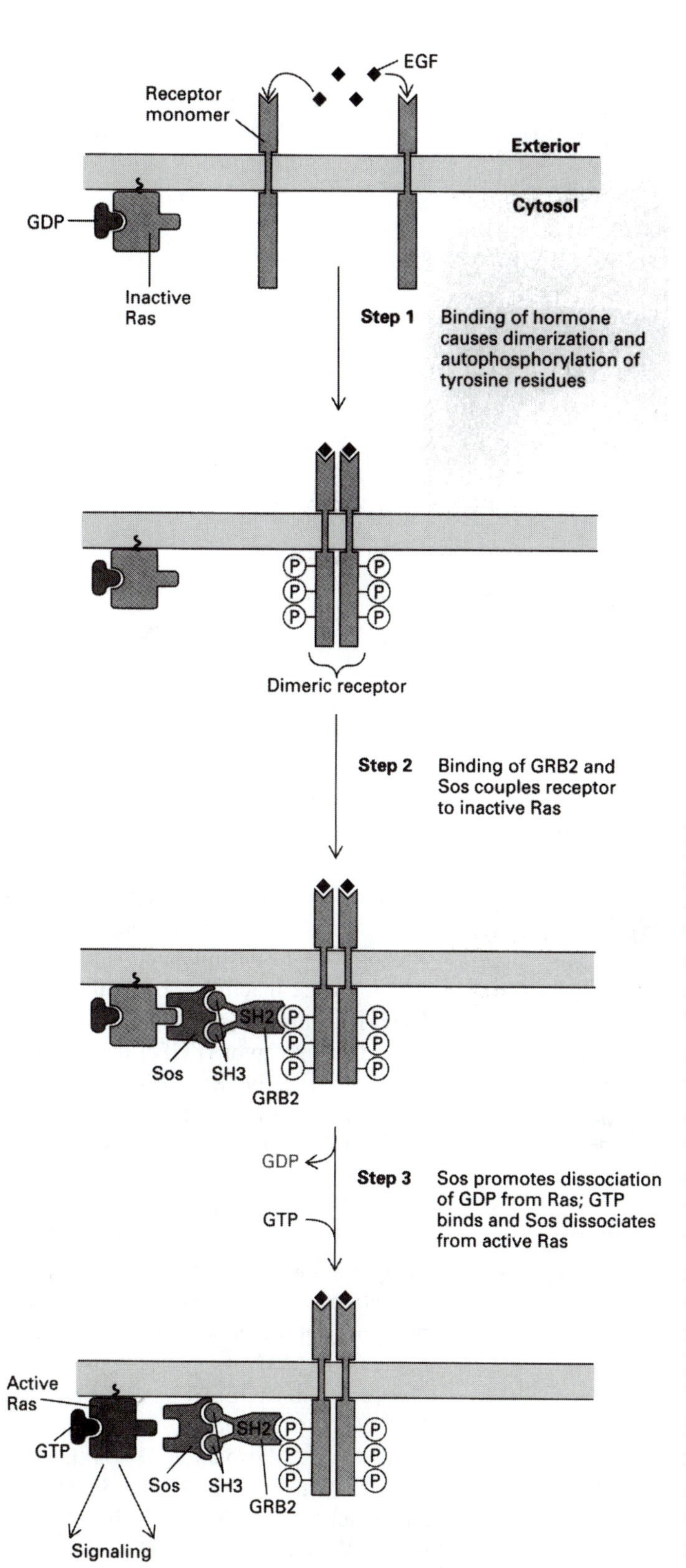

Figure 3–6 Activation of Ras following the binding of EGF to the EGFr. Binding of EGF causes the receptor monomers to dimerize and autophosphorylate tyrosine residues on its cytoplasmic domain (step 1). The SH2 domain of GRB2 binds to a specific phosphotyrosine on the activated EGF receptor dimers; the SH3 domains in GRB2 then bind Sos, which acts as a guanine nucleotide-exchange factor (GEF). Sos then interacts with the inactive Ras-GDP, which is associated with the plasma membrane (step 2). Exchange of GDP for GTP generates the active form of Ras (step 3). *Source:* From MOLECULAR CELL BIOLOGY by H. Lodish, A. Berk, S.L. Zipursky, P. Matsudaira, D. Baltimore, and J. Darnell © 1995 by Scientific American Books. Used with the permission of W.H. Freeman and Company.

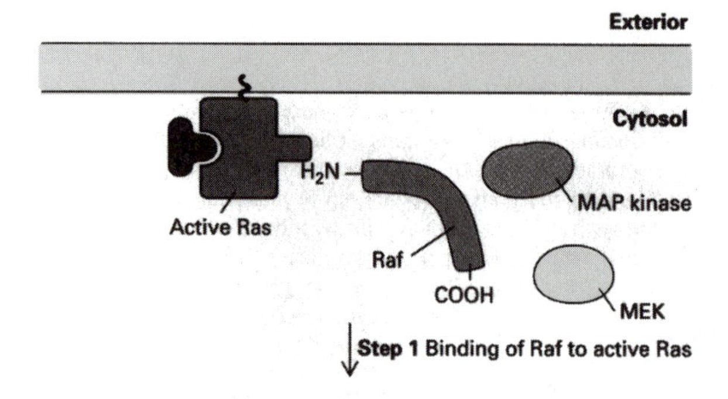

STIMULATED CELL

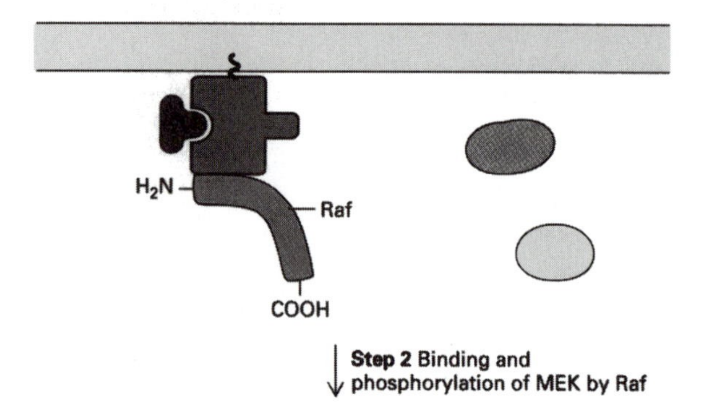

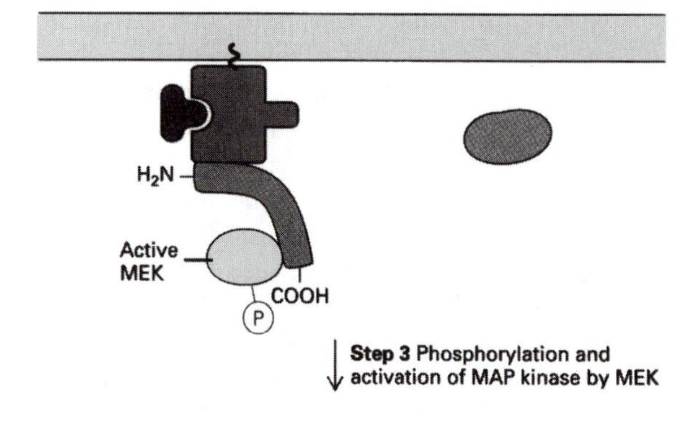

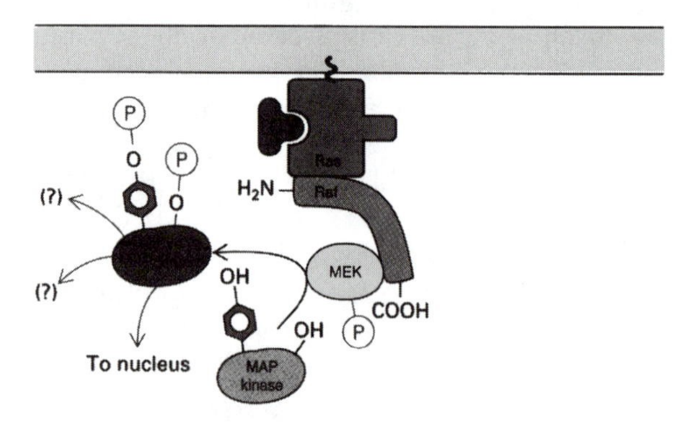

Figure 3–7 Kinase cascade that transmits signals downstream from activated Ras protein. In unstimulated cells, most Ras is in the inactive form with bound GDP. Binding of a growth factor, such as EGF, to its receptor (EGFr) leads to the formation of active Ras-GTP (see Figure 3–6). A signaling complex then is assembled downstream of Ras, leading to activation of MAP kinase by phosphorylation of threonine and tyrosine residues separated by a single amino acid. Phosphorylation at both sites is necessary for activation of MAP kinases. MAP kinases phosphorylate other proteins that enter the nucleus to activate gene expression. *Source:* From MOLECULAR CELL BIOLOGY by H. Lodish, A. Berk, S.L. Zipursky, P. Matsudaira, D. Baltimore, and J. Darnell © 1995 by Scientific American Books. Used with the permission of W.H. Freeman and Company.

tively—and phosphorylate pRB. Phosphorylation of pRB liberates E2F from the complex, freeing it to turn on the genes that code for the early proteins in late G_1. Phosphorylation of pRB by the cyclin D/E–cyclin-dependent kinase complexes marks the restriction point that separates the early G_1 phase from the late G_1 phase of the cell cycle. The early proteins, such as DNA polymerases and thymidine kinase, are involved in DNA synthesis and prepare the cell for commitment to the S phase. At the end of the G_1 phase, cyclin D and cyclin E are degraded.

Once the early genes are turned on, there is no going back, and the cell will enter the S phase, in which DNA is duplicated. Cyclin A begins to accumulate during the S phase, and its synthesis continues until the M phase. After the S phase, the cell enters the G_2 phase, in which the duplicated DNA is packaged into chromosomes. Cyclin B begins to accumulate, along with cyclin A, during the G_2 phase. During the M phase, the duplicated chromosomes are separated into two progeny cells. Cyclin A and cyclin B are degraded during the M phase. The end result is the faithful duplication of the genome and the formation of two progeny cells.

Regulation of the Cell Cycle

The observation that, after cell division, cells enter a resting state (G_0) or reenter the cell cycle depending on signals from the surrounding environment suggests that entry into and progression through the cell cycle is highly controlled. Exhibit 3–1 lists some of the factors involved in the regulation of the cell cycle (note that some of these factors are also involved in the activation of gene expression).

Transforming Growth Factor β, pRB, and the Cyclin-dependent Kinase Inhibitors

Since differentiated cells seldom enter the cell cycle and divide, it is assumed that the cell cycle is turned off. The shutting off is achieved through the interaction of inhibitory proteins, such as transforming growth factor β in the extracellular environment[19] and pRB in the nucleus. Transforming growth factor β induces the synthesis of the cyclin-dependent kinase inhibitor p15, which prevents the interaction of CDK4/6 with cyclin D, blocking entry into the G_1 phase of the cell cycle. Additional extracellular inhibitors induce the synthesis of the cyclin-dependent kinase inhibitor p27, which prevents CDK2 from binding to cyclin E, blocking progression through the cell cycle. In the resting cell, the tumor suppressor protein pRB is bound to E2F, the general transcription factor. This interaction keeps E2F trapped so that it cannot activate the genes that code for proteins necessary for entry into the S phase of the cell cycle. Thus, through the interaction of negative extracellular signals such as transforming growth factor β with their receptors, the cyclin-dependent kinase inhibitors p15 and p27 are activated, and the cyclin D and cyclin E cannot interact with their kinases and phosphorylate pRB. The end result is that pRB remains bound to E2F, the cell does not enter the S phase, and the cell remains in its resting state (G_0).

p53

The p53 protein is induced in response to ionizing radiation that can damage DNA. The p53 protein functions as the gatekeeper of DNA synthesis by regulating the expression of the gene that produces the cyclin-dependent kinase inhibitor p21. The p21 protein functions by inhibiting CDK2 at each step in the cell cycle (ie, during the G_1, S, and G_2 phases). The p53 protein, by acting on the gene that codes for p21, temporarily prevents DNA replication by halting the cell cycle at the G_1, S, and G_2/M interfaces until the DNA repair mechanisms have corrected any mistakes that occurred during the last round of DNA replication. If the damage is too great and cannot be repaired, the p53 protein sets programmed cell death (apoptosis) into motion so that the cell will be destroyed without causing an inflammatory response in the host.[20] If all is well with the DNA, the p53 gene product is degraded and the switch for the production of the p21 inhibitor protein is turned off, allowing the cyclin and cyclin-dependent kinase complexes to drive the cell through the cell cycle. In short, a functional p53 protein regulates the cell cycle by halting progression through the cell cycle at many checkpoints until it has determined that the DNA to be passed onto the progeny cells has been faithfully copied.

What occurs at the checkpoints when a cell contains damaged DNA due to physical or chemical agents? Cells have repair mechanisms that correct mistakes made during DNA synthesis and DNA repair.[21,22] These include site-specific repair mechanisms that recognize and remove a particular base and excision repair mechanisms that recognize physical distortions in the DNA double helix. These repair mechanisms involve (1) *excising* a damaged section of DNA from one strand of the DNA, (2) *resynthesizing* the excised region using DNA polymerase to copy the undamaged complementary strand, and (3) *ligating* the newly synthesized sequence of nucleotides to the neighboring base.

For example, when UV light causes thymine-thymine dimers in one strand of the DNA, the p53 protein is made and induces the p21 CDK2 inhibitor, which blocks the cell cycle at one of the checkpoints where CDK2 functions. In response to the UV damage, an N-glycosylase specific for that aberrant nucleotide and an apurinic/apyrimidinic (AP) endonuclease are induced in the cell carrying the damaged DNA. The glycosylase cleaves the N-glycosyl bond between the 5' pyrimidine and the dimer and the corresponding sugar. Then an AP endonuclease cleaves the phosphodiester bond 3' to the newly created AP site. The 3' phosphosugar and the 5' dimer that remain are removed by an exonuclease. Then the DNA strand is repaired by DNA polymerase, and the two nucleotides are ligated to complete the double strand.

The repair mechanism that uses site-specific N-glycosylases removes only the thymine-thymine dimer. Another repair mechanism recognizes bulky areas in the damaged double-stranded DNA and removes 5 to 8 nucleotides upstream and downstream from the site of damage on one strand of the double-stranded DNA. Then DNA polymerase 1 fills in the gap by copying the intact complementary strand, followed by ligation to complete the double helix.

A third DNA repair mechanism only removes the modification from the base. For example, methylation of the O^6 position of guanine is very mutagenic. A repair enzyme recognizes this defect and removes the methyl group from the O^6 position, inactivating the enzyme in the process.

These DNA repair mechanisms lead to the faithful copying of the DNA, leaving an intact piece of DNA that will function correctly in the cell and in any of its progeny cells. Thus, a number of DNA repair mechanisms are available to correct the damage that our cells undergo each day. The combination of a system to detect DNA damage present in eukaryotic DNA polymerases (proofreading), the activation of the genes for p53 and p21 to stop progression through the cell cycle at each checkpoint, and the ability to repair damaged DNA ensures the faithful replication of the genetic material that is passed onto progeny cells. These DNA repair mechanisms work in G_0 cells as well as in cells that are in the cell cycle.

As indicated, gene expression, DNA replication, cell division, and cell death are regulated through both positive and negative signals. Mistakes in DNA synthesis are repaired so that the genetic material will code for proteins that function correctly in the regulation of these processes.

SUMMARY

The main point to remember is that gene expression, DNA synthesis, and cell replication are highly regulated in normal eukaryotic cells. Their regulation is controlled by the presence of external growth factors, receptors on the plasma membrane and in the cytoplasm of particular cells, transcription factors in the cytoplasm, and components of the chromatin in the nucleus. When all of the components of the cell are working correctly, the cell will express only the appropriate genes and produce the proteins that are characteristic of that cell. Furthermore, the cell will only undergo DNA replication and cell division when it is proper for it to do so.

Discussion Questions

1. Discuss the role of the interaction of transcription factors with enhancers and promoters in the regulation of gene expression.
2. Discuss the flow of information from the nucleus to the cytoplasm and the roles of the various molecules required to make a protein in the cytoplasm.
3. Discuss the various DNA repair mechanisms present in eukaryotic cells.
4. Discuss the interaction of cyclin D and E with cyclin-dependent kinases in the entry of the cell into the G_1 phase of the cell cycle.
5. Discuss the role of p53 in the regulation of the cell cycle.
6. Discuss the role of pRB in the regulation of the cell cycle.

References

1. Lodish H, Berk A, Matsudaira P, Baltimore D, Zipursky SL, Darnell J. *Molecular Cell Biology.* 3rd ed. New York: WH Freeman & Co; 1995.
2. Cooper GM. *The Cell: A Molecular Approach.* Herndon, VA: ASM Press; 1996.
3. Lewin B. *Genes VI.* New York: Oxford University Press, 1997.
4. Tjian R. Molecular machines that control genes. *Sci Am.* February 1995:54–61.
5. Hill CS, Treisman R. Transcriptional regulation by extracellular signals: mechanisms and specificity. *Cell.* 80;1995:199–211.
6. Buratowski S. Mechanisms of gene activation. *Science.* 1995;270:1773–1774.
7. John S, Workman JL. Just the facts of chromatin transcription. *Science.* 1998;282:1836–1837.
8. Grant PA, Workman JL. A lesson in sharing? *Nature.* 1998;396:410–411.

9. Blackwood EM, Kadonaga JT. Going the distance: a current view of enhancer action. *Science.* 1998;281:60–63.
10. Evans RH, Hemmings BA. What goes up must come down. *Nature.* 1998;396:23–24.
11. Marx J. Taking a direct path to the genes. *Science.* 1992;257:744–745.
12. Samuel CE. Antiviral actions of interferon: interferon-regulated cellular proteins and their surprisingly selective antiviral activities. *Virology.* 1991;183:1–11.
13. Stillman B. Cell cycle control of DNA replication. *Science.* 1996;274:1659–1664.
14. Elledge SJ. Cell cycle checkpoints: preventing an identity crisis. *Science.* 1996;274:1664–1672.
15. Nasmyth K. Viewpoint: putting the cell cycle in order. *Science.* 1996;274:1643–1645.
16. Jacks T, Weinberg RA. The expanding role of cell cycle regulators. *Science.* 1998;280:1035–1036.
17. Weinberg RA. 1996. How cancer arises? *Sci Am.* September 1996;275:62–70.
18. Elion EA. Routing MAP kinase cascades. *Science.* 1998;281:1625–1628.
19. Sun P, Dong P, Dai K, Hannon GJ, Beach D. p53-independent role of MDM2 in TGF-β1 resistance. *Science.* 1998;282:2270–2272.
20. Raff M. Cell suicide for beginners. *Nature.* 1998;396:119–122.
21. Sancar A. DNA excision repair. *Annu Rev Biochem.* 1996;65:43–82.
22. Wood RD. Mismatch repair in eukaryotes. *Annu Rev Biochem.* 1996;65:135–168.

Chapter 4

Biology of Cancer Cells

James McSharry

This chapter begins by describing the basic molecular defects that characterize the cancer cell, including defects in the cellular machinery that regulates gene expression, DNA synthesis, and cell replication. It then describes the biological, chemical and physical causes of cancer and the manner in which they bring about these basic molecular defects. The biological causes of cancer include genetic predisposition, viral or bacterial infection, and immunodeficiency. The chemical causes include agents that disrupt the structure of the double helix of the DNA in chromosomes. The physical causes include ultraviolet light and X-rays. For the chemical and physical causes of cancer, the body has evolved repair mechanisms that fix the defects before they can be passed onto progeny cells. The chapter ends with a description of tumor promoters, agents that do not cause cancer but allow cells to replicate at inappropriate times. Constant cell replication can lead to chance mutations. The accumulation of mutations can turn a normal cell into a cancer cell. Eventually, the cancer cell can leave the original tumor and spread to distant sites in the body, which is the hallmark of cancer.

Cancer is a term given to a wide variety of different diseases that are characterized by unregulated gene expression, DNA replication, cell division, and cell death. However, the fundamental defects in all cancers are similar at the molecular level. The category a cancer falls into is determined by the type of cells involved, such as blood, bone, or brain cells. Cancer is caused by spontaneous or genetically acquired mutations in genes that code for proteins that regulate gene expression and the cell cycle. In a normal cell, the genes involved in the regulation of gene expression, DNA replication, cell division, and cell death are called *proto-oncogenes*. Their mutated counterparts in the cancer cell are called *oncogenes*. These mutated genes code for defective proteins (oncoproteins) that activate gene expression and initiate the cell cycle in an unregulated manner. The first two sections below describe some of the oncoproteins operational in cancer cells and their effects on gene expression, DNA replication, cell division, and cell death. The remainder of the chapter describes the biological, chemical, and physical causes of cancer and the role of tumor promoters in the genesis of cancer. The reader is referred to Chapter 3 for definitions of some of the terms used below.

DEFECTS IN GENE EXPRESSION

As discussed in Chapter 3, gene expression is highly regulated in normal differentiated cells. In contrast, gene expression is not well regulated in cancer cells.[1] For example, some cancer cells produce proteases (enzymes that degrade proteins) that destroy the basement membrane and angiogenic factors (peptides that allow new blood vessel formation) under circumstances that would be inappropriate for a normal differentiated cell. The lack of regulation in gene expression in cancer cells is due to the presence of oncogene products in cancer cells. Oncogenes were first discovered in the acutely transforming retroviruses, a group of RNA tumor viruses that efficiently and rapidly transform normal cells to cancer cells in culture and cause cancer in animals.[2,3] Since the discovery of oncogenes in these viruses, many cells obtained from human cancers have been shown to contain different oncogenes.[2] Exhibit 4–1 lists several classes of oncogene products that function in an unregulated manner in gene expression and in the cell cycle.

As discussed in Chapter 3, gene expression is regulated by the transfer of specific signals from the external environment through the cytoplasm into the nucleus, where they activate specific genes. Gene expression is regulated by the presence or absence of proteins in the environment (growth factors), on the cell surface (growth factor receptors), in the cytoplasm (transcription factors and steroid hormone receptors), and in the nucleus. In contrast, cancer cells contain oncogenes that code for oncoproteins that are

Exhibit 4–1 Examples of Defective Proteins Involved in Gene Expression and Cell Division

Growth Factors and Their Receptors
Defective epidermal growth factors (Sis)
Defective platelet-derived growth factor receptor (erbB)

Steroid Hormone Receptor
Defective thyroid hormone receptor (erbA)

Cytoplasmic Factors
Defective GTP- and GDP-binding protein (Ras) that binds GTP all of the time
Defective protein kinase (Src) that passes signals inappropriately

Transcription Factors
Defective Fos and Jun proteins that are not degraded rapidly
Overexpression of Myc, leading to increased cell division

Tumor Suppressor Proteins
The absence of pRB or p53 or mutations that inactivate these proteins, leading to uncontrolled cell growth

Cyclins
Defective cyclins D and E that are overexpressed in some cancers or that interact with their kinases inappropriately

Inhibitors of Cyclin-dependent Kinases
Defective cyclin-dependent kinase inhibitors p15, p16, p21, and p27 that do not inhibit the cyclin-dependent kinases from interacting with their corresponding cyclins

defective growth factors, growth factor receptors, transcription factors, and components of the chromatin. These modified proteins send signals between the external environment and the genes in the nucleus in an unregulated manner. Following are some examples.

Defective growth factors. Some cancer cells secrete defective growth factors such as the Sis oncoprotein, a modified platelet-derived growth factor (PDGF). *Sis* sends a continuous signal to cells to activate the genes involved in DNA replication and cell division, leading to unregulated cell growth and division.

Defective growth factor receptors. Some cancer cells have defective growth factor receptors. The epidermal growth factor receptor (EGFr) normally has an external ligand-binding portion, a transmembrane portion, and a cytoplasmic tail that brings the signal into the cell. Some cancer cells contain the oncogene product *erb* B, a defective EGFr. This oncogene product has lost the external ligand-binding portion of the receptor while retaining the transmembrane and cytoplasmic portions of the receptor. The tyrosine kinase associated with the cytoplasmic tail of the defective receptor is activated in an unregulated manner in the absence of an external signal from the extracellular environment. The activation signal is continuously passed to various cytoplasmic proteins that activate the cell in an unregulated manner.

Defective signals on the cytoplasmic side of the plasma membrane. In normal cells, signals are passed from the external environment through the plasma membrane to a set of proteins that reside on the cytoplasmic side of the plasma membrane. These include GRB, Sos, Ras, and Src. The oncogene *src* is present in Rous sarcoma virus, the first virus associated with solid tumors in chickens. The oncogene *ras* was the first oncogene discovered in human cancer cells.[1] Activation of the *ras* oncogene is the most common dominant mutation in human cancer. In normal resting cells, the protein Ras is bound to guanosine diphosphate (GDP), forming the inactive complex Ras-GDP. When GDP dissociates from Ras with the help of Sos, the Ras-GDP exchange factor (GEF), then guanosine triphosphate (GTP) binds to Ras to form the active kinase complex. The activated kinase passes signals down a cascade to phosphorylate other proteins that enter the nucleus and activate genes. In the normal cell, the Ras-GTP complex is short lived, with the GTP being rapidly dephosphorylated to GDP by the GTPase activating protein (GAP). In many cancer cells, the oncoprotein Ras is defective, having a valine in place of a glycine at amino acid position 12 in the peptide. The defective Ras oncoprotein fails to interact with the GTP/GDP exchange protein (GAP), resulting in a Ras protein that fails to release GTP from the complex. Under these circumstances, Ras always binds GTP. When a receptor tyrosine kinase is activated by an external signal, the signal is continuously passed from the plasma membrane through various cascades to the nucleus to activate genes involved in cell replication.

Defective transcription factors. Many human cancer cells contain oncogenes that code for defective transcription factors, such as the oncoproteins *Jun*, *Fos* and *Myc*. *Fos* and *Jun* dimerize to form the transcription factor AP1. In normal cells, *Jun* is very short lived. Once *Jun* becomes activated and turns on genes involved in the G_1 phase of the cell cycle, it rapidly degrades, turning the signal off. In many cancer cells, the gene that codes for *Jun* is mutated in such a way that the oncoprotein product is missing a portion of the protein. The defective oncoprotein *Jun* does not degrade rapidly and activates genes for longer time periods. The prolonged activity of *Jun* results in increased cell division. Many cancer cells overexpress the oncoprotein *Myc*, a protein that increases protein synthesis. Too much *Myc* leads to uncontrolled cell growth. Even too much of normal Myc can cause a cell to replicate out of turn. Some cancer cells have an oncogene that codes for a defective steroid hormone receptor. In normal cells, steroid hormones from the external environment enter the cytoplasm and bind to steroid hormone receptors. The steroid hormone–hormone receptor complex passes from the cytoplasm to the nucleus to initiate gene expression. In some cancers, the gene coding for the cytoplasmic steroid hormone receptor is mutated and makes a defective steroid hormone receptor, the oncogene product *erb* A. This defective hormone receptor moves from the cytoplasm to the nucleus to initiate gene expression without being bound by the steroid hormone. This leads to unregulated initiation of gene expression because the regulatory signals from the environment, such as steroid hormones, are not present.

As indicated in the above paragraphs, at each step of the signaling pathways—from peptides present in the external environment (*Sis*), to the cell surface receptors (*erb* B), to second messengers on the cytoplasmic side of the plasma membrane (*Ras* and *Src*), to transcription factors (*Jun, Fos,* and *Myc*) and steroid hormone receptors (*erb* A) in the cytoplasm, to the nucleus—there are known oncoproteins present in cancer cells that send signals for gene activation in an unregulated fashion. The end result is the inappropriate and unregulated expression of genes, one of the characteristics of the cancer cell.

DEFECTS IN DNA REPLICATION

Some differentiated cells, like nerve cells, do not replicate their DNA and do not divide under normal circumstances. Other differentiated cells usually replicate their DNA and divide only to replace dead cells. Therefore, normal cells are characterized by highly regulated DNA replication and cell division. In cancer cells, DNA replication and cell division are not regulated. Cancer cells move through the cell cycle in the usual manner (from stages G_1, S, G_2, through M), but cancer cells are always in the cell cycle and do not enter the resting state (G_0). Thus, cancer cells are characterized by the unregulated expression of the genes involved in DNA replication and cell division.

In the normal cell, progression through the cell cycle is regulated by cyclins, cyclin-dependent kinases, and cyclin-dependent kinase inhibitors. In cancer cells, the genes that encode cyclins, cyclin-dependent kinases, and cyclin-dependent kinase inhibitors are often mutated.[4] The mutations lead to the loss of regulation of DNA replication and cell division. For example, in the normal cell, the cyclin-dependent kinase inhibitor p16 prevents the cyclin-dependent kinases 4 and 6 from binding to cyclin D and phosphorylating the general transcription factor, E2F. The cyclin-dependent kinase inhibitor p16 is often mutated in the skin cancer melanoma.[5] Cyclin E is often mutated and overexpressed in breast cancer.[6] In short, the genes that encode proteins that prevent the cell from entering the S phase of the cell cycle are often mutated in cancer cells. Lack of these negative controls allows the cell to respond to signals for gene activation by entering the cell cycle, leading to uncontrolled DNA replication and cell division.

Tumor suppressor genes code for proteins that keep normal differentiated cells in the G_0 resting state and prevent them from entering the late G_1 and S phases of the cell cycle. The best-known tumor suppressor proteins are pRB and p53.[7,8] Underphosphorylated pRB binds to the general transcription factor E2F, preventing it from activating genes required for DNA synthesis in the late G_1 phase of the cell cycle. Many cancer cells contain mutations in the gene that codes for pRB, resulting in the loss or inactivation of the pRB protein. In the absence of pRB, E2F is free to bind to enhancers and promoters on genes necessary for DNA replication, leading to their activation. The cell is free to enter the S phase in an unregulated manner. Mutations in tumor suppressor genes that lead to the loss of function of tumor suppressor proteins often lead to cancer, because the inhibitors of DNA synthesis and cell replication are missing.

The p53 protein regulates the synthesis of p21, the cyclin-dependent kinase inhibitor that prevents cyclin-dependent kinase 2 from binding to cyclin E and blocking progression of the cell cycle at the checkpoints during the G_1, S, and G_2 phases. The majority of human cancers have mutations in the gene that codes for p53. Cells with such mutations fail to stop at the three checkpoints and consequently fail to repair mistakes in DNA that occur before they enter the S phase, after DNA synthesis but before they enter the G_2 phase, and before they enter the M phase. If mistakes in DNA replication do not get repaired, mutated DNA is passed onto progeny cells. Cancer cells are characterized by accumulation of mutations that have not been repaired because of the lack of a functional p53 as well as the lack of normal DNA repair mechanisms (see Chapter 3).

Thus, mutations in proto-oncogenes to form oncogenes that code for oncoproteins affect cell signaling pathways, allowing genes to be turned on in an unregulated fashion. Many oncogene products activate genes involved in progression through the cell cycle. Mutations in the tumor suppressor genes that inactivate the tumor suppressor proteins prevent the cell from being turned off in a regulated fashion. Thus, cancer cells tend to cycle all of the time. The end result of mutations in proto-oncogenes and tumor suppressor genes is unregulated DNA replication and cell division. With further cell division, the chance of additional mutations giving the cells a growth advantage can occur. Further mutations can lead to the ability to make inappropriate proteins, such as metalloproteinases and collagenases, allowing the cancer cells to pass from tissues through the basement membrane, pass through the walls of the lymphatic system, enter the bloodstream, and spread to a distant site (ie, to metastasize). Cancer cells that survive the trip through the circulation system can form a clot in a capillary, invade through the capillary wall, and invade the local tissue. Those cancer cells able to make angiogenesis factors can form a small tumor that then becomes vascularized and grows to a larger tumor, causing serious or even fatal metastatic disease.

FACTORS THAT CAUSE CARCINOGENIC MUTATIONS

As described above, cancer results from an accumulation of mutations in the genes that code for proteins that regulate gene expression, cell division, cell differentiation, and cell death. The development of cancer is a multistep process involving initiation, promotion, and progression. A permanent mutation in a gene (one that is not repaired by the cell's DNA repair mechanisms) is called an *initiating event*. In order for an initiated cell with a permanent mutation to form a small tumor, it must divide. The stimulation of an initiated cell to divide is called *promotion*. All cells in the tumor do not have the same characteristics. Therefore, the small tumor will contain cells in various stages of cancer.

The diversity of stages is called *tumor heterogeneity*. In order for the small tumor to grow and cause cancer, additional permanent mutations must accumulate in the tumor cells over time. The development of these mutations is called *progression*. On rare occasions, sufficient mutations have occurred in some of the cells of a small tumor to allow a localized tumor to grow, invade the circulation, and set up a tumor at a distant site. The formation of a tumor at a distant site is called *metastasis*. Most of the known causes of cancer in humans affect the genetic material directly or indirectly by causing mutations in genes. Therefore, they are called *initiating agents*. The mutations can be inherited in the germ cells or acquired through exposure to a wide variety of biological, chemical, and physical agents present in our environment. The remainder of this chapter discusses the mechanisms by which genetic predisposition and environmental factors induce initiating events that may lead to cancer.

Chemical and Physical Agents

Chemicals and radiation in our environment are the major sources of initiating agents.[9] Chemical carcinogens are mostly electrophils (chemicals that bind to negative charges on molecules) that can covalently bind to cellular DNA, leading to damaged DNA. If this damage in not repaired and is copied into mRNA, defective proteins could be produced, or if the damaged DNA is replicated, it could be passed to progeny cells. In some instances, known chemical carcinogens are nonelectrophils that are metabolized to electrophils by the cytochrome P-450 system present in most cells of the body, particularly in liver cells.

Physical carcinogens include free radicals produced in cells by normal metabolism, X-rays, gamma rays, and ultraviolet (UV) light. The types of damage caused by chemical and physical carcinogens to the DNA double helix include

- alkylation of DNA bases, which destroys the hydrogen bonding between bases
- covalent addition of planar compounds to the DNA helix (the correct base is replaced with the planar compound, changing the hydrogen bonding between bases)
- single- and double-strand breaks in the DNA caused by free radicals, X-rays, and gamma rays
- thymine-thymine dimers caused by UV light
- intrastrand, interstrand, and protein-DNA cross-links that inhibit proper DNA replication and transcription
- inhibition of methylation of bases

These changes weaken the DNA helix and lead to single- and double-strand breaks and faulty base pairing. If the DNA is still functional in replication, the cell containing the damaged DNA will replicate, incorrect base pairs will occur in the newly synthesized DNA, and the mutated DNA will be passed on to progeny cells.

Genetic alterations in tumor cells include

- subtle sequence changes, such as base substitutions or deletions or insertions of a few nucleotides

- alterations in chromosome number (eg, the loss or gain of whole chromosomes [aneuploidy])
- chromosome translocations involving the breaking and rejoining of different chromosomes
- gene amplification[10]

Mutation can result in the formation of oncogenes and mutated tumor suppressor genes, and transcription and translation of these mutated genes can result in the production of defective gene products (oncoproteins) that partially cause gene expression and cell replication to occur in an unregulated manner. Table 4–1 lists some chemical or physical carcinogens and their associated cancers.

Viruses

The second most common external source of cancer initiators consists of viruses. The fact that viruses can cause cancer in animals has been known since the early 1900s. In 1908 Ellerman and Bang showed that avian leukosis virus causes leukemia in chickens, and in 1911 Payton Rous showed that Rous sarcoma virus causes solid tumors in chickens[11] (59 years later, Payton Rous received the Nobel prize in Medicine or Physiology for this discovery). Bittner discovered mouse mammary tumor virus in the 1940s, and Ludwick Gross discovered the mouse leukemia viruses in the 1950s. Partly as a consequence, Heubner and Todaro were led to put forth the oncogene hypothesis of cancer, according to which "all vertebrate cells contain the information to produce RNA tumor viruses." In addition, because of the great success of the polio vaccination programs of the 1960s and the demonstration that viruses can cause cancer in animals, President Nixon signed the National Cancer Act into law in 1971. The underlying hope was that human cancer would be discovered to be caused by a virus and that a vaccine for this virus could be developed to eradicate cancer.

However, many years went by and several false starts were abandoned before the first virus that causes cancer in people was discovered. In the meantime, one of the genes of Rous sarcoma virus, the *src* gene, was shown to be the genetic element in the viral

Table 4–1 Carcinogens Known To Affect Humans

Carcinogen	*Site Affected*
Aromatic amines	Bladder
Asbestos	Bronchus, pleura
Benzene	Bone marrow
Soot, tars, and oils	Skin and lungs
Vinyl chloride	Liver
Cyclophosphamide	Liver
Diethylstilbestrol	Vagina
Aflatoxins	Liver
Tobacco smoke	Bronchus, mouth, pharynx, larynx, esophagus, bladder, pancreas

genome that was necessary and sufficient to cause cancer. Furthermore, a gene that was similar to the cancer-causing gene in Rous sarcoma virus was present in the genomes of chickens, mice, and man. Thus, the Heubner and Todaro hypothesis was confirmed.

In addition, the oncogene *src* in the virus was a mutation of the normal gene that is present in all vertebrates. The discovery of this was the first indication that cancer was a result of mutations in normal cellular genes. However, the viruses that cause cancer in chickens, mice, cats, and monkeys do not cause cancer in man. It was only in the late 1970s that human T-cell leukemia virus types I and II (HTLV-I and -II) were shown to cause cancer in humans.[12] HTLV-I and -II remain the only RNA viruses that have been shown to directly cause cancer in humans. In 1984, the human immunodeficiency virus (HIV) was shown to cause the acquired immune deficiency syndrome (AIDS).[13,14] HIV infection leads to a progressive decline in the absolute number of $CD4^+$ T cells, resulting in loss of immune surveillance and an increased incidence of a number of different cancers. However, HIV infection is not a direct cause of cancer. In fact, it kills the cells that it infects. By the late 1970s and early 1980s, a number of DNA and RNA viruses were discovered to be associated with human cancer. It is now clear that some of these viruses can cause cancer in people, and the molecular mechanisms involved in tumorigenesis are beginning to be elucidated. The viruses that cause cancer in people are listed in Table 4–2.

Five RNA viruses directly or indirectly cause cancer in humans. HTLV-1, HTLV-II, and HIV 1, and HIV 2 are retroviruses, so called because one of their structural proteins is an enzyme called reverse transcriptase (RNA-dependent DNA polymerase). For these viruses to replicate, they must bind to specific receptors and coreceptors on a cell's surface, fuse with the plasma membrane, enter the cytoplasm, and use the reverse transcriptase enzyme to copy their single-stranded RNA genomes into double-stranded DNA. The double-stranded DNA is then transported into the nucleus, where it becomes integrated into the host chromosome. This results in a permanent change in the genetic material of the host chromosome. Thus, integration of viral DNA is an initiating event.

Table 4–2 Viruses That Cause Cancer in Humans

Virus	*Disease*
RNA viruses	
Human T-cell leukemia virus type I (HTLV-I)	Adult T-cell leukemia (ATL)
Human T-cell leukemia virus type II (HTLV-II)	Hairy cell leukemia
Human immunodeficiency virus types 1 and 2 (HIV-1,2)	Acquired immune deficiency syndrome (AIDS)
Hepatitis C virus	Primary liver cancer
DNA viruses	
Hepatitis B virus	Primary liver cancer
Human papillomaviruses types 16, 18, etc.	Cervical cancer
Epstein-Barr virus	African Burkitt's lymphoma; nasopharyngeal carcinoma
Human herpes virus 8	Kaposi's sarcoma

Once the viral genetic material has become integrated into the host chromosome, it is called a *provirus* and will act as host genetic material. If the viral genes are transcribed by host DNA-dependent RNA polymerase II into messenger RNA and if the messenger RNA is translated into proteins, the viral gene products can cause the cell to grow in an inappropriate manner. For example, HTLV-I infects human $CD4^+$ T cells and codes for a protein called *tax,* which is a transactivator that binds to the promoter regions of HTLV-I genes as well as the promoter regions on a number of cellular genes, such as those that code for the T-cell growth factor, interleukin 2 (IL-2), and its growth factor receptor, the IL-2 receptor (IL-2r). The autocrine production of IL-2 and the IL-2r keep the T cell in the cell cycle replicating its DNA and producing more cells (promotion). As more HTLV-I infected cells replicate, additional mutations occur in the replicating cells (progression), which can cause the cell to become cancerous and cause disease, in this case T-cell leukemia.

Human immunodeficiency viruses (HIV-1 and -2), which infect and kill $CD4^+$ T helper lymphocytes, cause cancer in an indirect manner. The $CD4^+$ helper T cell is the central player in the immune system, because it provides cytokines (protein signals) that help both the humoral arm of the immune response (antibody-producing B cells) and the cell-mediated arm (cytotoxic T cells, NK cells, and macrophages) to function. Loss of $CD4^+$ helper T cells due to cell killing by HIV replication will eventually destroy the immune response, leading to a profound immunodeficiency. Immune surveillance is important for detecting and destroying single cancer cells before they get a chance to form a small tumor. The lack of a functional immune system (immune surveillance) will allow cancer cells to replicate unchecked (promotion) and lead to further mutations (progression) that may cause many different kinds of cancers. For example, persons with AIDS have an increased risk of developing cancers of the lung and of cervical and lymphoid organs.[15]

Hepatitis C virus causes primary liver cancer by infecting and killing hepatocytes. Since liver cells can replace themselves if damaged, chronic hepatitis C virus infection leads to chronic cell damage and chronic cell replacement. Chronic cell division increases the chance of mutation. Eventually, accumulated chance mutations (initiating events) in the proto-oncogenes and tumor suppressor genes will lead to cells that grow out of control (promotion) and mutate further (progression) to form tumor cells that gain the ability to grow into a tumor, metastasize, and cause serious clinical disease.

In summary, RNA viruses such as HTLV-I and -II cause cancer directly by integrating their genomes into the host DNA and expressing a transacting factor (tax) that causes the inappropriate expression of a number of normal cellular genes involved in cell replication, leading to unregulated cell growth. Unregulated cell growth of $CD4^+$ T cells leads to mutations that can lead to cancer (T-cell leukemia). HIV-1 and -2 cause cancer indirectly by killing $CD4^+$ helper T cells, leading to profound immunosuppression, which allows spontaneously formed cancer cells to replicate unchecked by the immune surveillance system. Hepatitis C virus infection kills hepatocytes, leading to continuous cell growth to replace dead cells. The increased cell growth leads to mutations in the proto-oncogenes and tumor suppressor genes, allowing unregulated cell growth that eventually results in primary liver cancer.

Of the four DNA viruses that cause cancer in humans, the papillomaviruses and Epstein-Barr virus (EBV) are initiating agents that incorporate their genetic information into the host chromosome. Papillomavirus types 16 and 18 cause cancer of the uterine cervix, as do some other genotypes, but less frequently.[16] When the virus infects the cells of the cervix, portions of the viral genetic information are incorporated into the host chromosome. Two of the papillomavirus genes that become incorporated into the host chromosome code for protein products E6 and E7. The E6 protein binds to p53, causing it to be degraded by means of the ubiquitin protein degradation pathway. The E7 protein binds pRB protein, preventing it from interacting with the general transcription factor (E2F). The end result of papillomavirus 16 or 18 infection of the cervix is the loss of function of two major tumor suppressor gene products, p53 and pRB. The normal inhibitors of DNA synthesis are not present, and, in the presence of tumor promoters, the cell divides out of control (promotion). Further mutations in other genes involved in cell growth and division (progression) can lead to cancer.

EBV infects B lymphocytes and nasopharyngeal epithelial cells, resulting in the integration of portions of the EBV genome into the host chromosome.[17] Expression of certain genes leads to the production of proteins that allow the cell to ignore the normal controls on cell division and replicate indefinitely. The term *immortal* is used to describe a cell that, when well nourished, will undergo DNA replication and cell division indefinitely. An immortal cell is *not* a cancer cell. However, in the presence of tumor promoters and severe immune suppression, such as occur in malaria and AIDS, the cells will replicate (promotion) and accrue further mutations (progression) until they cause cancer. For example, in Africa, where malaria is prevalent, EBV infection causes Burkitt's lymphoma. Worldwide, EBV is associated with lymphoma in immunosuppressed AIDS patients. In each case, the EBV-infected cell is allowed to grow out of control because immune surveillance is not operable, owing to the profound immunosuppression caused by malaria and AIDS.

Hepatitis B virus (HBV) destroys hepatocytes leading to their replacement by cell replication. Chronic HBV infection causes primary cancer of the liver.[18] Increased division of normal cells (promotion) leads to increased chance of random mutations (progression). If some of these mutations occur in genes that code for proteins involved in the regulation of the cell cycle (proto-oncogenes and tumor suppressor genes), then, over a number of years, increased cell replication can lead to primary liver cancer. Further mutations in genes that code for proteins that control the cells' location can lead to cells that leave their place of origin, invade the local lymphatics, and spread to distant sites to cause cancer (metastasis).

Finally, the newly discovered human herpes virus 8, or Kaposi's sarcoma herpes virus (KSHV), has been closely associated with Kaposi's sarcoma in both HIV-infected and non-HIV-infected patients. Currently, it is not entirely clear how KSHV causes Kaposi's sarcoma, but cancer may be caused by the growth factors synthesized by viral gene products in KSHV-infected cells.[19]

As indicated, a number of viruses can cause cancer in humans. In some cases, the viral genetic material is inserted whole or in part into the host chromosome, causing a permanent change in the host genetic material (an initiation event). Once such an event occurs, the cell is induced to grow by any number of factors, and the growing cell accumulates more genetic changes—changes that can lead to cancer. A few viruses, such as HBV and hepatitis C virus (HCV), cause cancer by killing cells that are replaced by normal cell replication. Increased and prolonged cell replication characteristic of chronic infection with HBV or HCV leads to random mutations (an initiating event). Through further cell replication caused by tumor promoters and accumulation of enough genetic changes (progression), the cell may become cancerous. HIV causes cancer indirectly by causing immunosuppression. The lack of immune surveillance leads to cancer because cancer cells are not removed by this important immune mechanism. Promotion and progression of randomly initiated cells can lead to cancer in this environment.

Other Microorganisms

Schistosoma haematobium and *Helicobacter pylori* are closely associated with bladder cancer and stomach cancer, respectively. *S. haematobium* is a blood fluke, one of the flatworms that causes infections in humans.[20] *S. haematobium* is endemic in Africa and the Middle East, where it causes infections of the bladder and ureter. Chronic infection is associated with cancer, possibly because of the granulomas formed in the bladder that cause constant irritation of the bladder wall and resultant cell proliferation. With chronic cell proliferation comes mutation and eventually cancer. *H. pylori* is a gram-negative rod that lives within the mucus layer that overlays the gastric mucosal epithelium.[21] Its association with peptic ulcers and stomach cancer is well established. The body's attempt to repair the damaged gastric mucosa causes constant cell replication that could lead to cancer.

There are no known oncogenes in these organisms. However, constant irritation of the infected area may cause cell destruction, followed by constant renewal of damaged tissue. The increase in cell division to repair tissue damage over time can lead to the occurrence of chance mutations. If these mutations are not detected and repaired by the DNA polymerase editing functions and repair mechanisms, a cell could end up with an initiating event that, through promotion, could eventually progress to cancer. Thus, even microorganisms that do not have oncogenes can induce chronic cell replication that can lead eventually to cancer.

INHERITED MUTATIONS

Mutations in the germ cells can lead to hereditary cancers. These include (1) germ-line mutations that affect tumor suppressor genes (dominant mutations leading to a specific cancer), (2) germ-line mutations that affect the genes involved in DNA repair mechanisms (inherited mutagenic disorders), and (3) germ-line mutations that lead to defects in the immune system (inherited immune deficiency diseases).

Dominant Mutations Leading to a Specific Cancer

A small percentage of all cancers (5–10%) are due to the inheritance of one or more mutated genes that are carried in the germ cells of a parent and passed onto an offspring. As a result, all cells of the offspring show an abnormal karyotype, predisposing the individual to a particular type of cancer. Although the inherited cancers that lead to a specific clinical syndrome are called dominant inherited mutations, they are actually recessive mutations; both alleles of the gene must be defective in order to demonstrate the phenotype.

Each cancer that is known to be inherited also occurs in a noninherited or spontaneous form. The spontaneous forms of such cancers are much more prevalent than the hereditary forms. Hereditary cancer is distinguished from nonhereditary cancers by

- detection at an earlier age (eg, pediatric tumors such as retinoblastoma and Wilms' tumor)
- multifocal lesions within one organ (eg, more than one tumor in the same eye in retinoblastoma)
- bilateral tumors (eg, tumors in both eyes in retinoblastoma or both kidneys in Wilms' tumor)
- the development of multiple primary cancers in the same patient that are not the result of metastasis (eg, the "family cancer syndrome," where a person will have breast, ovarian, colon, and endometrial cancers and usually at a younger age than other people get any of these cancers)

Hereditary cancer is the result of two or more mutations, the first mutation occurring in one allele of a particular gene in the germ line and later mutations occurring in the second allele of the same gene in somatic cells. The end result is the complete loss of a gene or its function through deletion or point mutation of both alleles. For example, in retinoblastoma, a hereditary pediatric cancer of the eye, one allele of the RB gene is mutated in the germ line (initiation), and a second mutation (initiation) occurs in the other allele of the RB gene in a somatic cell in the retina. The loss or inactivation of both alleles of the RB gene results in the absence of the pRB tumor suppressor in the cell. The lack of a major tumor suppressor protein, such as pRB, will allow the cell to enter the cell cycle whenever the cell gets an appropriate or inappropriate signal to undergo DNA replication and cell division. If tumor promoters are around to stimulate cell division, the cell will continue to divide in an unregulated fashion, because the inhibitory signal for cell replication (pRB) is missing. With continued growth and cell division (promotion), the chance of mutations occurring in other genes is greatly increased (progression). As the dividing cell accumulates mutations in genes involved in the regulation of gene activation and cell replication, the cell will grow out of control, eventually leading to cancer. Because the first mutation has occurred before birth, the chance of getting the second mutation that sets up the cell to become cancerous is increased. Inherited cancers are relatively rare, but they have taught us a lot about the genetic causes of cancer.

Each of the cancers known to be inherited also occurs sporadically through two somatic mutations in the same allele (initiation) at a later age. These so-called spontaneous tumors usually only occur in one member of a paired organ. However, the genetic defect is the same in both the inherited and sporadic kinds of cancer, except that the genetic defect occurs randomly in both alleles of the same genes in somatic cells. For example, sporadic retinoblastoma occurs much more frequently than inherited retinoblastoma, but it occurs at a later age and usually involves only one eye; both the inherited and sporadic forms of retinoblastoma involve the loss or inactivation of both alleles of the RB gene. Of particular interest is that the majority of the inherited genetic defects that predispose to cancer involve mutations in tumor suppressor genes. Thus, when the tumor suppressor gene product is defective or missing, the cell is predisposed to grow. If other mutations occur, such as the accumulation of mutations in proto-oncogenes changing them into oncogenes, then the cell is on its way toward cancer. Table 4–3 lists some dominant inherited human cancers and the tumor suppressor gene that is lost or inactivated in each disease.

Inherited Mutagenic Disorders

Inherited defects in the genes that encode proteins that are involved in DNA repair can lead to an increase in the incidence of cancer among patients carrying these mutations. Normal cells have DNA repair systems that are induced into action by a wide variety of chemical or physical agents that cause DNA damage. They function by identifying the damaged section of DNA, removing the damage, copying the undamaged strand of DNA to replace the damaged area, and closing the gap between the bases. Individuals with inherited disorders that affect the DNA repair mechanisms, such as xeroderma pigmentosum, ataxia-telangiectasia, Fanconi's anemia, and Bloom syndrome, experience a significantly increased risk of developing various forms of cancer. These inherited diseases are characterized by defects in the genes that code for enzymes that repair damaged DNA. For example, exposure to UV light causes thymine-thymine dimers in DNA. Normal cells have a system for repairing genetic damage that involves excision of the thymine-thymine dimer from the affected strand of the double-stranded DNA (see "Regulation of the Cell Cycle" in Chapter 3). Patients with xeroderma pigmentosum have lost the ability to repair UV-damaged DNA because they have a defect in the enzyme (an endonuclease) involved in the first step of the DNA repair process. A similar situation occurs with patients with ataxia-telangiectasia, who have defects in the genes required to repair DNA damaged by ionizing radiation. Thus, persons who inherit defects in genes that code for proteins involved in the various DNA repair mechanisms are at increased risk for cancer. In patients with inherited mutagenic disorders DNA-damaging agents (initiating events) cause defects in the DNA that are not repaired. When the unrepaired DNA replicates and the cell divides, the DNA damage accumulates. The accumulation of defective genes involved in gene regulation and DNA replication leads to increased cell replication (promotion) and the accumulation of additional mutations (progression), which can lead to cancer.

Table 4–3 Dominant Inherited Human Cancers

Cancer	*Tumor Suppressor Gene*
Familial polyposis of the colon	APC and DCC
Multiple endocrine adenomatosis syndrome	RET
Neurofibromatosis	NF1, NF2
Retinoblastoma	RB
Wilms' tumor	WT1
Familial breast cancer	BRCA-1, BRCA-2
Pancreatic cancer	DPC4

Inherited Immunodeficiency Syndromes

Inherited defects in genes that regulate the immune system can predispose a person to cancer. Examples of inherited immune deficiency diseases include Bruton's agammaglobulinemia, thymic hypoplasia (DiGeorge syndrome), immunodeficiency with thrombocytopenia and eczema (Wiskott-Aldrich syndrome), and severe combined immunodeficiency syndrome. Since immune surveillance destroys cancer cells expressing a mutated phenotype, individuals with inherited defects in the immune system are at increased risk for lymphoreticular tumors and leukemia. Thus, predisposition to cancer can be inherited if there are germ-line (prezygotic) mutations in tumor suppressor genes, the genes that are involved in DNA repair, and genes involved in the proper functioning of the immune system. These mutations are initiation events. Cell growth and division of the initiated cell (promotion) and further mutations in the growing and dividing initiated cell (progression) can lead to cancer.

A wide variety of factors—from an inherited predisposition to cancer to viruses that integrate their genomes into the host chromosome to chemical and physical agents that affect the genome—can initiate a process that could lead to cancer. Once the initiated cancer cell begins to replicate through the effects of tumor promoters, it gains the potential to further mutate. As additional mutations occur in the genes that code for proteins that regulate DNA replication and cell division, the tumor cell progresses toward cancer. Eventually, some cells in the tumor might acquire additional mutations that allow tumor cells to leave the original site and metastasize to a distant site, invade tissues at the distant site, create a tumor there, and cause metastatic cancer.

TUMOR PROMOTERS

If a chemical or physical carcinogen causes permanent damage to cellular DNA, and the mutation is viable, nothing will happen unless the cell begins to divide. Tumor promoters are biological, chemical, or physical entities that cause cells to divide. They are not mutagenic by themselves but amplify the effects of low doses of carcinogens. Further, they increase the likelihood of a tumor only if a mutagenic (initiation) event has occurred and the cell is exposed to the tumor promoters for a prolonged period. The action of tumor promoters is reversible at the early stages of promotion and is not additive. There is probably a threshold for the doses of the tumor promoters. Tumor promoters stimulate cell division by activating the cyclic AMP/adenyl cyclase and inositol phosphate-diacyl glycerol-protein kinase C systems. Tumor promoters can activate these systems in the absence of growth factors and growth factor receptors. Therefore, the gene activation and cell division can occur in an unregulated manner. If the cell is mutated, then a cell with a defect will undergo DNA replication and divide. A wide variety of chemicals are tumor promoters, including the artificial sweetener saccharine. Others include the following:

- phorbol-12-tetradeconoate-13-acetate (TPA)
- phorbol-12-myristate-13-acetate (PMA)
- benzoyl peroxide
- diacyl glycerol

Once the mutated cell begins to divide (promotion), the chance of additional mutations increases. Eventually, the cell accumulates a number of mutations in tumor suppressor genes and proto-oncogenes, allowing the cell to grow in an unregulated fashion. With increased cell replication, the cell accumulates more mutations (progression). Some of these mutations code for proteins that enable the tumor to grow, invade the local tissue, enter the lymphatics, metastasize, and invade distant organs. Angiogenesis factors can enable a very tiny tumor to become vascularized and grow into a sizable tumor, while the genes for metalloproteinases and collagenases may be expressed inappropriately, allowing the tumor cells to invade adjacent tissues and the lymphatics, spread to the bloodstream, and begin to circulate throughout the body.

In summary, some biological and physical carcinogens are initiators. Some chemicals known to interact with DNA are initiators, but most chemicals only enhance cell growth and replication and therefore are tumor promoters. Some viruses change the genetic content of the cell and are tumor initiators, but others, such as HBV and HCV, induce the infected cells to grow and are therefore tumor promoters. Tumor initiators directly affect DNA, leading to mutations that include the loss of a gene product or the production of defective gene products. Functional defective gene products involved in the regulation of gene expression, DNA replication, cell division, and cell death can cause the cells to express genes under inappropriate circumstances and to replicate the DNA and divide at inappropriate times. Promotion and progression of these mutated cells can lead to cancer.

SUMMARY

Cancer cells have defects in the molecular machinery that regulates gene expression, DNA synthesis, and cell division. These defects are caused by mutations in the genes that encode the proteins that carry out the functions of the cell. The mutations are caused by biological, chemical, and physical agents. Viruses, bacteria, and genetic predisposition are common biological causes of cancer. There are no repair mechanisms to fix biological causes of cancer. Chemical and physical causes of cancer interfere with the structure of the DNA in our chromosomes. Eukaryotic cells have evolved several repair mechanisms that will fix the DNA damage caused by these agents. If the damage is not repaired, then further mutations can occur, and a mutated cell can grow into a tumor and eventually lead to disease.

Discussion Questions

1. Discuss the effects of physical and chemical carcinogens on the structure and function of DNA.
2. Discuss the role that mutations in tumor suppressor genes play in the initiation of cancer.
3. Describe the role of RNA tumor viruses in the initiation of cancer.
4. Discuss the role of infection with human immunodeficiency virus (HIV) and immune surveillance in the initiation of cancer in AIDS patients.
5. Discuss the role of oncogenes in the initiation of cancer.
6. Discuss the role of tumor promoters in the etiology of cancer.

References

1. Perkins AS, Stern DF. Molecular biology of cancer: oncogenes. In: DeVita VD, Hellman S, Rosenberg SA, eds. *Cancer: Principles and Practice of Oncology.* 5th ed. Philadelphia: Lippincott-Raven Publishers; 1997:79–105.
2. Bishop JM. Cellular oncogenes and retroviruses. *Annu Rev Biochem.* 1985;52:301–354.
3. Varmus HE. The molecular genetics of cellular oncogenes. *Annu Rev Genet.* 1984;18:553–612.
4. Sherr CJ. Cancer cell cycles. *Science.* 1996;274:1672–1677.
5. Serrano M. The tumor suppressor protein $p16^{INK4a}$. *Exp Cell Res.* 1997;237:7–13.
6. Prall OW, Rogan EM, Sutherland RL. Estrogen regulation of cell cycle progression in breast cancer cells. *J Steroid Biochem Mol Biol.* 1998;65:169–174.
7. Weinberg RA. The retinoblastoma protein and cell cycle control. *Cell.* 1995;81:323–330.
8. Weinberg RA. How cancer arises. *Sci Am.* September 1996;275:62–70.
9. Yuspa SH, Shields PG. Etiology of cancer: chemical factors. In: DeVita VD, Hellman S, Rosenberg SA, eds. *Cancer: Principles and Practice of Oncology.* 5th ed. Philadelphia: Lippincott-Raven Publishers; 1997:185–200.
10. Lengauer C, Kinzler KW, Vogelstein B. Genetic instabilities in human cancers. *Nature.* 1998;396:643–649.
11. Nevins JR, Vogt PK. Cell transformation by viruses. In: Fields BN, Knipe DM, Howley PM, eds. *Fundamental Virology.* 3rd ed. Philadelphia: Lippincott-Raven Publishers; 1996:267–309.
12. Yoshida M. Host HTLV-I interaction at the molecular level. *AIDS Res Hum Retroviruses.* 1994;10:1193–1197.
13. Barre-Sinousi F, Chermann JC, Rey F, et al. Isolation of a T lymphotropic retrovirus from a patient at risk for acquired immunodeficiency syndrome (AIDS). *Science.* 1983;220:868–871.
14. Gallo RC, Salahuddin SZ, Popovic M, et al. Frequent detection and isolation of cytopathic retroviruses (HTLV-III) from patients with AIDS and at risk for AIDS. *Science.* 1984;224:500–503.
15. Remick SC, Harper GR, Adullah MA, McSharry JJ, Ross JS, Ruckdeschel JC. Metastatic breast cancer in a young patient seropositive for human immunodeficiency virus. *J Natl Cancer Inst.* 1991;83:447–448.
16. Howley PM. Papillomaviridae: the viruses and their replication. In: Fields BN, Knipe DM, Howley PM, eds. *Fundamental Virology.* 3rd ed. Philadelphia: Lippincott-Raven Publishers; 1996:947–978.
17. Kieff E. Epstein-Barr virus and its replication. In: Fields BN, Knipe DM, Howley PM, eds. *Fundamental Virology.* 3rd ed. Philadelphia: Lippincott-Raven Publishers; 1996:1109–1162.
18. Tiollais P, Buendia M-A. Hepatitis B virus. *Sci Am.* April 1991:116–123.
19. Gallo RC. The enigmas of Kaposi's sarcoma. *Science.* 1998;282:1837–1839.
20. Mahmoud AAF. Trematodes (schistosomiasis) and other flukes. In: Mandell GL, Bennett JE, Dolan R, eds. *Principles and Practice of Infectious Diseases.* 4th ed. New York: Churchill Livingston; 1995:2538–2544.
21. Blaser MJ. *Helicobacter pylori* and related organisms. In: Mandell GL, Bennett JE, Dolan R, eds. *Principles and Practice of Infectious Diseases.* 4th ed. New York: Churchill Livingston; 1995:1956–1964.

Chapter 5

Laboratory Experimental Studies

Philip C. Nasca

Scientific evidence concerning the carcinogenicity of various environmental exposures comes from a number of sources, including laboratory experiments. The current chapter reviews the various experimental approaches currently being used to assess the carcinogenic potential of various compounds.

A large number of chemicals are commonly used in settings in which human exposure can easily occur. Potentially harmful chemicals are used in industrial applications of various chemicals and medical therapies and are contained in many consumer products. The magnitude of the problem suggests the need to utilize screening methods that can identify chemicals likely to be human carcinogens in a timely and efficient manner. These methods include using animal models, performing short-term in vitro tests, and selecting chemicals for short- and long-term testing based on their structural similarities to known mutagenic or carcinogenic agents. The strengths and weaknesses of these various approaches are discussed in this chapter. The chapter also includes a description of the International Agency for Research on Cancer guidelines for assessing the extent to which the available experimental and epidemiological data support the classification of a compound as a carcinogen.

In 1978, it was estimated that more than 63,00 chemicals were commonly used in settings in which human exposure is possible.[1] The number of such chemicals has grown considerably since that time, as has the magnitude of the effort needed to identify chemicals likely to be human carcinogens.[2] Opportunities for human exposure to carcinogenic chemicals include industrial applications of various chemicals, treatment by means of medical therapies, and utilization of consumer products. Epidemiological research has made significant contributions to our understanding of the relation between various chemicals or chemical mixtures and human cancers. However, the number of chemicals that have been studied in human populations is small, and uncertainties plague some studies owing to poor exposure measurement and uncontrolled confounding.[3] Findings from experimental studies are also needed to help define the universe of chemicals that pose a carcinogenic risk to humans.

Experimental research includes studies of the carcinogenic effects of chemicals in various animal models. The long-term nature of the animal studies and the associated expense, however, prevent testing more than a small fraction of the chemicals that require testing. The carcinogenic potential of a particular chemical can also be assessed through so-called short-term studies, which are designed to determine if the chemical acts as a mutagen in one or more in vitro systems. Since most animal and human carcinogens are mutagens, chemicals that are shown to be mutagenic in these test systems may also be carcinogenic. Chemical structural analysis has also been used to determine good candidates for testing. Chemicals are selected for short- and long-term studies based on their structural similarities to known carcinogenic agents.

This chapter focuses on the strengths and weaknesses of these various approaches, the criteria that are used to help interpret data from these studies, and the classification systems that have evolved from these data. New developments in the field of experimental carcinogenesis and the use of these approaches for classifying chemicals as human carcinogens are also discussed. These testing programs and subsequent classification activities are conducted by a number of agencies, including the National Toxicology Program (NTP) of the National Institute of Environmental Health and Safety, the GENETOX program of the US Environmental Protection Program (EPA), and the International Agency for Research on Cancer (IARC). These agencies have not only supported testing programs but have also developed guidelines for interpreting experimental data and ranking chemicals and other naturally occurring substances in terms of their possible carcinogenicity.

ANIMAL TESTING

Background

Most animal testing involves the administration of suspect chemicals or complex mixtures of chemicals to various strains of mice, rats, and hamsters. Animals are randomized to treatment and control groups and are administered measured doses of the chemical or placebo. Among the strengths of these studies are their ability to control and accurately determine exposure levels and their ability to control selection bias and confounding through randomization. The use of inbred animals also serves to control for confounding by genetic factors. Among their weaknesses are their long duration and the associated expense, which limit the number of chemicals that can be tested in any given year. Concerns have also been raised about extrapolating data from animal models to humans. While appropriate cautions must be taken when interpreting the data, the utility of findings from animal studies has been clearly demonstrated. Of the 53 chemicals classified as human carcinogens by IARC in 1989, all were found to be carcinogenic in animals.[4,5] There is also a close correspondence between long-term animal studies and epidemiological studies regarding the anatomic site of the cancer produced by a particular chemical exposure. Similar routes of exposure frequently produce the same cancer in both animals and humans.

General Methods

The suspect chemicals may be administered to test animals in various ways, including orally, through inhalation, through subcutaneous or intramuscular injection, through topical application directly to the skin, and through implantation in the trachea, pleura, vagina, and oral cavity, among other locations. The amount of the chemical administered may be the maximum tolerated dose (MTD), which is the highest dose that can be given for the duration of the study without shortening the longevity of the test animals as a result of noncarcinogenic toxic effects.[2] The MTD may cause some minor toxic effects, such as necrosis, which leads to significant tissue regeneration, possibly making it difficult to interpret the neoplastic effects of the chemical.

In order to determine if a dose-response relation exists between the putative chemical and tumor incidence, the animals may be divided into subgroups whose dosage levels vary. For example, the dosage for one subgroup may be the MTD and for others the MTD diluted by factors of 2, 4, and 8. The treatments may begin in utero or when the animals are six weeks of age, and they usually continue until the animals reach 24 or 30 months of age. The follow-up periods are usually in the range of from 3 to 6 months following the end of the dose period.

In studies of transplacental carcinogenesis, female animals are bred and treated with the suspect chemical. The potential for the chemical to cross the placenta and cause cancer in utero is determined by examining tumor incidence in the offspring at the time of birth. Two animal species are usually involved in the bioassays, and the experiments usually involve equal numbers of male and female animals. When the animals are sacrificed, both external and histologic examinations are conducted of 30 organs and tissues. The difficulty of separating benign from malignant neoplasms in rodents has prompted some regulatory agencies to strongly suggest the involvement of a board-certified pathologist who has experience in judging the nature of these animal tumors.[6,7]

Evaluating Study Results

A number of statistical methods are used to analyze data from long-term animal studies. Animals may die prior to study termination as a result of nonneoplastic causes, making it necessary to use life-table or actuarial methods of analysis. Tumors that do not cause the death of the animal but are detected only at autopsy pose additional statistical challenges. The various statistical approaches that can be used to analyze data from long-term animal studies are described in detail by Peto et al.[8]

A number of qualitative criteria have been developed to evaluate long-term animal studies, including the conditions under which the chemical was tested. These criteria involve the route of administration and animal characteristics such as species, strain, sex, and age. The consistency of findings across several studies is of vital importance. Consistent observation of increased tumor incidence in a specific target organ among the same or different species or strains of animals provides strong evidence that a chemical is an animal carcinogen. The tested chemicals may produce a wide range of neoplastic endpoints, from relatively benign tumors to multiple malignant tumors to both benign and malignant tumors observed in the same animals. Benign tumors may be endpoints in themselves or may represent a premalignant form of the cancers observed in these animals. The interpretation of study results is sometimes complicated by the extent to which the toxic properties of the chemical produce significant or unusual growth or weight gain differences between treated animals and control animals.[9]

Quantitative criteria also play a role in assessing the extent to which existing studies implicate a chemical as an animal carcinogen. As in epidemiological studies, a marked increase in the incidence of specific tumors among treated animals and the observance of a dose-response relation in all or most studies provide strong evidence of carcinogenicity. The dose-response relations may vary considerably depending on the species, strain, sex, and age of the test animals and the route of administration. Evidence of carcinogenicity may also be provided by an increased incidence of multiple tumors at the same anatomic site and by a significant reduction in the latent period (time between first treatment and the first appearance of the tumor).[9]

Transgenic Mouse Models

Animal studies have a number of strengths and a number of weaknesses. The weaknesses include high cost and problems in interpreting study results. As regards the first weakness, animal studies are expensive and time consuming, usually taking two years to complete. As regards the second, highly inbred rodent strains are used to reduce the potential confounding effects of genetic variability, but the reduction in genetic variability leads to two problems that can interfere with the interpretation of study results. Inbred species tend to produce specific patterns of "spontaneous" tumors that occur with a high incidence in the absence of chemical exposures. This propensity to develop a high incidence of specific tumors is observed from generation to generation in untreated animals and thus represents an underlying heritable risk. This risk may be largely independent of the chemical exposures being tested. Investigators must consider the background incidence rates for various spontaneous tumors when interpreting results for inbred rodent species.

In addition, the use of highly inbred rodent species leads to a significant reduction in potential tissue responses to the chemicals being tested and an increase in strain- and sex-specific responses to particular chemicals. The observation that a particular chemical is associated with an increased incidence of specific cancers in several strains or species and in both sexes is strong evidence that the chemical is an animal carcinogen and also strong evidence that the chemical may be a human carcinogen. When tumor development is limited to specific strains or sexes, the evidence that the chemical is a carcinogen is weakened.[10] To help overcome these problems, experimental scientists have been developing new animal studies that utilize transgenic mouse models.

Transgenic mice are produced when specific genes are added to or deleted from the animals' normal genetic makeup.[11] In the case of experimental carcinogenesis, scientists add modified genes that create a predictable response to various carcinogenic chemicals.[12] Multiple copies of these modified genes (inducible oncogenes) are added to the genomes of the transgenic mice, forming multiple tissue-specific target cells for various chemicals. Tissue responses to chemical carcinogens can be made more predictable by deleting various tumor suppressor genes from the normal genome of the mice. These tumor suppressor genes usually provide protection for animals that are sensitive to the genotoxic effects of various chemicals. Many transgenic mouse models have been proposed, and much of the current research in this area is focused on discovering the models best able to identify known carcinogenic agents.[12]

SHORT-TERM TESTING

Background

Due to the limited number of chemicals that can be tested in long-term animal studies, alternative approaches have been developed for more rapid screening of chemicals for carcinogenic potential. Various in vitro test systems have been developed to determine if the chemicals in question are genotoxic. Current models of cancer causation suggest a multistep process involving initiating and promoting agents, environmental and heritable cofactors that can enhance the carcinogenic effects of these agents, and other factors that contribute to tumor progression. Environmental agents often initiate cancer by producing permanent damage to the host DNA through mechanisms such as point mutations and chromosomal translocations.

Ames Test

In 1973, Bruce Ames and his colleagues developed a simple test system for detecting the mutagenic activity of chemicals in bacteria.[13] The test was designed to determine if a chemical is mutagenic (a finding of mutagenicity suggests the chemical could have carcinogenic effects). The Ames test used a mutated gene of *Salmonella* bacteria that normally controls the metabolism of the amino acid histadine. Bacteria that contain this mutated gene cannot grow in vitro unless histadine is added to the culture medium. The experiment involves adding the histadine-dependent bacteria and the suspect chemical to an agar solution. Mutagenic chemicals will create a mutation in some of the histadine-dependent bacteria, causing them to now become histadine-independent, thus allowing them to grow even though histadine has not been added to the agar solution. These histadine-independent bacteria will grow very rapidly and will form colonies of cells that are readily detectable among the vast majority of histadine-dependent bacteria, which will fail to grow on the agar.

Many chemicals are initially found in an inactive form and need to be activated by enzymes before they can act as mutagens. The Ames test was further refined by adding mammalian liver extract, which is rich in these enzymes, to the agar solution.[11] The test now involves numerous strains of *Salmonella* bacteria and associated gene mutations. Ames conducted a series of validation studies designed to test a number of known human and animal carcinogens for mutagenicity. Some of the substances tested were known chemical carcinogens, such as benzo[*a*]pyrene, whereas others were powerful carcinogens that occur in nature, such as aflatoxin. These early validation studies showed sensitivity and specificity of 90% or better.[14,15]

Other In Vitro Test Systems

Tests that use mammalian cells have also been developed. The cells employed in these tests include mouse lymphoma cells, Chinese hamster ovarian and lung cells, and human lymphoblasts. Further, in vitro tests have been designed to detect a number of chromosomal aberrations. A number of cancers are associated with chromosomal translocations, in which part of one arm of a chromosome is interchanged with part of one arm of another chromosome. These translocations are nonrandom and occur in predictable locations on the affected chromosomes. Burkitt's lymphoma, a form of lymphatic cancer that has been causally related to infection with the Epstein-Barr virus, frequently contains chromosomal translocations. Approximately 75% of cases of Burkitt's lymphoma show chromosomal translocations between the long arms of chromosomes 8 and 14; less frequent translocations between the long arm of chromosome 8 and the short arm of chromosome 2 or the long arm of chromosome 22 also occur. These translocations occur at a point on the chromosome where genes for the human immunoglobulins and the c-*myc* oncogene are located[16–18] (see "Epstein-Barr Virus" in Chapter 12). Nonrandom translocations, including the Philadelphia chromosome, have also been detected in certain forms of leukemia.[19]

Loss or gain of a chromosome may also be associated with various forms of cancer. An increased incidence of acute lymphocytic leukemias has been observed in children with Down's syndrome, who have three number 21 chromosomes instead of the normal two.[20] These tests are also designed to detect sister chromatid exchanges and micronuclei. In addition, short-term tests have been developed to detect DNA synthesis occurring at an unscheduled point in the cell cycle and to look for the effects of chemicals on cellular DNA repair mechanisms. Finally, chemicals are tested in vitro to determine their ability to alter the morphology and growth patterns of normal mammalian cells.

Evaluation of Short-Term Tests

Recently, investigators performed four short-term in vitro tests on 114 chemicals that had been tested through the NTP program for carcinogenicity in long-term animal studies.[21–23] The four short-term tests included the *Salmonella* mutagenesis assay (SAL), tests designed to detect the induction of chromosomal aberrations (ABS) and sister chromatid exchanges (SCE), and a test designed to detect a point mutation at the *tk* locus in L5178Y mouse lymphoma cells (MOLY). These validation studies were designed to determine if any of the four tests performed better than the others. The investigators were also interested in determining if complementary testing with the ABS, SCE, and MOLY tests would provide significant improvements in sensitivity without concomitant loss of specificity as compared with SAL testing alone. Finally, the investigators attempted to determine if various combinations of the four tests would outperform the SAL test alone in determining the carcinogenicity or lack of carcinogenicity of a particular chemical.[21]

Of the 114 chemicals tested in long-term animal experiments, 67 were found to be carcinogenic. The results of the validation studies are summarized in Table 5–1. The sensitivity ranged from 48% to 72%, with the SAL test showing the lowest sensitivity. Conversely, the SAL test had the highest level of specificity (91%) and the highest positive predictive value (89%). Concordance between the short-term results and the findings from the long-term animal studies was not significantly different among the four tests, ranging from 59% to 66%. Given that the four tests show equal concordance rates, the technical simplicity, low cost, and large reference literature associated with the SAL test suggest that it should play a primary role in short-term testing. The results of the studies also show that, whereas the addition of other short-term testing slightly improves sensitivity, it results in a significant loss of specificity. In addition, no combination of the four short-term tests showed improved predictability when compared with SAL testing alone. When the analysis was limited to chemicals judged to be highly potent animal carcinogens, the concordance rate observed for the SAL test (73%) was significantly higher than the concordance rates for the ABS test (55%), the SCE test (53%), and the

Table 5–1 Operational Characteristics of In Vitro Genetic Tests

	Test							
	SAL		*ABS*		*SCE*		*MLA*	
	+	–	+	–	+	–	+	–
Carcinogenesis								
+	32	35	35	32	46	21	48	19
–	4	43	13	34	26	21	28	19
Significance of association, *p*	<0.0001		0.007		0.105		0.127	
Sensitivity, %	48		52		69		72	
Specificity, %	91		72		45		40	
Positive predictivity, %	89		73		64		63	
Negative predictivity, %	55		52		50		50	
Concordance, %	66		61		59		59	

Key: SAL = *Salmonella* (Ames) mutagenesis assay; ABS = induction of chromosome aberrations; SCE = sister chromatid exchange; MLA = induction of mutations at the *tk* locus in L1578Y mouse lymphoma cells.

Source: Reproduced with permission from *Environmental Health Perspectives*, Vol. 100, R.W. Tennant and E. Zeiger, Genetic Toxicology: Current Status of Methods of Carcinogen Identification, pp. 307–315, 1993.

MOLY test (52%).[23] Subsequent studies of similar design have led to the same conclusions regarding the relationships between the four short-term tests.[24,25]

The SAL sensitivity and specificity rates observed in these studies are clearly lower than the initial results reported for this test.[14,15] The differences can probably be attributed to the larger number of noncarcinogenic agents included in more recent studies and the inclusion of animal carcinogens that are not mutagens. The difficulty of predicting nongenotoxic animal carcinogens from in vitro tests is not limited to the SAL test. Lee et al[26] compared results for 48 nongenotoxic carcinogens and 29 noncarcinogens identified through rodent studies with results obtained from in vitro studies of chromosomal aberrations and sister chromatid exchanges. When the results for both in vitro tests were combined, sensitivity and specificity were found to be low (56.3% and 51.7%, respectively). The overall accuracy rate was only 54.5%.

Classification of a chemical as an animal carcinogen is based on an observed increased incidence of selected tumors in treated animals. However, the chemical may act as a tumor promoter in conjunction with a tumor initiator or it may act as an initiator operating through a mechanism that does not involve genotoxicity. Chemicals that do not directly react with DNA may still affect DNA replication, repair, or gene metabolism through indirect pathways, including by increasing the amount of DNA damage caused by free radicals. Animal carcinogens that are not mutagenic tend to be associated with an increased incidence of a single tumor in a single species, whereas mutagenic carcinogens tend to produce a broader spectrum of tumor types in several species. These results suggest the existence of different causal pathways for mutagenic and nonmutagenic carcinogenic agents. Identifying nonmutagenic carcinogens currently presents special difficulties because of the low likelihood of detecting them with existing short-term tests and the failure to discover a common set of structural or physical traits that might predict carcinogenicity in chemicals.[23]

STRUCTURE-ACTIVITY RELATIONSHIPS

Another approach to screening large numbers of chemicals for carcinogenic potential is to determine the molecular structural-activity relationships (SARs) that characterize animal and human carcinogens. The SAR data are then used to build a database that serves as a template for identifying chemicals likely to be good candidates for short- and long-term testing. Early SAR approaches were developed to deal with congeneric compounds that possessed a common molecular structure and similar modes of action. The 300 carcinogenic and noncarcinogenic compounds contained in the NTP database are significantly more heterogeneous (as regards molecular structure and modes of action), making development of highly predictive systems more difficult.[27]

A number of approaches have been developed during the past decade to help predict carcinogenicity based on SARs. Three structural-relation systems use available data from rodent testing, input from expert chemists, published data on mutagenicity testing, and data on in vivo toxicity and maximum tolerated dose in the construction of the database.[28–30] Seven prediction methods do not directly use findings from long-term rodent experiments in the development of the initial database.[31–37] These systems use a variety of methodologies, including measuring electrophilic reactivity to discriminate between carcinogenic and noncarcinogenic compounds, predicting interactions with cytochrome P-450 and the Ah receptor, and utilizing rules developed by an expert panel of chemists for predicting carcinogenesis.[27]

Several of these systems use computer-based and statistical methodologies to develop automated approaches to screening large numbers of chemicals for SARs that might reasonably predict carcinogenic activity. One system, called PROGOL, uses a machine-learning methodology called inductive logic programming (ILP).[27] Logical statements are created that describe chemical structures based on relations between atoms and bonding connections.

Automated systems have also been developed using artificial intelligence theory and statistical methods, such as the computer-automated structure evaluation (CASE) program and its extension, the multiple computer-automated structure evaluation (MULTICASE) program.[38] These programs begin with the development of a learning database that contains the chemical structures of biologically active compounds and data on biological activity derived from mutagenic studies. The CASE program breaks the molecular structure of each chemical into fragments and then catalogs the fragments according to level of biological activity (based on the original source of the fragment). A statistical analysis is performed to assign a probability of biological activity to each fragment and to provide an estimate of potency. The MULTICASE program is similar, but it conducts additional statistical analyses designed to arrange active molecular fragments into descriptive categories called biophores. Chemicals are placed into groups of compounds that share common biophores. These activities create a learning database that can then be used as a template to compare the structural characteristics of compounds that have not been included in the database or have not been subjected to mutagenic or long-term testing.[38]

In 1992, Klopman and Rosenkranz[39] measured the ability of the CASE and MULTICASE programs to predict mutagenicity by comparing predictions based on chemical structure with actual data from *Salmonella* mutagenicity testing. Two databases containing results from *Salmonella* mutagenicity testing were used. The GENETOX program of the EPA was used as the learning set for this study. Once the CASE and MULTICASE programs "learned" the GENETOX database, they used this database to predict the mutagenic activity of 114 compounds that were contained in the NTP dataset but were absent from the GENETOX learning set. The CASE and MULTICASE programs were able to correctly predict mutagenic activity 84% and 86% of the time, respectively. Sensitivity and specificity were reported as 88.5% and 83.0% for the CASE program and 95.1% and 81.1% for the MULTICASE program. These investigators point out that the MULTICASE results approach the 85% interlaboratory variability observed for *Salmonella* mutagenicity testing under carefully controlled conditions.

More recently, the NTP has been conducting a predictive-toxicology evaluation (PTE) project in which several predictive approaches have been tested against results for 39 compounds tested by the NTP in long-term carcinogenesis bioassays.[40] Given that this group of chemicals included both mutagenic and nonmutagenic compounds, it is perhaps not surprising that the accuracy of the in vivo test predictions was lower than that observed when the testing was restricted to mutagenic compounds. Systems that do not include findings from animal testing in their databases showed accuracy rates that ranged from a low of 49% for the CASE method to 64% for the PROGOL method. The three methods that do utilize animal testing data did better, with accuracy rates ranging from 67% to 77%.[27]

Lee et al[26] also used an inductive learning program to discriminate between nongenotoxic carcinogens and chemicals that had not been identified as carcinogens in long-term studies. This computerized program correctly predicted carcinogenicity for nongenotoxic chemicals between 70% and 80% of the time.

CLASSIFICATION OF SUBSTANCES AS CARCINOGENS

IARC has published criteria for evaluating and classifying data from long-term animal studies.[9] The criteria used to classify compounds based on animal testing are shown in Exhibit 5–1. A chemical is classified as an animal carcinogen if it is consistently associated with an increased tumor incidence in multiple experiments using different species or strains of animals. The presence of a dose-response or other suggestive features, such as decreased age at onset, is also considered. A compound may be classified as showing limited evidence of carcinogenicity when only a few studies have been performed or when existing studies have suffered from various methodological limitations, such as inadequate doses, inadequate duration of exposure or length of follow-up, and low statistical power due to small sample sizes.

The large number of short-term tests makes it difficult to establish a rigid set of criteria for the data from these types of test. Therefore, IARC has suggested a number of general principles that apply to all in vitro testing. These general principles, which are shown in Exhibit 5–2, relate to establishing the validity of the in vitro test as regards long-term testing approaches and providing opportunities for testing a wide range of doses over a sufficient duration of exposure. The guidelines also stress the importance of

Exhibit 5–1 IARC Classification of Evidence for Carcinogenicity in Experimental Animals

- *Sufficient evidence* of carcinogenicity is provided when there is an increased incidence of malignant tumors
  (a) in multiple species <u>or</u>
  (b) in multiple experiments (preferably with different routes of administration or using different dose levels) <u>or</u>
  (c) to an unusual degree with regard to incidence, site or type of tumor, or age at onset <u>with</u>
  (d) additional evidence being provided by the observation of a dose-response.
- *Limited evidence* of carcinogenicity is available when the data suggest a carcinogenic effect but the data are limited because
  (a) the studies only involve a single species or strain <u>or</u>
  (b) the experiments are restricted by inadequate dosage levels, inadequate duration of exposure to the agent, inadequate period of follow-up, poor survival, too few animals, or inadequate reporting <u>or</u>
  (c) the neoplasms produced often occur spontaneously and , in the past , have been difficult to classify as malignant by histological criteria alone (eg, lung adenomas and adenocarcinomas and liver tumors in certain strains of mice).
- *Inadequate evidence* of carcinogenicity is available when, because of major qualitative or quantitative limitations, the studies cannot be interpreted as showing either the presence or absence of a carcinogenic effect.
- *No evidence* of carcinogenicity applies when several adequate studies are available which show that, within the limits of the tests being used, the chemical or complex mixture is not carcinogenic.

Source: Reprinted with permission from *Silica and Some Silicates*, IARC Monographs on the Evaluations of Carcinogenic Risks to Humans, No. 42, © 1987, International Agency for Research on Cancer.

providing an appropriate metabolic system for ensuring that the compound will be tested under biologically active conditions. The roles of dose-response and independent confirmatory studies in judging the potential carcinogenicity are also emphasized.

A scheme for classifying evidence of carcinogenicity based on human studies is shown in Exhibit 5–3. The definitions given are similar to those for long-term animal studies (Exhibit 5–1). Evidence of carcinogenicity is termed *sufficient* if a causal relation has been established between a particular cancer and the exposure in question. Criteria that are used to firmly establish a causal relation are discussed in detail in Chapter 9 (on tobacco use). Briefly, an environmental exposure is likely to be causally related to a specific cancer when the magnitude of the association is large and it can be demonstrated that the exposure is measured with reasonable accuracy. Strong evidence of a causal relation is provided when findings of similar magnitude are reported from studies conducted by independent investigators in different populations. The existence of a dose-response relation, adequate control of selection bias at the design phase, and adequate control of confounding through the use of sound data collection and analysis methods also lend credence to a purported causal relation. *Limited* evidence of carcinogenicity occurs when existing epidemiological studies have not been able to clearly eliminate

Exhibit 5–2 IARC Guidelines for Short-term Tests

- The test should be valid with respect to known animal carcinogens and noncarcinogens.
- The experimental parameters under which the chemical or complex mixture is tested should include a sufficiently wide dose range and duration of exposure to the agent and an appropriate metabolic system is employed.
- Appropriate controls should be used.
- The purity of the compound should be assured , or in the case of complex mixtures, the source and representativity of the sample being tested should be specified.

Source: Reprinted with permission from *Silica and Some Silicates*, IARC Monographs on the Evaluations of Carcinogenic Risks to Humans, No. 42, © 1987, International Agency for Research on Cancer.

alternative explanations for the observed association. These alternative explanations include chance or bias.

SUMMARY

Determining the potential carcinogenicity of the large number of chemicals to which humans are potentially exposed is a daunting task requiring a number of complementary approaches. Epidemiological studies, long-term animal assays, short-term in vitro testing, and structure-activity analysis all have a role to play.

Epidemiological research studies will continue to serve an important function in the investigation of carcinogenicity because of their focus on human populations. Much of our knowledge about chemical carcinogenesis in humans has come from epidemiological studies of cancer incidence and mortality in occupationally exposed populations.

Exhibit 5–3 IARC Classification of Evidence Regarding the Carcinogenicity of Chemicals in Humans

- *Sufficient evidence* of carcinogenicity indicates that there is a causal relationship between the exposure and human cancer.
- *Limited evidence* of carcinogenicity indicates that a causal interpretation is credible, but that alternative explanations, such as chance, bias, or confounding, could not adequately be excluded.
- *Inadequate evidence* of carcinogenicity, which applies to both positive and negative evidence, indicates that one of two conditions prevailed: (a) there are few pertinent data or (b) the available studies, while showing evidence of an association, do not exclude chance, bias, or confounding.
- *No evidence* of carcinogenicity applies when several adequate studies are available which do not show evidence of carcinogenicity.

Source: Reprinted with permission from *Silica and Some Silicates*, IARC Monographs on the Evaluations of Carcinogenic Risks to Humans, No. 42, © 1987, International Agency for Research on Cancer.

Cancers that occur as a result of medical treatments have also provided valuable insights. Examples include the transplacental induction of vaginal and uterine cancers in young women who were exposed in utero to the drug diethylstilbestrol and the occurrence of second primary cancers among patients treated with antineoplastic drugs. Relationships between various lifestyle factors, such as cigarette smoking and alcohol abuse, and various cancers have provided some of the most compelling evidence concerning chemical carcinogenesis. Despite the importance of these contributions, only a fraction of the chemicals that require testing can be the focus of epidemiological research.

Long-term testing has identified a large number of chemical compounds that are carcinogenic in animals and thus pose a potential threat to human populations. Long-term animal studies allow for accurate exposure measurement and excellent control over various potential biases through randomization. The use of inbred animals also helps in controlling for confounding by genetic factors. However, animal studies are expensive and take four to six months to complete, and caution must be used in extrapolating the findings to humans. The newest model for long-term animal testing includes the use of transgenic mice, whose genes are altered (specific genes are added to or deleted from the normal genome) in order to help predict cellular response to carcinogenic chemicals.

The development of short-term in vitro test systems has provided a rapid means of testing larger numbers of compounds. These systems appear to be fairly accurate in detecting carcinogens that are genotoxic, but they are less effective in detecting carcinogens that may act through alternate mechanisms.

Finally, a number of systems have been developed to utilize data on structural-activity relations to help predict which chemicals are likely to be carcinogens. These automated systems show promise for screening large numbers of chemicals and identifying those compounds that should be given priority for testing through the use of in vitro and in vivo test systems. The new computerized approaches to structure-activity analysis hold promise, and additional research should be conducted in this area.

Discussion Questions

1. Discuss the strengths and weaknesses of using animal models to determine if a compound is a carcinogen.
2. Discuss the advantages of using transgenic mouse models to determine if a compound is an animal carcinogen.
3. Discuss the strengths and weaknesses of using short-term testing to determine if a compound is a potential carcinogen.
4. Discuss the conceptual basis for using molecular structural-activity relationships (SARs) to identify possible animal or human carcinogens.
5. Discuss the guidelines developed by the International Agency for Research on Cancer to help classify compounds as animal carcinogens in light of available experimental data.
6. Discuss the guidelines developed by the International Agency for Research on Cancer to help classify compounds as human carcinogens in light of available experimental and epidemiological data.
7. Discuss the guidelines developed by the International Agency for Research on Cancer to help assess the scientific validity of short-term testing results.

References

1. Maugh TH. Chemicals: how many are there? *Science.* 1978;199:162.
2. Tomatis L, Kaldor JM, Bartsch H. Experimental studies in the assessment of human risk. In: Schottenfeld D, Fraumeni JF Jr, eds. *Cancer Epidemiology and Prevention.* 2nd ed. New York: Oxford University Press; 1996:11–27.
3. Kaldor J. The role of epidemiological observation in elucidating the mechanisms of carcinogenesis. In: Vainio H, Magee PN, McGregor DB, McMichael AJ, eds. *Mechanisms of Carcinogenesis in Risk Identification.* Lyon, France: International Agency for Research on Cancer; 1992:601–608.
4. Krewski D, Goddard MJ, Zielinski JM. Dose-response relationships in carcinogenesis. In: Vainio H, Magee PN, McGregor DB, McMichael AJ, eds. *Mechanisms of Carcinogenesis in Risk Identification.* Lyon, France: International Agency for Research on Cancer; 1992:579–599.
5. Tomatis L, Aitio A, Wilbourn J, Shuker L. Human carcinogens so far identified. *Jap J Cancer Res.* 1989;80:795–807.
6. Sontag JA, Page NP, Saffiotti U. *Guidelines for Carcinogenic Bioassay in Small Rodents.* Bethesda, MD: Department of Health, Education and Welfare; 1976. National Cancer Institute Carcinogenesis Technical Report Series; DHEW publication No. 76-801.
7. Haseman JK, Huff JE, Zeiger E, McConnell EE. Comparative results of 327 chemical carcinogenicity studies. *Environ Health Perspect.* 1987;74:229–235.
8. Peto R, Pike MC, Day NE, et al. Guidelines for simple sensitive significance tests for carcinogenic effects in long-term animal experiments. In: *Long-term and Short-term Screening Assays for Carcinogens: A Critical Appraisal.* Lyon, France: International Agency for Research on Cancer. 1980:311–426. IARC Monographs on the Evaluation of the Carcinogenic Risk of Chemicals to Humans, suppl 2.
9. *Silica and Some Silicates.* Lyon, France: International Agency for Research on Cancer; 1987. IARC Monographs on the Evaluation of the Carcinogenic Risk of Chemicals to Humans, No. 42.
10. Tennant RW. Evaluation and validation issues in the development of transgenic mouse carcinogenicity models. *Environ Health Perspect.* 1998;106(suppl 2):473–476.
11. Varmus H, Weinberg RA. *Genes and the Biology of Cancer.* New York: Scientific American Library; 1993:61–65.
12. Tennant RW, Stasiewicz S, Mennear, J, et al. Genetically altered mouse models for identifying carcinogens. *IARC Sci Publ.* 1999;146:123–150.
13. Ames BN, Durston WE, Yamasaki E, Lee FD. Carcinogens are mutagens: a simple test system combining liver homogenates for activation and bacteria for detection. *Proc Natl Acad Sci USA.* 1973;70:2281–2285.
14. McCann J, Choi E, Yamasaki E, Ames BN. Detection of carcinogens as mutagens in the *Salmonella*/microsome test: assay of 300 chemicals. *Proc Natl Acad Sci USA.* 1975;72:5135–5139.
15. Purchase IF, Longstaff E, Ashby J, et al. Evaluation of six short-term tests for detecting organic chemical carcinogens and recommendations for their use. *Nature.* 1976;264:624–627.
16. Manilov G, Manilov Y. A marker band on one chromosome no. 14 in Burkitt's lymphoma. *Heriditas.* 1971;68:300.
17. Zech L, Haglund AN, Nilsson K, Klein G. Characteristic chromosomal abnormalities in biopsies and lymphoid cell lines from patients with Burkitt's lymphoma. *Int J Cancer.* 1976;17:47–56.
18. Yunis JJ, Oken MM, Kaplan ME, et al. Distinctive chromosomal abnormalities in histologic sub-types of non-Hodgkin's lymphoma. *N Eng J Med.* 1982;307:1231–1236.
19. Le Beau MM. Molecular biology of cancer. In: DeVita VT Jr, Hellman S, Rosenberg SA, eds. *Cancer: Principles and Practice of Oncology.* Philadelphia: Lippincott-Raven Publishers; 1997:106–108.
20. Weinstein HJ, Tarbell NJ. Leukemias and lymphomas of childhood. In: DeVita VT Jr, Hellman S, Rosenberg SA, eds. *Cancer: Principles and Practice of Oncology.* Philadelphia: Lippincott-Raven Publishers; 1997:2145–2146.
21. Tennant RW, Margolin BH, Shelby MD, et al. Prediction of chemical carcinogenicity in rodents from in vitro genetic toxicity assays. *Science.* 1987;236:933–941.
22. Zeiger E, Haseman JK, Shelby MD, et al. Evaluation of four in vitro genetic toxicity tests for predicting rodent carcinogenicity: confirmation of earlier results with 41 additional chemicals. *Environ Mol Mutagen.* 1990;16(suppl 18):1–14.
23. Tennant RW, Zeiger E. Genetic toxicology: current status of methods of carcinogen identification. *Environ Health Perspect.* 1993;100:307–315.
24. Zeiger E. Genotoxicity database. In: Gold LS, Zeiger E, eds. *Handbook of Carcinogenic Potency and Genotoxicity Databases.* Boca Raton, FL: CRC Press; 1997:687–729.

25. Zeiger E. Identification of rodent carcinogens and noncarcinogens using genetic toxicity tests: premises, promises, and performance. *Regul Toxicol Pharmacol.* 1998;28:85–95.
26. Lee Y, Buchanan BG, Mattison DM, et al. Learning rules to predict rodent carcinogenicity of non-genotoxic chemicals. *Mutation Res.* 1995;328:127–149.
27. King RD, Srinivasan A. Prediction of rodent carcinogenicity bioassays from molecular structure using inductive logic programming. *Environ Health Perspect.* 1996;104(suppl 5):1031–1040.
28. Tennant RW, Spalding J, Stasiewicz S, Ashby J. Prediction of the outcome of rodent carcinogenicity bioassays currently being conducted on 44 chemicals by the National Toxicology Program. *Mutagenesis.* 1990;5:3–14.
29. Bahler D, Bristol DW. The induction of rules for predicting chemical carcinogenesis in rodents. In: Hunter L, Searles D, Shavlick J, eds. *Intelligent Systems for Molecular Biology—93.* Cambridge, MA: AAI/MIT Press; 1993:29–37.
30. Jones TD, Easterly CE. On the rodent bioassays currently being conducted on 44 chemicals: a rash analysis to predict test results from the National Toxicology Program. *Mutagenesis.* 1991;6:507–514.
31. Muggleton SH. Inverse entailment and Progol. *New Generation Computing.* 1995;13:245–286.
32. Bakale G, McCreary RD. Prospective K_e screening of potential carcinogens being tested in rodent bioassays by the US National Toxicology Program. *Mutagenesis.* 1992;7:91–94.
33. Benigni R. QSAR prediction of rodent carcinogenicity for a set of chemicals currently bioassayed by the US National Toxicology Program. *Mutagenesis.* 1991;6:423–425.
34. Sanderson BM, Earnshaw CG. Computer prediction of possible toxic action from chemical structure. *Hum Exp Toxicol.* 1991;10:261–273.
35. Lewis DFV, Ionnides C, Parke DV. A prospective toxicity evaluation (COMPACT) on 40 chemicals currently being tested by the National Toxicology Program. *Mutagenesis.* 1990;5:433–436.
36. Enslein K, Blake BW, Borgstedt HH. Prediction of probability of carcinogenicity for a set of ongoing NTP bioassays. *Mutagenesis.* 1990;5:305–306.
37. Rosenkranz HS, Klopman G. Prediction of the carcinogenicity in rodents of chemicals currently being tested by the US National Toxicology Program. *Mutagenesis.* 1990;5:425–432.
38. Zhang YP, Sussman N, Macina OT, et al. Prediction of the carcinogenicity of a second group of organic chemicals undergoing carcinogenicity testing. *Environ Health Perspect.* 1996;104(suppl 5):1045–1050.
39. Klopman G, Rosenkranz HS. Testing by artificial intelligence: computational alternatives to the determination of mutagenicity. *Mutation Res.* 1992;272:59–71.
40. Bristol DW, Wachsman JT, Greenwell A. The NIEHS Predictive-Toxicology Evaluation Project. *Environ Health Perspect.* 1996;104(suppl 5):1001–1010.

Chapter 6

Biomarkers and Epidemiological Studies of Cancer

Philip C. Nasca

Although biomarkers have been used for many years in epidemiological research, recent advances in fields such as cellular biology, molecular genetics, and toxicology have provided the cancer epidemiologist with a new array of tools. This chapter reviews the various types of biomarkers employed in epidemiological studies of cancer. The biomarkers discussed include those that help researchers to assess the extent to which chemical and biological agents in the environment interact with cellular components, those that are used to assess preclinical changes in target tissues, and those that are used to measure inherited susceptibility to the effects of chemical and biological agents in the environment. The chapter also presents some methodological issues surrounding the collection of biological specimens for molecular-epidemiological studies and the analysis and interpretation of data from studies designed to assess gene-environment interactions. The chapter concludes with a discussion of the development and maintenance of biological specimen banks and the emerging ethical issues concerning the use of biomarkers in epidemiological research.

A biomarker is a biochemical measure used to detect genetic, cellular, or molecular alterations. The use of biomarkers in epidemiological research is not new. Epidemiologists have for many years used serological testing to establish prior infection with various biological agents. Since many of these agents can cause subclinical infections, the use of clinical history alone can lead to misclassification of infected and noninfected individuals. A well-known example from cardiovascular disease epidemiology is the relation between serum cholesterol measurements and the increased risk of ischemic heart disease. The ability to measure serum cholesterol provided some of the earliest insights into the etiology of this condition. Further refinements in measurement allowed investigators to characterize the nature of the relationship in greater depth by establishing the different roles of high- and low-density lipoproteins in arthrosclerosis.

Significant advances in cellular biology, immunology, toxicology, and other life sciences have provided epidemiologists with an expanded array of tools for linking biological, chemical, and more traditional epidemiological data. This chapter presents a brief overview of a classification system for biomarkers commonly being used in epidemiological research and provides specific examples of biomarkers used in cancer epidemiology. Some of the methodological issues posed by the use of biomarkers are discussed. Additional topics include the development and use of biological specimen banks and the ethical issues that arise from the inclusion of biomarkers in epidemiological research.

TYPES OF BIOMARKERS

During the last half of the 20th century, epidemiological research studies have played a major role in identifying a number of chemical and biological agents in the environment that are causally linked to various cancers. For example, tobacco, alcohol, ionizing and solar radiation, occupational chemicals, exogenous and endogenous hormones, and viruses have been found to be carcinogenic. In addition, although the exact nature of the relation between dietary factors and cancer is still uncertain, it is likely that diet plays an important role in cancer etiology. During this same time period, advances in molecular biology provided significant insights into the cellular mechanisms involved in carcinogenesis. It is now clear that malignant transformation arises from a sequence of events involving acquired and inherited mutations of the cellular DNA and that genetic susceptibility and promotional factors contribute to carcinogenesis.

Combining traditional epidemiological approaches and biological measures of exposure and effect has offered additional insight into the continuum between initial exposure and the development of frank malignancy.[1] A standard set of terms has been developed for classifying various measures of dose, early biological effect, and susceptibility to environmental agents[1,2] (Figure 6–1). Classical epidemiological methods have been successful in identifying broad associations between external agents and various can-

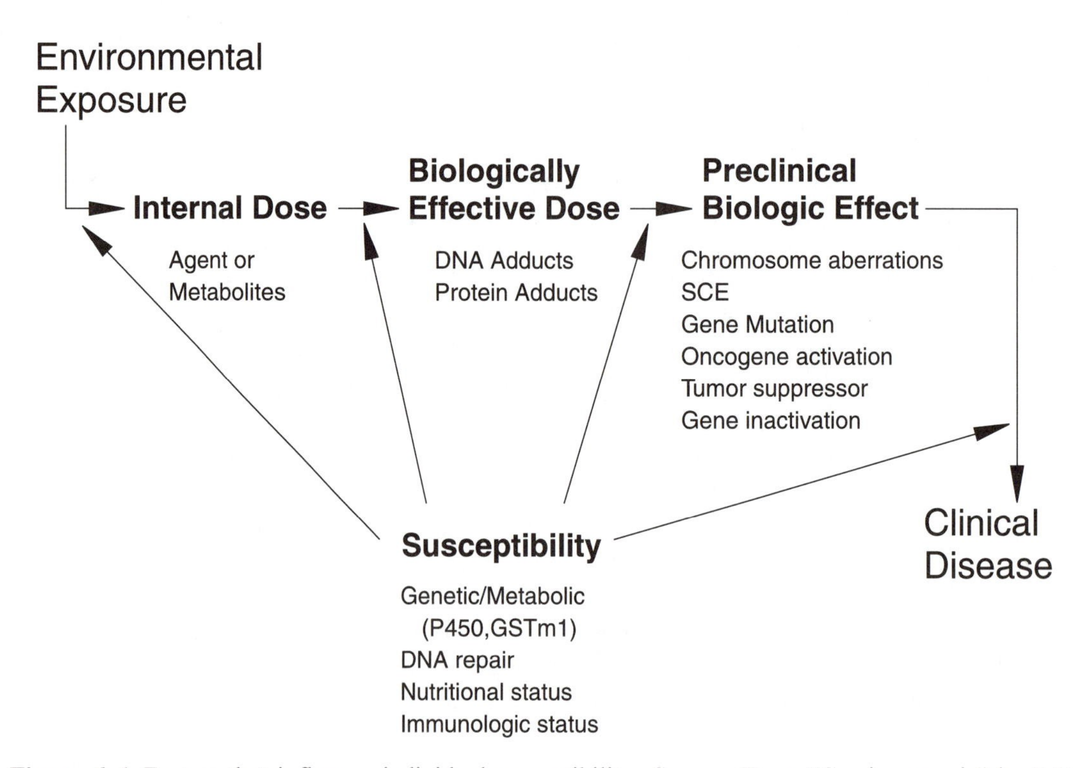

Figure 6–1 Factors that influence individual susceptibility. *Source:* From "Carcinogenesis" by F.P. Perera and R. Santella in *Molecular Epidemiology: Principles and Practices*, P.A. Schulte and F.P. Perera, eds., copyright © 1993 by Academic Press, reproduced by permission of the publisher.

cers. The incorporation of various types of biomarkers provides opportunities for improving our understanding of how these external agents operate in human tissues to create a series of cellular events leading to frank malignancy. Biomarkers have also been useful in evaluating the relation between external agents and genetic susceptibility to the effects of these agents.

INTERNAL DOSE

Traditional epidemiological tools such as questionnaires and medical records are important for measuring the external dose of a particular environmental exposure. Since these epidemiological measures rely on human recall, a certain amount of exposure misclassification can be expected to occur. The magnitude and direction of the misclassification can vary from exposure to exposure and may be related to the type of exposure information the investigator is attempting to collect. Biological measurements can be helpful in determining the accuracy of epidemiological exposure assessments. Biomarkers that are used to confirm exposure data are referred to as markers of internal dose. A number of markers of internal dose have already been discussed in previous chapters; these are summarized in Table 6–1. In several types of marker of internal dose, the investigator examines the extent to which the marker correlates with the epidemiological measure. The accuracy of epidemiological exposure data can be assessed by measuring body burden levels of the actual compound or one of its stable metabolites in human tissues. Cotinine, a metabolite of nicotine, in blood, urine, or saliva, is a good marker of recent exposure to cigarette smoke.[3]

In an effort to overcome the potential for recall bias inherent in the use of food frequency questionnaires, investigators have measured the levels of various micronutrients in serum, plasma, red cells, subcutaneous fat, and hair and nails. In order to establish a temporal relationship between the marker (micronutrient) levels and later disease, stored samples are often used in the analysis. Although this approach has some appeal, serum marker levels are highly regulated by the body, tend to show large fluctuations over time, and may not accurately represent long-term dietary intake. In addition, markers do not exist for most dietary components of current interest to investigators. The limitations of markers for determining long-term dietary patterns need to be recognized, and investigators should not abandon gathering important dietary data by means of standardized food frequency questionnaires.[4]

Serum markers can be very valuable in determining if a known carcinogenic agent present in certain foodstuffs is actually internalized by exposed individuals. Strong correlations have been reported between levels of the potent carcinogen aflatoxin in urine and dietary intake of foods frequently contaminated with the mold that produces the toxin.[5] Other studies have shown two potent carcinogens, benzene and radioactive lead-210, are found in cigarette smoke. Analysis of breath[6] and urine[7] samples showed that benzene and benzene metabolites occur at higher levels in smokers than in nonsmokers. Similar studies showed that smokers are significantly more likely than nonsmokers to have lead-210 detected in bone and soft tissue.[8,9] Another study showed that cotinine is found more often in the cervical mucus of smokers than in that of nonsmokers.[10] A link-

Table 6–1 Examples of Markers of Internal Dose

Biomarker	*Source of Exposure*	*Biologic Sample*	*Measurement*
Cotinine	Cigarette smoke	Serum, urine, saliva	Higher levels in smokers compared to nonsmokers
Vitamin levels	Diet	Serum	Serum levels of Vitamins A, E , C, and D linked with risk for various cancers
Selenium	Diet	Hair, toe nails	Levels of selenium linked with risk for lung cancer
Levels of benzene and benzene metabolites	Cigarette smoke	Urine, breath concentrations	Higher levels of benzene and metabolites in smokers compared to nonsmokers
Levels of lead-210	Cigarette smoke	Bone, soft tissues	Higher levels of lead-210 in smokers compared to nonsmokers
Aflatoxin	Contaminated food	Urine	Higher levels of aflatoxin in urine of exposed compared to nonexposed
Bacterial mutations	Cigarette smoke	Cervical fluids	Samples from smokers more likely to be mutagenic in Ames test
Mean cell volume, high-density lipoprotein, alkaline phosphatase	Alcohol	Serum	Marker levels correlate with alcohol consumption levels
DNA sequences	HPV	Cervicovaginal lavage	Polymerase chain reaction identifies HPV types 16 and 18 associated with intraepithelial neoplasia

age between a chemical in the environment and the mutagenic potential of an exposed person's bodily fluids is evidence that the person received an internal dose. Smokers are significantly more likely than nonsmokers to produce fluids from the uterine cervix that are mutagenic in bacterial test systems.[11]

Biomarkers include not only chemicals and their metabolites but also biological agents and factors that have been shown to be related in a predictable way to levels of exposure to certain chemicals. For example, studies have shown that high-density lipoprotein,[12] mean cell volume, and alkaline phosphatase[13] are related to daily consumption of alcohol. Newer molecular tools, such as polymerase chain reaction (PCR) techniques, have been used to improve our ability to confirm a previous infection with a virus and even to subtype the virus with a high degree of accuracy. PCR techniques for detecting specific DNA sequences in cervicovaginal lavage samples are far superior to other methods of identifying patients who have been infected with HPV types 16 and 18. The ability to firmly establish infection with these subtypes has led to a clear understanding of the role of HPV in cervical neoplasia.[14]

BIOLOGICALLY EFFECTIVE DOSE

An association between an environmental agent and a particular cancer is more likely to be causal if it can be shown that the agent not only enters the body but interacts biologically with host tissues. Examples of markers of biologically effective dose are shown in Table 6–2. Consider the first biomarker listed. Adducts are created when reactive chemicals form stable complexes with macromolecules such as cellular DNA or proteins. These complexes are held together by the presence of one or more covalent bonds between the environmental chemical and the target DNA or protein.[15] The binding of a chemical or its active metabolite to DNA can cause gene damage or mutations that, if the genes are not repaired, can have a critical effect on cell growth and proliferation. An attempt is often made to correlate data on adduct formation with data from epidemiological exposure histories.[3] Because it is usually not feasible to sample cells from the healthy tissue of the target anatomic site (eg, a lung), it is often necessary to sample surrogate tissues that are more readily accessible. Investigators often look for adducts in hemoglobin from red blood cells. The extent to which these surrogate measures accurately represent the level of adducts in actual target tissue is currently being studied in relation to various exposures.[15] It has been shown that hemoglobin and DNA adducts associated with tobacco carcinogens can be detected in the blood of smokers and snuff users and can be related to the level of smoking.[16–18] Finally, metabolites of a known lung carcinogen have been quantified in the urine of cigarette smokers.[19]

A particular environmental exposure may also cause alterations in a physiological system, leading to increased or decreased production of various substances. As indicated in Table 6–2, investigators have attempted to link exposure to alcohol[20–30] and tobacco[31,32] to

Table 6–2 Examples of Markers of Biologically Effective Dose

Biomarker	*Source of Exposure*	*Biologic Sample*	*Measurement*
DNA and protein adducts	Cigarette smoke	Serum	More common in smokers than nonsmokers
Estrogen and androgen levels	Cigarette smoke	Serum, urine	Examine hormone levels in relation to daily smoking levels
Estrogen levels	Alcohol	Serum, urine	Higher levels in alcohol drinkers than nondrinkers

increased levels of estrogens and androgens. Although more research is needed, existing data suggest that alcohol consumption increases the level of biologically available estrogen, which is a known risk factor for breast cancer. In other words, estrogen may be an intermediate in the causal pathway between alcohol and breast cancer.

PRECLINICAL BIOLOGIC EFFECT

The likelihood that an association between an environmental agent and a cancer is causal in nature is increased if it can be shown that the agent is linked to preclinical biological effects that are predictive of cancer. Several examples of this type of biomarker are shown in Table 6–3. A variety of gross cytogenetic markers and point

Table 6–3 Early Biologic Effect or Response

Compound Analyzed	*Exposure Source*	*Biologic Sample*	*Population*
Single strand breaks	Styrene	WBC	Workers
Unscheduled DNA synthesis	Propylene oxide	WBC	Workers
Sister chromatid exchange	Various industrial exposures, radiation, air pollution	WBC	Workers, residents
Micronuclei	Organic solvents, heavy metals, cigarette smoke, betel quid	WBC, oral mucosa	Workers
Chromosomal aberrations	Various industrial exposures, radiation, air pollution	WBC	Workers, residents
DNA hyperploidy	Aromatic amines	Bladder and lung cells	Workers
HPRT mutation	Chemotherapeutic agents, radiation	WBC	Patients, workers
GPA mutation	Chemotherapeutic agents, radiation	RBC	Patients, Japanese atom bomb survivors
Mutation in tumor suppressor genes	AFB_1	Tumor tissue	Patients
Oncogene activation	PAH, cigarette smoke	Serum	Workers, cancer patients

Key: AFB_1 = aflatoxin B_1, GPA = glycophorin A, HPRT = hypoxanthine guanine phosphoribosyl transferase, PAH = polycyclic aromatic hydrocarbons, RBC = red blood cells, WBC = white blood cells

Source: From "Carcinogenesis" by F.P. Perera and R. Santella in *Molecular Epidemiology: Principles and Practices*, P.A. Schulte and F.P. Perera, eds., copyright © 1993 by Academic Press, reproduced by permission of the publisher.

mutations are used to detect early preclinical effects of exposure to industrial chemicals, cigarette smoke and other lifestyle-related substances, radiation, and chemotherapeutic agents.[33] Cigarette smoke has been linked with specific cytological lesions[34] and increased leukocyte counts,[35–39] which are associated with adult onset leukemias. Specific patterns of oncogene expression or deletions of certain suppressor genes have been linked to exposure to the human papillomavirus (HPV) and Epstein-Barr virus (EBV).

Because biological effect markers may be caused by a number of chemicals, it is necessary to collect external exposure histories using standard epidemiological methods. White and red blood cells are most often used as surrogate biological materials for sampling in these studies. These markers of early biological effect may also serve as useful intermediate endpoints in chemoprevention studies, and they may lead to early disease detection once disease pathogenesis is understood better.[33]

The use of biological effect markers may also lead to a more finely discriminating classification of disease. Rhabdomyosarcomas are uncommon cancers of the striated muscles in children. These tumors are classified histopathologically as either alveolar or embryonal. Alveolar rhabdomyosarcomas are associated with a poorer prognosis, and thus accurate histopathological diagnoses are needed. However, the histopathological criteria used to separate alveolar from embryonal tumors are subtle, and no immunohistochemical marker for these tumor types has been identified.[40] The differentiation of these tumor types is now aided by the identification of two nonrandom chromosomal translocations that occur almost exclusively in alveolar tumors.[40,41]

MARKERS OF SUSCEPTIBILITY

The carcinogenic potential of an environmental agent may vary depending on the genetic makeup of the host. Markers of susceptibility indicate if an individual is more or less susceptible to the effects of a particular carcinogenic exposure. Examples of markers of susceptibility are shown in Table 6–4. Alcohol has been shown to be a potent carcinogen and is related to cancers of the oral cavity and aerodigestive tract. Acetaldehyde is a metabolite of alcohol and an established animal carcinogen. A human gene that codes for the enzyme aldehyde dehydrogenase 2 has been identified. In individuals with the normal form of the gene, the enzyme helps to eliminate acetaldehyde from the body, whereas the mutated form of the gene inactivates the enzyme, prolonging tissue exposure to the carcinogen. Esophageal cancer risk has been shown to be higher in alcohol drinkers who carry the mutant form of the gene than in alcohol drinkers who carry the wild form of the gene.[42–44]

Individuals who have impaired immune systems may be more susceptible to the carcinogenic effects of certain viruses than patients who have normally functioning immune systems. Patients who suffer from inborn immunodeficiency disorders or whose immune systems has been suppressed by drugs or HIV infection experience dramatically increased risks of developing non-Hodgkin's lymphoma, probably as a result of the reactivation of latent EBV.[45] A patient whose immune system has been depressed by HIV infection may also be predisposed to suffer increased risks for cancers of the uterine cervix and anal canal in the presence of HPV infection.[46–49] HIV-infected men are at higher risk for Kaposi's sarcoma, and their tumors appear more virulent than those ob-

Table 6–4 Examples of Markers of Susceptibility

Type of Susceptibility	*Cancer Relation*
Aldehyde dehydrogenase 2; normal gene codes for enzyme that eliminates the carcinogen acetaldehyde; mutant form inactivates the enzyme	Acetaldehyde; metabolite of alcohol shown to be carcinogenic in animals; esophageal cancer risk increased in alcohol drinkers who carry the mutant form of the gene
N-acetyltransferase; fast acetylators detoxify carcinogens more rapidly than slow acetylators	Slow acetylators tend to experience higher risks of bladder cancer in males with occupational exposures to carcinogens
O^6-alkyldeoxyguanine-DNA alkyltransferase; variability of repair system activity among individuals	Associated with an increased risk of lung cancer
Patients with the inherited disorder xeroderma pigmentosum have faulty repair systems and cannot repair utraviolet radiation damage to DNA	Associated with an excess risk of skin cancer due to ultraviolet radiation
Immunodeficiency caused by inherited disorder or acquired through HIV infection or exposure to immunosuppressive drugs	Increased risk of non-Hodgkin's inherited lymphomas associated with reactivated Epstein-Barr virus
Immunodeficiency caused by inherited disorder or acquired through HIV infection or exposure to immunosuppressive drugs	Increased risk of cancer of the uterine cervix and anal canal associated with human papillomavirus
Depression of cytotoxic T-cell clones associated with malarial infection	Increased risk of Burkitt's lymphomas associated with Epstein-Barr virus
Genetic variability in degree to which a carcinogen can bind to cellular receptor sites	Breast cancers are classified as estrogen positive or negative

served in immunocompetent patients. A yet-to-be-identified cofactor is suspected to act in conjunction with the immunosuppressive properties of HIV to cause these tumors.[50] In the case of Burkitt's lymphoma, malarial infection tends to depress cytotoxic T-cell clones, which help to control EBV expression. In the absence of normal immunological controls, it is thought that EBV virus leads to a number of changes at the cellular level that lead to tumor development.[51]

Most chemicals are not biologically active when they enter the body. They need to be converted into biologically active forms before they can interact with host DNA to cause mutations. Cytochrome P-450 enzymes act as catalysts in the oxidation process that turns biologically inactive environmental chemicals into substances capable of interacting with DNA. Since cytochrome P-450 enzyme production is under genetic control, individuals vary greatly in their ability to activate various procarcinogens and thus in their risk of developing different forms of cancer. Some evidence suggests that alcohol can activate cytochrome P-450 enzyme activity in liver, lung, esophageal, and intestinal tissues, possibly increasing the chance that other carcinogens might be more readily activated.[52,53] In this example, an external exposure may affect genetically determined susceptibility factors, and these factors may in turn affect the action of other environmental carcinogens.

One of the best known examples of the relationship between environmental exposures and genetic susceptibility involves the acetylation detoxification reaction. The *N*-acetylation detoxification process uses the enzyme *N*-acetyltransferase to help purge the body of various environmental carcinogens. Individuals can be classified as slow or fast acetylators based on genotyping or through phenotypic testing. Slow acetylators are homozygous for the slow form of the gene, and fast acetylators are either heterozygous or homozygous for the fast form of the gene. Males who are slow acetylators and have been exposed to a variety of carcinogenic agents in occupational settings experience a higher risk of developing bladder cancer. In addition, studies that measured biomarkers of biologically effective dose and susceptibility in the same individuals have been carried out, and higher numbers of DNA adducts have been observed in association with cigarette smoking among individuals who are slow acetylators. The strong association between cigarette smoking and bladder cancer observed in earlier epidemiological studies is further strengthened by the observation that higher levels of biological interaction between the environmental agent and the cellular targets occur in individuals who detoxify the agent less efficiently. Additional studies that focus on phenotypes for chemical activation and detoxification and the ability to repair DNA damage in the same individuals are needed.[33]

Another important focus of future research is the relation between cancer risk and the capacity to repair DNA damage caused by exposure to a carcinogen. The O^6-alkyldeoxyguanine-DNA alkyltransferase DNA repair enzyme system repairs DNA damage caused by *N*-nitroso compounds in cigarette smoke and various pollutants. The activity of this repair system varies as much as 180-fold between individuals.[54] Inborn genetic disorders are also associated with faulty DNA repair systems and increased risks for certain cancers. Xeroderma pigmentosum is an autosomal recessive syndrome associated with an unusually high incidence of skin cancers. This increased skin cancer risk has been traced to a significantly reduced ability to repair DNA damage caused by exposure to UV radiation.[55]

The efficiency with which various substances bind to receptor sites in the cellular nucleus represents another form of genetic susceptibility. The ability of a carcinogen to bind to receptor sites affects the probability that the substance will interact biologically with the cell.[54] Breast cancers are now routinely tested to determine if the tumor has estrogen or progesterone receptors. The information as to the kind of receptor is used by the physician to develop a therapeutic plan for the breast cancer patient. Factors that affect estrogen production might be expected to be more strongly associated with estrogen receptor–positive breast cancers. In one study of alcohol and breast cancer risk, an association was observed primarily in estrogen receptor–positive tumors.[56] This effect has also been observed in some animal studies.[57] However, a second epidemiological study found the opposite effect, and additional studies are needed to clarify the relationship between type of receptor and cancer.[58]

SOME METHODOLOGICAL ISSUES

Although biomarkers have the potential to enhance classical approaches to exposure measurement, the limitations of biomarker measurements in epidemiological studies of cancer need to be recognized. An induction period of 10–30 years has been observed between first exposure to an external agent and the initial diagnosis of adult onset cancers. Since most of the currently available biomarkers, such as DNA adducts and micronutrients in sera, aid in the measurement of recent exposures only, the most etiologically relevant exposures may not be detectable by these markers.[5,59] Even in the case of a chemical with a longer half-life, investigators need to collect data on external exposures and assume that no new exposures have occurred or that exposure patterns have remained stable over time.[59]

The temporal relationship between biological measurements and disease onset needs to be established. Findings from case-control studies are suspect given that the biomarkers may be a result of the disease process and not related to its cause. The rarity of most cancers and the expense associated with analyzing biological samples make the cohort approach infeasible in most situations.

Another approach is to use a nested case-control design. Samples are drawn on all cohort subjects and frozen until such time as a sufficient number of cohort subjects have developed the cancer of interest. The diseased cohort subjects become the cases. A sample of cohort members who have not developed the cancer of interest are selected to serve as controls. Only specimens for the cases and controls are analyzed. This approach minimizes the cost of the study while ensuring that the exposure was measured a number of years prior to development of the cancer. This approach assumes, however, that baseline measurements accurately represent exposure patterns over the entire time period, from first exposure to disease onset.[59] For example, an investigator might want to examine breast cancer risk in relation to hormone levels. Several serum samples could be drawn from female cohort members to measure hormone levels at several points in the menstrual cycle. The measurements could then be used to represent the typical hormonal patterns of women at baseline. The assumption would be that these patterns are maintained over a period of years, and the validity of this assumption could be tested in smaller methodological studies done prior to launching an expensive cohort study.

Many studies involving biomarkers fail to take confounding variables into account. Pearce et al[59] show that the use of biomarkers may actually introduce confounding, because the measurements reflect the total exposure to a substance from a number of external sources and these sources may be associated with different risk factors for the cancer.

Many studies that depend on biomarkers include small numbers of subjects and thus have limited statistical power to detect small to moderate effects. Also, biomarker measurement usually involves the use of an invasive specimen-collection procedure. It may also bring with it other burdens, such as special handling and storage requirements, time demands, and dietary demands (eg, fasting). The additional burdens for cases and controls—that is, beyond those usually associated with an epidemiological interview—can decrease the response rate and increase the risk of selection bias.

Data concerning the reliability of a biomarker is critical to interpreting study findings. Various trace elements, including selenium, arsenic, and iron, have been suspected as playing a role in the development of selected cancers. Investigators have utilized toenail clippings for trace element sampling because toenail clippings are easier to collect and store than blood, and toenails are less prone to external contamination than hair or fingernails. In addition, measures of trace elements in blood may vary from day to day, and trace element sampling of toenail clippings usually better reflects long-term trace element exposure (this is important given the long induction period associated with adult onset cancers).

A reliability study by Garland et al[60] was designed to determine the reproducibility of trace element measurements in toenail clippings over a period of six years. A total of 127 women provided two samples six years apart. Correlation coefficients were 0.48 and 0.54 for selenium and arsenic, respectively, and the correlation coefficients for other trace elements ranged from 0.26 for copper to 0.58 for zinc. This level of random in-person variability would lead to underestimating the true magnitude of the association between a trace element exposure and a cancer. The investigators investigated the potential effect of such variability in a hypothetical case-control study in which a true odds ratio of 3.0 is observed when the highest quintile of exposure is compared to the remaining 4 exposure quintiles. Using the level of reproducibility observed in the sample of 127 women, the investigators calculated that the odds ratio would be attenuated to 2.15 for toenail arsenic and 1.67 for toenail copper. These calculations clearly show how random variability in the biomarker can lead to serious underestimation of the true measure of effect.

INTERPRETATION OF FINDINGS

The following example of a susceptibility gene illustrates some of the strengths and weaknesses of studies that use biomarkers. The glutathione S-transferase (GST) enzyme system plays an important role in determining an individual's ability to metabolize various carcinogens, including benzo[*a*]pyrene, styrene, ethylene oxide, halomethanes, and methyl bromide.[33] Each member of this family of enzymes is under the control of different genes. Deletion of these genes results in a lack of enzyme activity and reduced elimination of carcinogenic substances. Two of the enzymes, GSTM1 and GSTT1, have been extensively studied in relation to several known carcinogens and their associated DNA adducts. Detection of DNA adducts is expected to be related to the presence or absence of normal GSTM1 and GSTT1 enzymatic activity. Other studies have been designed to assess the extent to which the absence of GST activity is related to preclinical biological markers, including sister chromatid exchanges, lymphocyte micronuclei, urine mutagenicity, loss of heterozygosity, and specific somatic mutations involving the p53 tumor suppressor gene and K-*ras* oncogene.[33,61]

Rebbeck[61] recently conducted an in-depth review of the literature concerning the molecular epidemiology of GST in terms of Bradford Hill's criteria for assessing causality in epidemiological research. This review, which provides a useful bridge between classical and molecular epidemiology, is summarized below. The existing evidence concerning a possible etiologic role for GSTM1 or GSTT1 in various cancers was evaluated in terms of biological plausibility, temporal relationship, dose-response, magnitude of effect, and consistency across studies. The possibility that GSTM1 and GSTT1 are causally related to cancer susceptibility is supported by the observation that increased risk for cancer has always been found among persons who are homozygous for the inactive genotypes. Molecular epidemiological studies have shown significant interactions between GSTM1 and GSTT1 and known carcinogenic agents such as cigarette smoke. The fact that these enzymes metabolize these same carcinogens adds to the biological plausibility of the findings. Rebbeck also points out that, since the genes controlling production of these enzymes are inherited in the germ line, their temporal relationship to exposure and subsequent disease is established. A dose-response relationship has been observed in most studies between disease risk and the interaction between GSTM1 and cigarette smoking. In addition, dose-response relationships have been observed between disease risk and the presence of more than one susceptibility genotype in the same individual. Although the magnitude of the excess cancer risk associated with GSTM1 and GSTT1 alone is seldom more than twofold, interactions of GSTM1 and GSTT1 with other susceptibility genes or established carcinogens produce substantially larger effects. Although some consistency across studies has been observed for lung cancers, particularly in Japanese populations, studies of bladder, stomach, and colorectal cancers have delivered less consistent results.

This lack of consistency may reflect the lack of a causal connection or may result from a number of methodological problems that limit interpretation of the data. These problems are not unique to studies of GSTM1 and GSTT1 but apply generally to many areas of this emerging branch of epidemiological research. Rebbeck points out that many of the studies are conducted using hospital or clinic patients as case and control subjects and offer little information concerning inclusion or exclusion criteria for study subjects, patient characteristics, or tumor pathology. Most importantly, measures of effect are seldom adjusted for standard confounders, such as age, race, and sex. The failure to adjust for potential confounding in the face of small to moderate measures of effect is a serious concern. These studies also tend to have small numbers of case and control subjects and thus lack the statistical power to detect small effects. Finally, given that multiple alleles are often examined, the possibility that positive studies might result from multiple comparisons requires careful consideration.

BIOLOGICAL SPECIMEN BANKS

Winn et al[62] summarized some of the characteristics of existing biologic specimen banks and the issues that need to be considered when developing a new repository. A biological specimen bank is designed to store biological specimens for later analysis in a manner that maintains the stability of the samples and permits their efficient retrieval. The number of biological specimen banks is growing. In 1990, the International Agency for Research on Cancer listed 205 specimen banks in its *Directory of On-going Research in Cancer Epidemiology*. The 1996 edition of the directory[63] lists 345 specimen banks dealing in cells in culture, red cells, red cell membranes, serum, and plasma. Various types of tissues, urine, viable and nonviable white cells, whole blood, saliva, nails, freeze-dried fecal samples, seminal plasma, and exfoliated cervical cells are also collected.

Some banks store specimens on individuals who have already developed disease. The National Cancer Institute's serum immunodiagnostic bank on cancer patients and the Centers for Disease Control and Prevention's serum bank on disease outbreaks are prime examples. The samples are analyzed to help characterize and study the natural history of disease. Other banks include persons who do not have clinical disease when the specimens are obtained. Individuals are followed over time, thus allowing for the establishment of temporal relationships between biomarkers and disease endpoints. Winn et al[62] emphasize the need to design specimen banks in a manner that anticipates new developments in laboratory analysis and incorporates the collection of important patient data. These authors make the point that, while startup costs for specimen banks can be high, high utilization rates make these banks more cost-efficient than standard approaches to collecting biological specimens for inclusion in epidemiological studies.

In creating a specimen bank, attention must be given to developing standard protocols for ensuring that specimens are maintained under stable conditions and free from contamination. Equal attention must be paid to establishing standardized approaches for collecting the specimens. The complexity of specimen collection, processing, and storage should not be underestimated. The National Heart Lung and Blood Institute recently published guidelines for drawing blood and processing and storing sera for genetic studies.[64] These guidelines cover DNA extraction from blood samples and the alternative approach of using immortalized cell lines, and they also describe alternatives to the collection of anticoagulated blood, such as buccal cavity swabs and dried blood spots. Similar protocols have been developed by the Centers for Disease Control and Prevention for the Third National Health and Nutrition Examination Survey (NHANES III) DNA Bank.[65]

ETHICAL ISSUES

The banking of biological specimens for later inclusion in epidemiological studies has created an efficient and scientifically sound resource for conducting studies of gene-environment interactions, and new molecular techniques have allowed researchers to characterize the relationships between various environmental exposures and genetic susceptibility in ever greater detail. These new research methods have also raised a number of difficult ethical issues that have received extensive coverage in the medical literature. Below is a brief overview of some of the complex issues that arise from the inclusion of biomarkers in epidemiological research.

Biological specimens, like epidemiological data, are collected from subjects who sign approved informed consent forms. Such informed consent forms lay out in great detail what data or specimens will be collected, how the data and specimens will be used, who has access to the data, and how the data will be secured. However, new laboratory techniques are constantly emerging, and it has been difficult to develop informed consent procedures that anticipate all future research needs. For example, the NHANES III study provided for the collection of blood specimens for banking, but its informed consent form lacked provisions for genetic testing. After extensive review, it was decided that identifying information collected at the time of initial specimen collection could not be used to link genetic testing with other data sources. The investigators were permitted to proceed with "anonymized" testing, in which identifying information is permanently stripped from the samples before testing. (In anonymous testing, identifying information is not gathered at the time of specimen collection.)[66]

A second ethical issue involves the potential effects that genetic results might have on the subjects. Concerns exist that the identification of highly penetrant genes that predict serious disease can lead to psychological harm, social stigmatization, and loss of insurance coverage. Because of the possibility of such types of harm, close attention must be paid to the development of informed consent forms, and pre- and posttest counseling may be required.[66,67] Informed consent forms must provide study participants with a clear explanation of the purposes of the test and its expected use in the proposed research. Practical aspects of the test must also be addressed. For instance, the researchers should give participants a clear description of the actual testing procedure and any associated risks and should make sure participants understand the limits of the test, including the degree of uncertainty associated with using test results to predict cancer risk.[68]

Vineis and Schulte[69] have reviewed the scientific and ethical issues related to genetic screening to identify workers who might have an increased susceptibility to various industrial carcinogens. These authors utilized the *N*-acetyltransferase phenotype as an example of the scientific and ethical difficulties that are likely to arise from using genetic screening for the purpose of protecting workers. First, they point out that, although the polymorphic phenotypes can be distinguished, some misclassification is unavoidable. While a certain amount of misclassification can be tolerated in an etiologic study, the current level of misclassification would need to be reduced in order to protect individual workers. The phenotype has been a useful research tool for investigating gene-environment interactions, but results from various studies have been variable, and the use of this approach for predicting an individual's cancer risk is questionable. Most importantly, use of genetic screening, as these authors point out, has the potential to bar workers from employment opportunities and ignores other proven public health approaches to cancer prevention.

In addition to a number of legislative approaches being considered by the US Congress,[67] scientific groups have been developing guidelines for investigators involved in the genetic testing of human subjects. In 1997, the Task Force on Informed Consent of the Cancer Genetics Studies Consortium[70] issued a consensus statement on the process of subject education and the contents of informed consent forms based on the type of testing to be performed. The psychological and social implications of genetic testing, privacy and confidentiality issues, options for medical follow-up, and tissue storage and reuse are also discussed in this document. The discussion here provides only a glimpse of the complex ethical issues that arise when using biomarkers in epidemiological studies.

SUMMARY

The use of biomarkers to measure exposure and susceptibility is not new. However, new molecular biological techniques have improved the accuracy of exposure measurements and the ability of researchers to identify susceptibility genes that modify an individual's response to carcinogens. Improvements in exposure accuracy have been particularly noteworthy in viral studies, where polymerase chain reaction techniques can now be used to confirm infection with specific viral subtypes. The data gained by means of these techniques have been extremely valuable in establishing a causal relationship between HPV and cervical neoplasia, for example. New molecular techniques have also proven useful for identifying specific ways in which these agents alter the expression of cellular genes or lead to the deletion of certain tumor suppressor genes. The detection of adducts can confirm that a putative agent, initially measured through a questionnaire, actually interacts with the subject's DNA, while various cytogenetic studies are helpful in detecting early preclinical effects of exposures to carcinogenic agents. The identification of susceptibility phenotypes such as *N*-acetyltransferase offers opportunities for investigating relationships between inherited susceptibility and environmental exposures. Investigating interactions between two environmental exposures, such as exposures to HPV and HIV, has also been facilitated by the use of improved laboratory techniques.

Although the use of biomarkers holds promise for future research, caution is necessary in interpreting study findings. The inclusion of biomarkers in epidemiological research does not eliminate the need to apply the same standards of good epidemiological practice that apply to more classical approaches. Many studies that have included biomarkers have suffered from potential selection biases, a failure to adequately control for confounding, low statistical power, lack of consistency across studies, and a failure to establish a temporal relationship between the exposure measurement and the disease. The use of nested case-control designs, the establishment of guidelines for specimen collection and storage, and the creation of biological specimen banks are helping to improve the quality of these studies. Finally, no matter how scientifically valid, these studies introduce a number of complex ethical issues that still need to be resolved.

Discussion Questions

1. Define *marker of internal dose* and describe two examples of internal dose markers that have been used in cancer research.
2. Define *marker of biologically effective dose* and describe two examples of the use of this type of marker in cancer research.
3. Define *marker of preclinical biologic effect* and describe two examples of the use of this type of marker in cancer research.
4. Define *susceptibility marker* and describe two examples of the use of this type of marker in cancer research.
5. Discuss two or three methodological issues that should be considered when developing a protocol for collecting biological specimens.
6. Discuss two to three methodological issues that should be considered when developing a plan to analyze and interpret data on gene-environment interactions.
7. Discuss some of the issues involved in the development of biological specimen banks.
8. Discuss two to three ethical issues that arise when using biomarkers in epidemiological research.

References

1. Schulte PA. A conceptual and historical framework for molecular epidemiology. In: Schulte PA, Perera FP, eds. *Molecular Epidemiology: Principles and Practices.* San Diego: Academic Press; 1993:1–36.
2. Hulka BS. Overview of biological markers. In: Hulka BS, Wilcosky TC, Griffith JD, eds. *Biological Markers in Epidemiology*. New York: Oxford University Press; 1990:1–15.
3. US Department of Health and Human Services. *The Health Benefits of Smoking Cessation: A Report of the Surgeon General.* Rockville, MD: US Department of Health and Human Resources, Public Health Service, Centers for Disease Prevention and Health Promotion, Office on Smoking and Health; 1990. UDHHS (PHS) publication No. 90-8416.

4. Willett WC. Diet and nutrition. In: Schottenfeld D, Fraumeni JF Jr, eds. *Cancer Epidemiology and Prevention.* 2nd ed. New York: Oxford Press; 1996:438–461.
5. McMichael AJ. "Molecular epidemiology": new pathway or travelling companion? *Am J Epidemiol.* 1994;140:1–11. Invited commentary.
6. Wallace L, Pellizzari E, Hartwell TD, et al. Exposures to benzene and other volatile compounds from active and passive smoking. *Environ Health.* 1987;42:272–279.
7. Ong CN, Lee BL, Shi CY, et al. Elevated levels of benzene related compounds in the urine of cigarette smokers. *Int J Cancer.* 1994;59:177–180.
8. Holtzman RB, Ilcewica FH. Lead-210 and polonium-210 in tissues of cigarette smokers. *Science.* 1966;153:1259–1260.
9. Blanchard RL. Concentrations of 210 P_b and 210 P_o in human soft tissues. *Health Phys.* 1967;13:625–632.
10. McCann MF, Irwin DE, Walton LA, et al. Nicotine and cotinine in the cervical mucus of smokers, passive smokers, and non-smokers. *Cancer Epidemiol Biomarkers Prev.* 1992;1:125–129.
11. Holly EA, Petrakis NL, Friend NF, et al. Mutagenic mucus in the cervix of smokers. *J Natl Cancer Inst.* 1986;76:983–986.
12. Giovannucci E, Colditz G, Stampfer MJ, et al. The assessment of alcohol consumption by a simple self-administered questionnaire. *Am J Epidemiol.* 1991;133:810–817.
13. Poikolainen K, Karkkainen P, Karkkainen J. Correlations between biological markers and alcohol intake as measured by diary and questionnaire in men. *J Stud Alcohol.* 1985;46:383–387.
14. Schiffman MH. New epidemiology of human papillomavirus infection and cervical neoplasia. *J Natl Cancer Inst.* 1995;87:1345–1347.
15. Goldring JM, Lucier GW. Protein and DNA adducts. In: Hulka BS, Wilcosky TC, Griffith JD, eds. *Biological Markers in Epidemiology.* New York: Oxford University Press; 1990:78–104.
16. Perera FP, Santella RM, Brenner D, et al. DNA adducts, protein adducts, and sister chromatid exchange in cigarette smokers and non-smokers. *J Natl Cancer Inst.* 1987;79:449–456.
17. Carmella SG, Kagan SS, Kagan M, et al. Mass spectrometric analysis of tobacco-specific nitrosamine hemoglobin adducts in snuff dippers, smokers and non-smokers. *Cancer Res.* 1990:50:5438–5445.
18. Foiles PG, Akerkar SA, Carmella SG, et al. Mass spectrometric analysis of tobacco-specific nitrosamine DNA adducts in smokers and non-smokers. *Chem Res Toxicol.* 1991;4:364–368.
19. Carmella SG, Akerkar S, Hecht SS. Metabolites of the tobacco-specific nitrosamine 4-(methylnitrosamino)-1-(3-pyridyl)-butanone in smoker's urine. *Cancer Res.* 1993;53:721–724.
20. Mendelson JH, Mello NK, Cristofaro P, Ellingboe J. Alcohol effects on luteinizing hormone releasing hormone-stimulated anterior pituitary and gonadal hormones in women. *J Pharmacol Exp Ther.* 1989;50:902–909.
21. Mendelson JH, Mello NK, Cristofaro P, et al. Alcohol effects on naloxone-induced stimulated luteinizing hormone, prolactin and estradiol in women. *J Stud Alcohol.* 1987;48:287–294
22. Mendelson JH, Mello NK, Cristofaro P, Skupny A. Alcohol effects on naltrexone-induced stimulation of pituitary, adrenal, and gonadal hormones during early follicular phase of the menstrual cycle. *J Clin Endocrinol Metab.* 1988;66:1181–1186.
23. Mendelson JH, Luka SE, Mello NK, et al. Acute alcohol effects on plasma estradiol levels in women. *Psychopharmacology.* 1988;4:464–467.
24. Mendelson JH, Mello NK, Ellingboe J. Acute alcohol intake and pituitary gonadal hormones in normal human females. *J Pharmacol Exp Ther.* 1981;218:23–26.
25. Valimaki M, Harkonen M, Ylikahri R. Acute effects of alcohol on female sex hormones. *Alcohol Clin Exp Res.* 1983;7:289–293.
26. Becker U, Gluud C, Bennett P, et al. Effect of alcohol and glucose infusion on pituitary-gonadal hormones in normal females. *Drug Alcohol Depend.* 1988;22:141–149.
27. Ginsburg ES, Walsh BW, Shea BF, et al. Effect of acute ethanol ingestion on prolactin in menopausal women using estradiol replacement. *Gynecol Obstet Invest.* 1995;39:47–49.
28. Dorgan JF, Reichman ME, Judd JT, et al. *Cancer Causes Control.* 1994;5:53–60.
29. Hankinson SE, Willett WC, Manson JE, et al. Alcohol, weight and adiposity in relation to estrogen and prolactin levels in postmenopausal women. *J Natl Cancer Inst.*1995;87:1297–1302.
30. Reichman ME, Judd JT, Longcope C, et al. Effects of alcohol consumption on plasma and urinary hormone concentrations in premenopausal women. *J Natl Cancer Inst.* 1993;85:722–727.

31. Key TJ, Pike MC, Brown JB, et al. Cigarette smoking and urinary estrogen excretion in pre-menopausal and post-menopausal women. *Br J Cancer.* 1996;74:1313–1316.
32. Khaw KT, Tazuke S, Barrett-Connor E. Cigarette smoking and levels of adrenal androgens in post-menopausal women. *N Engl J Med.* 1988;318:1705–1709.
33. Perera FP, Santella R. Carcinogenesis. In: Schulte PA, Perera FP, eds. *Molecular Epidemiology: Principles and Practices.* San Diego: Academic Press; 1993:277–300.
34. Crane MM, Keating MJ, Trujillo JM, et al. Environmental exposures in cytogenetically defined subsets of acute non-lymphocytic leukemia. *JAMA.* 1989;262:634–639.
35. Wald N. Smoking and leukemia. *BMJ.* 1988;297:638.
36. Howell RW. Smoking habits and laboratory tests. *Lancet.* 1970;2:152.
37. Corre F, Lelluch J, Schwartz D. Smoking and leukocyte counts: results of an epidemiologic survey. *Lancet.* 1971;2:632–634.
38. Friedman GD, Siegelaub AB, Seltzer CC, et al. Smoking habits and the leukocyte count. *Arch Environ Health.* 1973;26:137–143.
39. Petitti DB, Kipp H. The leukocyte count: associations with intensity of smoking and persistence of effect after quitting. *Am J Epidemiol.* 1986;123:89–95.
40. Barr FG, Chatten J, D'Cruz CM, et al. Molecular assays for chromosomal translocations in the diagnosis of pediatric soft tissue sarcomas. *JAMA.* 1995;273:553–557.
41. Barr FG, Nauta LE, Davis RJ, et al. In vivo amplification of the *PAX3-FKHR* and *PAX7-FKHR* fusion genes in alveolar rhabdomyosarcoma. *Hum Mol Genet.* 1996;5:15–21.
42. Yokoyama A, Muramatsu T, Ohmori T, et al. Esophageal cancer and aldehyde dehydrogenase-2 genotypes in Japanese males. *Cancer Epidemiol Biomarkers Prev.* 1996;5:99–102.
43. Yokoyama A, Muramatsu T, Ohmori T, et al. Multiple primary esophageal and concurrent upper aerodigestive tract cancer and the aldehyde dehydrogenase-2 genotype of Japanese alcoholics. *Cancer.* 1996;77:1986–1990.
44. Yokoyama A, Ohmori T, Muramatsu T, et al. Cancer screening of upper aerodigestive tract in Japanese alcoholics with reference to drinking and smoking habits and aldehyde dehydrogenase-2 genotype. *Int J Cancer.* 1996;68:313–316.
45. Kinlen LJ. Immunologic factors, including AIDS. In: Schottenfeld D, Fraumeni JF Jr, eds. *Cancer Epidemiology and Prevention.* Philadelphia: Saunders; 1997:532–545.
46. Caussy D, Goedert JJ, Palefsky J, et al. Interaction of human immunodeficiency and papilloma viruses: association with anal epithelial abnormality in homosexual men. *Int J Cancer.* 1990;46:214–219.
47. Wright TC Jr, Sun XW. Anogenital papillomavirus infection and neoplasia in immunodeficient women. *Obstet Gynecol Clin North Am.* 1996;23:861–893.
48. Hillemanns P, Ellerbrock TV, McPhillips S, et al. Prevalence of anal human papillomavirus infection and anal cytologic abnormalities in HIV-seropositive women. *AIDS.* 1996;10:1641–1647.
49. Sun XW, Kuhn L, Ellerbrock TV, et al. Human papillomavirus infection in women infected with the human immunodeficiency virus. *N Engl J Med.* 1997;337:1343–1349.
50. Rabkin CS. Epidemiology of AIDS-related malignancies. *Curr Opin Oncol.* 1994;6:492–496.
51. Kafuko GW, Burkitt DP. Burkitt's lymphoma and malaria. *Int J Cancer.* 1970;6:1–9.
52. Garro AJ, Lieber CS. Alcohol and cancer. *Annu Rev Pharmacol Toxocol.* 1990;30:219–249.
53. Garro AJ, Espina N, Lieber CS. Alcohol and cancer. *Alcohol Health and Research World.* 1992;16:81–86.
54. Perera FP. Molecular epidemiology: insights into cancer susceptibility, risk assessment, and prevention. *J Natl Cancer Inst.* 1996;88:496–509.
55. Swift M. Single gene syndromes. In: Schottenfeld D, Fraumeni JF Jr, eds. *Cancer Epidemiology and Prevention.* Philadelphia: Saunders; 1982:475–482.
56. Nasca PC, Lie S, Baptiste MS, et al. Alcohol consumption and breast cancer: estrogen receptor status and histology. *Am J Epidemiol.* 1994;140:980–988.
57. Singletary K. Ethanol and experimental breast cancer: a review. *Alcohol Clin Exp Res.* 1997;21:334–339.
58. Gapstur SM, Potter JD, Drinkard C, Folsom AR. Synergistic effect between alcohol and estrogen replacement therapy on risk of breast cancer differs by estrogen/progesterone receptor status in the Iowa Women's Health Study. *Cancer Epidemiol Biomarkers Prev.* 1995;4:313–318.
59. Pearce Neil, de Sanjose S, Boffetta P, et al. Limitations of biomarkers of exposure in cancer epidemiology. *Epidemiology.* 1995;6:190–194.

60. Garland M, Morris JS, Rosner BA, et al. Toenail trace element levels as biomarkers: reproducibility over a 6-year period. *Cancer Epidemiol Biomarkers Prev*. 1993;2:493–497.
61. Rebbeck TR. Molecular epidemiology of the human glutathione S-transferase genotypes GSTM1 and GSTT1 in cancer susceptibility. *Cancer Epidemiol Biomarkers Prev*. 1997;6:733–743.
62. Winn DM, Reichman ME, Gunter E. Epidemiologic issues in the design and use of biologic specimen banks. *Epidemiol Rev*. 1990;12:56–70.
63. Sankaranarayanan R, Wahrendorf J, Demaret E, eds. *Directory of On-going Research in Cancer Epidemiology*. Lyon, France: International Agency for Research on Cancer; 1996.
64. Austin MA, Ordovas JM, Eckfeldt JH, et al. Guidelines of the National Heart, Lung, and Blood Institute Working Group on Blood Drawing, Processing, and Storage for Genetic Studies. *Am J Epidemiol*. 1996;144:437–441.
65. Steinberg KK, Sanderlin KC, Chin-Yih O, et al. DNA banking in epidemiologic studies. *Epidemiol Rev*. 1997;19:156–162.
66. Holtzman NA, Andrews LB. Ethical and legal issues in genetic epidemiology. *Epidemiol Rev*. 1997;19:163–174.
67. Bondy M, Mastromarino C. Ethical issues of genetic testing and their implications in epidemiologic studies. *Ann Epidemiol*. 1997;7:363–366.
68. Geller G, Botkin JR, Green MJ, et al. Genetic testing for susceptibility to adult-onset cancer: the process and content of informed consent. *JAMA*. 1997;227:1467–1474.
69. Vineis P, Schulte PA. Scientific and ethical aspects of genetic screening of workers for cancer risk: the case of the *N*-acetyltransferase phenotype. *J Clin Epidemiol*. 1995;48:189–197.
70. Geller G, Botkin JR, Green MJ, et al. Genetic testing for susceptibility to adult-onset cancer: the process and content of informed consent. *JAMA*. 1997;277:1467–1474.

Chapter 7

Epidemiological Studies of Genetic Factors for Cancer

Wei Zheng

This chapter covers some of the fundamental concepts and principles used in epidemiological studies on genetic factors related to cancer. Also described in this chapter are some basic DNA analysis techniques and epidemiological methods commonly used in the study of genetic factors. Some examples from previous studies are described to help readers to understand the concepts and methodology discussed herein.

One of the major successes of cancer epidemiological research over the last half century has been the identification of many environmental risk factors for cancer.[1] Environmental factors broadly construed also include lifestyle factors, such as cigarette smoking, dietary habits, physical activity, and reproductive patterns. The rapid advances in recombinant DNA technology over the last decade have made the importance of genetic factors in cancer etiology increasingly evident. We now know that cancer cases related to the previously identified hereditary cancer syndromes, such as Li-Fraumeni syndrome, familial adenomatous polyposis, hereditary nonpolyposis colon cancer, and familial breast and ovarian cancers, make up only a small percentage of the cancer cases caused by genetic factors. A large proportion of the cancers previously thought to be attributable to environmental factors alone are now believed to occur as a result of interaction between inherited susceptibility factors and environmental exposures.[2] The role of genetic and environmental interaction in the occurrence of several common malignancies has been clearly demonstrated in many recent epidemiological studies, as reviewed by Strong and Amos[3] and Caporaso and Goldstein.[4] The study of gene-environment interaction has become one of the major themes in genetic epidemiology, a rapidly developing discipline that integrates the principles and methodology of genetics and epidemiology.[5] This chapter reviews the principles and methods used in epidemiological studies of cancer-related genetic factors and discusses methodologic issues that arise in studies using genetic biomarkers.

FUNDAMENTAL CONCEPTS OF HUMAN GENETICS

To understand the role of genetic factors in the etiology of cancer and the study designs used to evaluate these factors, some basic concepts of human genetics are useful.

I would like to thank Drs. Kim Creek, Jason Moore, and Thomas Sellers for their helpful comments and suggestions in the preparation of this chapter.

As described in Chapter 3, deoxyribonucleic acid (DNA) is the carrier of genetic information transmitted from parent to offspring. Human nuclear DNA is organized into 22 pairs of autosomal chromosomes and 2 sex-specific chromosomes, X and Y. There are two copies of each autosome in the cell nucleus, and each parent donates one copy to each pair. Females carry two X chromosomes, while males carry one each of the X and Y chromosomes.

The basic unit of genetic information is the gene, and each gene is located in a particular position on a chromosome, called a *locus.* A particular form of a gene is referred to as an *allele.* At a given locus, there may exist two or more forms of a gene with different DNA sequences (alleles). A pair of chromosomes may contain the same allele at a given locus (homozygosity) or different alleles (heterozygosity). Some nucleotide changes may lead to an altered function and/or production of the gene products, while others may not be of any functional significance.

Human *N*-acetyltransferase-2 (NAT2) is a good example to illustrate this concept. NAT2 is an important enzyme in the metabolism of heterocyclic amines, which are well-established animal carcinogens that are formed during high-temperature cooking of animal foods.[6] Nucleotide changes at 11 positions of the 870 base pair coding region of the *NAT2* gene have been identified thus far.[7,8] Seven of these substitutions result in amino acid changes, while the other four are silent. (To say they are silent means that, although the substitutions occurred in a nucleic acid, the changes did not lead to a change in the coded amino acid. This can happen because most amino acids can be encoded with more than one combination of nucleic acids.) A combination of one to four of these nucleotide substitutions gives rise to 25 variant *NAT2* alleles. Some of these alleles, such as *NAT2*12A, *12B, *12C,* and **13,* encode proteins with the high *O*-acetylation capacity of heterocyclic amines, similar to that encoded by the wild-type allele *NAT2*4*. Other alleles, however, give rise to different forms of enzymes with reduced catalytic activity. In a recent study of the relationship between the *NAT2* gene and breast cancer among Iowa women, 10 of the 26 alleles were found in 561 cases and controls, and the most common (wild-type) allele, *NAT2*4,* was identified only in approximately 25% of the chromosomes examined.[9] The *NAT2* gene is a good example of a polymorphic gene for which the most common allele has a frequency of less than 99% in the general population.

Each person inherits one copy of a gene from each parent to form his or her own genotype for that gene. The alleles at a given locus may or may not be the same. Homozygous individuals have two copies of the same allele, while heterozygous individuals have two different alleles. For an autosomal gene with k alleles, there exist $k(k+1)/2$ distinct genotypes. For example, for a gene with three alleles (*A1, A2*, and *A3*), there exist six possible genotypes, including three homozygous genotypes (*A1/A1, A2/A2*, and *A3/A3*) and three heterozygous genotypes (*A1/A2, A1/A3*, and *A2/A3*). The phenotype of an individual, such as the activity of a given enzyme or the onset of cancer, depends on his or her genotype and the penetrance of the gene. The term *penetrance* is used in genetic epidemiology to describe the probability of displaying a phenotype given a specific genotype. Many factors, including certain environmental exposures, may affect the penetrance of a particular gene. Indeed, most cancer occurs as a result of the joint effects of multiple genes (polygenic effects) or the effects of gene-environment interaction (multifactorial effects).

For single-gene defects, the inheritance patterns within a family can be described using the following four Mendelian transmission models: autosomal dominant, autosomal recessive, X-linked dominant, and X-linked recessive.[5] Autosomal dominant disorders occur with higher frequency within a family than autosomal recessive disorders, since one copy of the mutant gene is sufficient to cause the disease. All affected individuals usually have at least one affected parent, and about 50% of the offspring from matings of an affected heterozygote with a normal individual are affected. Autosomal recessive disease occurs only in individuals who are homozygous for the mutation (ie, both chromosomes carry the defective gene). Since heterozygotes for the defective gene have one normal allele, they are phenotypically normal. X-linked recessive diseases occur usually only in males, since females have two X chromosomes and are at a low risk for inheriting a defective gene in both chromosomes from their parents. X-linked dominant disorders, however, occur in both males and females, since one copy of the abnormal gene is sufficient to cause disease.

Of these inheritance models, autosomal dominant transmission is probably the most common type for hereditary cancer syndromes, such as those involving tumor suppressor genes.[3] Retinoblastoma is a good example of this paradigm, for about 50% of the offspring of parents with hereditary retinoblastoma eventually develop this rare malignancy. This transmission pattern is consistent with the autosomal dominant model.[3] At the somatic level, however, mutation or deletion of both copies of the *Rb1* gene is required for the malignant transformation of the cells, a feature of the autosomal recessive genotype. This seemingly contradictory paradigm can be explained by the two-hit model proposed by Knudson in the early 1970s,[10] approximately 15 years before the *Rb1* gene was cloned.[11] In hereditary retinoblastoma, children usually inherit one copy of the defective *Rb1* gene from their parents. The tumor, however, will not occur until the second copy of the gene is mutated or deleted in a somatic cell owing to an environmental insult or chance event. In very rare cases, two mutations occur in the same somatic cell. In the general population, the incidence of retinoblastoma is about 1 in 20,000 children.[12] In families with hereditary retinoblastoma, 50% of children will inherit the defective *Rb1* gene, and of these 90% will develop retinoblastoma. Compared to sporadic cases, cases with an inherited predisposition have cancer diagnosed at an earlier age and have a higher frequency of bilateral retinoblastoma.[10]

The Li-Fraumeni syndrome is another good example of an autosomal dominant disorder. This syndrome is characterized by a germ-line mutation of the *p53* tumor suppressor gene and by familial clustering of a variety of cancers, including childhood sarcomas, young-onset breast cancer, and brain tumors.[13] As in the case of hereditary retinoblastoma, susceptible individuals, although phenotypically normal at birth, are usually heterozygous for the mutant *p53* gene. The tumor cells become homozygous for this defective gene when the normal allele is lost or mutated. Because of the time required for the second mutation, penetrance of mutant genes among carriers increases with age in most hereditary cancer syndromes. For mutant *p53* carriers, the risk of cancer has been estimated to be 50% by the age of 45 years and 90% by age 65.[3]

HIGH-PENETRANCE MUTANT GENES VERSUS LOW-PENETRANCE POLYMORPHIC GENES

Most hereditary cancer syndromes are caused by the mutation or deletion of genes involved in critical cell functions, such as DNA repair, proliferation, cell cycle control, and apoptosis. Mutations of these genes usually result in altered function or altered production of gene products. Carriers of these mutant genes have a very high risk of developing cancer. For example, the risk of developing breast cancer among women who carry defective breast cancer susceptibility genes *BRCA1* and *BRCA2* has been estimated to be as high as 60% by age 50 and 80% by age 70.[14]

Although these mutant genes give rise to an extremely high risk of cancer, they are rare in the general population and thus have a low population attributable risk. In addition, not all mutant gene carriers will develop cancer during their lifetime, supporting the notion that environmental factors and other genes may be involved in the development of cancer even among individuals with a very strong genetic predisposition. It has been estimated that only about 1% of cancer cases are caused by germ-line mutations of these highly penetrant cancer genes.[12] Hereditary cancer syndromes are usually characterized by an early age of onset, the occurrence of multiple tumors, and a Mendelian pattern of inheritance within the family. Substantial progress has been made over the last decade in the identification of the genes that are responsible for major hereditary cancer syndromes. Many of these genes have been cloned or mapped to specific locations within the human genome.[15] Table 7–1 lists some examples of these highly penetrant genes for major hereditary cancer syndromes in humans.

Table 7–1 Examples of High-penetrance Genes Responsible for Hereditary Cancer Syndromes

Syndrome	*Gene (Chromosome)*	*Tumor Type*
Retinoblastoma	*RB1* (13q14)	Retinoblastoma, osteosarcoma
Wilms' tumor	*WT1* (11p13-14)	Kidney
Neurofibromatosis type 1	*NF1* (17q11)	Neurofibrosarcomas, leukemia
Neurofibromatosis type 2	*NF2* (22q11-13)	CNS
Li-Fraumeni	*p53* (17p13.1)	Breast, sarcoma, leukemia, brain, and others
Familial breast-ovary	*BRCA1* (17q21-3) *BRCA2* (13q12-13)	Breast, ovary
Von Hippel-Lindau	*VHL* (3p)	Renal cell and others
Familial melanoma	*p16/CDKN2A* (9p21)	Melanoma
Gorlin's syndrome	*PTCH* (9q22)	Basal cell, fibrosarcoma, and others
Ataxia telangiectasia	*ATM* (11q22-q23)	Lymphoma, leukemia, breast, and others
Familial adenomatous polyposis	*APC* (5q21)	Colorectum
Xeroderma pigmentosa	*XP(A-G)* (9q34.1), many others	Skin, adrenal
Hereditary non-polyp colorectal	*hMSH2* (2p22) *hMLH1* (3p21) *hPMS1* (2q31-33) *hPMS2* (7p22)	Colorectum
Multiple endocrine neoplasia type 1	*MENI* (11q13)	Carcinoids, pancreas, parathyroid
Multiple endocrine neoplasia type 2	*RET* (10q11.2)	Medullary thyroid, phaeochromocytoma

Source: Data from N. Caporaso and A. Goldstein, Issues Involving Biomarkers in the Study of the Genetics of Human Cancer, in *Application of Biomarkers in Cancer Epidemiology*, P. Toniolo, et al., eds., IARC Scientific Publication No. 142, © 1997, International Agency for Research on Cancer and D.T. Bishop, Genetic Predisposition to Cancer: An Introduction, in *Genetic Predisposition to Cancer*, R.A. Eeles, eds., pp. 3–15, © 1996.

While the high-penetrance mutant cancer genes described above may "predetermine" the development of cancer among carriers, other groups of genes only moderately elevate the risk of cancer, in many cases just by increasing the person's susceptibility to environmental carcinogens.[16] Many low-penetrance genes are involved in the metabolism of endogenous or exogenous compounds, and their genetic variations are correlated with the function of gene products, the production of gene products, or both. For example, catechol-*O*-methyltransferase (COMT), an enzyme that adds a methyl group to catechol estrogens in a detoxification pathway, is encoded by a polymorphic gene. A *G→A* transition in exon 4 of the gene results in a valine to methionine substitution in the gene product.[17] In individuals homozygous for this variant allele, the activity of the enzyme is substantially reduced. Genetic polymorphism of the *COMT* gene has recently been reported to be associated with the risk of breast cancer in some epidemiological studies.[18–20]

Sometimes a susceptibility gene may encode only one of several enzymes involved in similar metabolic pathways. Cytosolic glutathione *S*-transferases (GSTs) are a family of important enzymes involved in the cellular detoxification of many carcinogens.[21,22] These enzymes catalyze the conjugation of diverse electrophilic compounds (such as carcinogens) with glutathione, in most cases giving rise to less reactive metabolites that are more readily excreted from cells. In humans, there are four classes of cytosolic GST isoenzymes: α, μ, π, and θ. Some enzymes overlap considerably in substrate specificity. For example, GST-μ and -π can both detoxify carcinogenic polycyclic aromatic hydrocarbons, such as benzo[*a*]pyrene, while GST-θ can detoxify smaller reactive hydrocarbons, such as ethylene oxide and diepoxybutane.[23] The *GSTM1* gene (encoding GST-μ) is absent in about 50% of Caucasians, whereas the *GSTT1* gene (encoding GST-θ) is absent in about 15% of Caucasians. The absence of the *GSTM1* and *GSTT1* genes has been reported to increase the risk of several common cancers, including cancers of the lung, bladder, and breast.[22,24,25]

Although low-penetrance genes usually do not give rise to obvious familial clustering, they may contribute significantly to the number of cancer cases in the general population because of their high prevalence. As mentioned earlier, homozygous deletion in the *GSTM1* gene is very common in the general population and is present in about 50% of Caucasians and Asians. In a recent meta-analysis of 12 case-control lung cancer studies with a total of 1,593 case subjects and 2,135 control subjects, absence of the *GSTM1* gene was found to be associated with a small increased risk of lung cancer (OR = 1.41, 95% CI = 1.23–1.61).[26] If the association is causal, *GSTM1* gene deletion could account for about 17% of lung cancer cases in the general population. Table 7–2 compares some of the major characteristics of high-penetrance mutant cancer genes with major characteristics of low-penetrance polymorphic genes.

BASIC DNA ANALYSIS TECHNIQUES IN MOLECULAR EPIDEMIOLOGICAL STUDIES

Much of the recent progress in our understanding of the genetic basis of the etiology of human cancer is attributable to the remarkable advances in recombinant DNA technology that have occurred over the last decade. In particular, the invention of the polymerase chain reaction (PCR) technique and the application of this technique in DNA

Table 7–2 Comparison of High- and Low-Penetrance Genes

	High Penetrance	*Low Penetrance*
Role	Tends to be "causal," ie, necessary and sufficient for disease	Allele alters susceptibility; neither necessary nor sufficient for disease cause
Example	*BRCA1* (breast/ovary) *APC* (polyposis coli) *RB* (retinoblastoma)	*CYP1A1* (lung) *CYP2D6* (lung) *GST-M1* (lung, bladder)
Frequency in population	Low to rare	Often common
Familial hereditary pattern	Clear	Equivocal
Strength of association	High	Low to moderate
Absolute risk of disease	High	Low
Population attributable risk	Low	High
Gene-environment interaction	Secondary and variable	Primary and implicit
Role of environmental exposure	Secondary and variable	Critical

Source: Reprinted with permission from N. Caporaso and A. Goldstein, Issues Involving Biomarkers in the Study of the Genetics of Human Cancer, in *Application of Biomarkers in Cancer Epidemiology*, P. Toniolo, et al., eds., pp. 237–250, IARC Scientific Publications No. 142, © 1997, International Agency for Research on Cancer.

analysis have made it feasible and cost-efficient to determine individual genotypes in epidemiological studies of cancer. This section presents a brief overview of DNA-analysis techniques commonly used in molecular epidemiological studies. Readers are referred to *Molecular Biology of the Cell*[27] and *Recombinant DNA,*[28] two excellent reference books, for more details.

The PCR technique is used to amplify specific nucleotide sequences *in vitro* so that the amplified DNA fragment is the dominant DNA molecule in the reaction tube, making further analysis easier. This technique is used when part of the nucleotide sequence of a given DNA fragment is already known. The known part of the sequence is used to design two synthetic DNA oligonucleotides, one complementary to one strand of the DNA double helix and the other complementary to the other strand, with the two lying on opposite ends of the region to be amplified. These oligonucleotides serve as primers for *in vitro* DNA synthesis and determine the ends of the final DNA fragment (PCR product).

The basic PCR reaction mixture contains double-stranded template DNA, specific primers, deoxynucleoside triphosphates (dNTPs), thermostable DNA polymerase (such as *Taq*), and cofactors (Mg^{++} and K^{+}). The first step in the PCR cycle is to separate the double-stranded DNA template at a high temperature (typically at 95°C); the process of separation is called *denaturing*. Next, the reaction mixture is cooled rapidly to 45–65°C to allow the gene-specific primers to anneal to the template, then it is heated to 72°C to allow the DNA polymerase to synthesize a complementary strand from the 3' ends of each primer. This extension results in two molecules of double-stranded DNA, each of which has one strand with its 5' end defined by its specific primer. These reactions are repeated for a second cycle. At the end of the second cycle, four double-stranded DNA molecules are formed, including two single strands with both ends defined by the primers. At the end of the third cycle, 8 molecules of double-stranded DNA are formed, including 8 single strands with both ends defined by the primers. With the repetition of this cycle, the DNA fragments with both ends defined by the primers are accumulated exponentially and soon dominate the population of the DNA molecules in the tubes (see Figure 7–1). In an ideal system, with doubling at each cycle, after 30 cycles there would be a billionfold increase in product (2^{30}=1,073,741,824). In reality, the efficiency of the process is usually less than perfect, and 25–30 cycles usually net a multimillionfold increase.

The length of time required for each PCR cycle depends on many factors, including the length of the DNA fragment to be amplified. Typically, a cycle takes 3 to 5 minutes, and the whole process takes less than a few hours. Theoretically, the PCR technique can detect a single copy of a gene in a sample. In practice, 25–50 ng of DNA is typically used

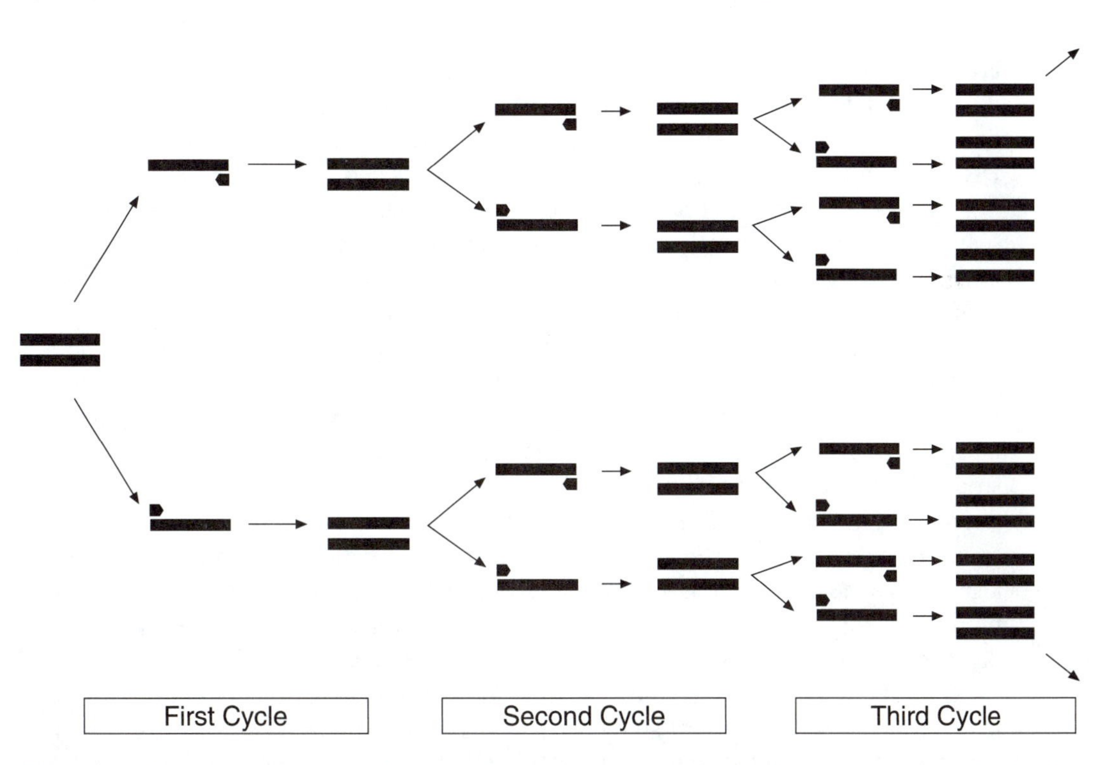

Figure 7–1 PCR amplification. PCR produces an amount of DNA that doubles in each cycle of DNA synthesis. Three cycles of reaction produce 16 DNA chains, 8 of which have both their ends defined by the primers. After three more cycles, 240 of the 256 DNA chains will be defined by the primers. *Source:* Copyright 1994 From *Molecular Biology of the Cell, 3rd Edition* by B. Alberts, et al., eds. Reproduced by permission of Taylor & Francis, Inc., http://www.routledge-ny.com.

to serve as a template. Because PCR amplification requires only a small amount of DNA and can be highly automated, it has been widely used in molecular epidemiological studies of genetic factors.

Gel electrophoresis is commonly used in DNA analyses to separate and identify DNA fragments of different sizes. Each nucleotide in a nucleic acid molecule carries a single negative charge, and when an electric field is applied, the molecule will migrate toward the positive electrode. The supporting gels through which DNA molecules migrate are prepared using polyacrylamide or agarose. Polyacrylamide is used to separate smaller molecules, whereas agarose is used for larger ones. The pore size of a gel can be adjusted based on the concentration of polyacrylamide or agarose so that it is small enough to retard the migration of the DNA molecules of interest. Because of the retaining effect of the gel, large molecules migrate more slowly than small molecules, and for a linear DNA fragment the rate of migration depends primarily on the size of the molecule. Polyacrylamide gels have a much greater resolving power than agarose gels. They have the ability to separate molecules of DNA whose lengths differ by as little as 0.2% (eg, fragments of 500 nucleotides or less that differ by a single nucleotide). For large DNA molecules, however, the pores in polyacrylamide gels are too small to permit them to pass, and agarose gels with various concentrations are then normally used.

The DNA bands on gels are invisible unless the DNA is labeled or stained. One commonly used sensitive method to visualize DNA is to stain the gels with ethidium bromide, a dye that binds tightly to double-stranded DNA and fluoresces brightly under ultraviolet light. An even more sensitive method is to incorporate a radioisotope (eg, ^{32}P) into the DNA molecules and then use autoradiography to detect the radioisotope-labeled DNA molecules. An example of gel electrophoresis is shown in Figure 7–2.

Restriction enzymes (endonucleases) are important tools in molecular biology research (those used are mostly obtained from bacteria). Each of these enzymes recognizes a specific DNA sequence, usually four to eight nucleotides, and always cuts the DNA at a specific site within or adjacent to the recognition sequence. For example, *Eco*R I recognizes the sequence of *GAATTC* and digests the phosphodiester bond between *G* and *A* to yield two DNA fragments, —*G* and *AATTC*—. *Eco*57 I recognizes the sequence of *CTGAAG* and cuts the DNA at a site 16 nucleotides downstream of the recognition sequence. When one or more nucleotides in the recognition sequence of a particular restriction enzyme is altered, this enzyme will no longer be able to cut the DNA strands at the restriction site. Sometimes, a single nucleotide change can create a new restriction site. A deletion or an insertion in a DNA sequence lying between two restriction sites can also change the size of the DNA fragment after restriction enzyme digestion. The polymorphisms that are reflected in the length of DNA fragments after restriction enzyme digestion are referred to as *restriction fragment length polymorphisms (RFLPs),* and PCR-RFLP–based assays have been used widely in molecular epidemiological studies to determine the genotypes of study participants for polymorphic candidate genes.

For example, cytochrome P-450-1B1 (CYP1B1) is an important enzyme in the metabolism of estrogens and certain mammary carcinogens, such as polycyclic aromatic hydrocarbons and heterocyclic aromatic amines. This enzyme is genetically polymorphic, and the variations in the *CYP1B1* gene may be related to the risk of breast cancer.[29] A *G* to *C* transversion at exon 3 of the *CYP1B1* gene results in a valine (*GTG*) to leucine

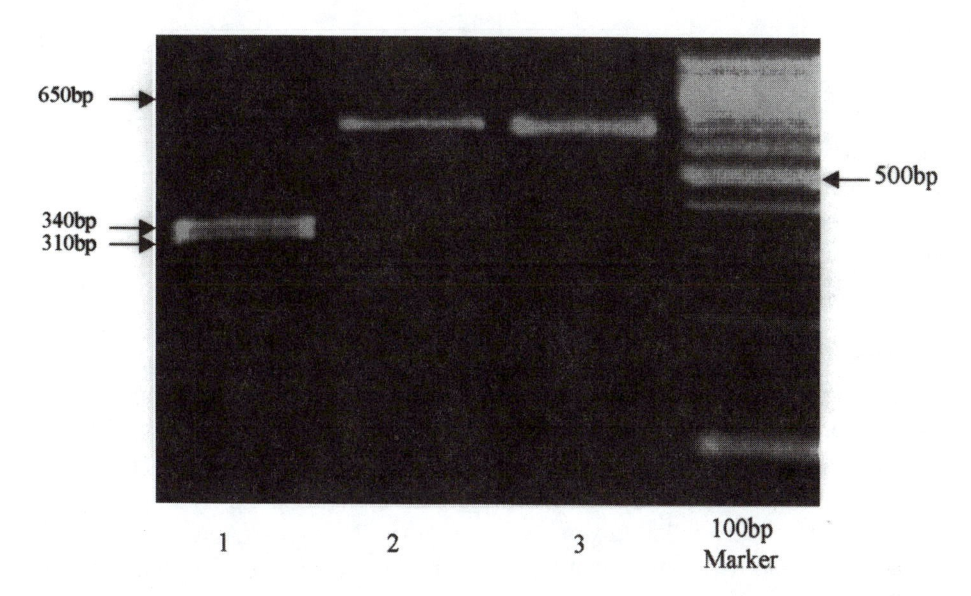

Figure 7–2 Gel electrophoresis following RFLP analysis of the 650-bp *CYP1B1* product. Representative genotypes are shown in Lane 1 (homozygous for the *Leu* allele), Lane 2 (heterozygous for the *Leu* allele), and Lane 3 (homozygous for the *Val* allele). *Source:* Reprinted with permission from W. Zheng, et al., Genetic polymorphism of Cytochrome p450-1B1 and Risk of Breast Cancer, *Cancer Epidemiology Biomarkers Prevention,* Vol. 9, pp. 147–150, © 2000, American Association for Cancer Research.

(*CTG*) substitution in codon 432. This change creates an *Eco*57 I restriction site, facilitating the detection of this polymorphism in epidemiological studies.

To study the relation of this polymorphism to breast cancer risk, one could design a PCR protocol to amplify a DNA fragment of the gene that contains the polymorphic site. The PCR products would then be digested by the *Eco*57 I enzyme, which recognizes and cuts the DNA molecules that contain the *CTGAAG* sequence, the *Leu* allele. When the *Leu* allele is present in the DNA molecule of one chromosome but absent from the DNA molecule of the other homologous chromosome, two shorter fragments would be produced from the chromosome with the *Leu* allele after *Eco*57 I digestion, but the fragment would not be cut in the case of the other chromosome. Samples that are homozygous for the *Leu* allele would only have the shorter fragments and those homozygous for the *Val* allele would only have the longer fragments. These fragments could then be separated and identified using electrophoresis, and the genotype for each individual could thus be determined. Figure 7–2 shows an electrophoresis analysis of a 650–base pair DNA fragment from exon 3 of the *CYP1B1* gene.[29] The DNA molecules with the *Leu* allele were cut into two pieces of 310 and 340 base pairs, while those with the *Val* allele remain at 650 base pairs. Using this PCR-RFLP–based assay, the genotype of the *CYP1B1* gene for each individual could be determined.

DNA sequencing is also used in some molecular epidemiological studies to determine the nucleotide sequence of a given candidate gene. Currently, this technique is more often employed to detect gene mutations than to detect polymorphisms, since it is more expensive and time consuming than the RFLP-based assays. There are two common DNA sequencing methods, a chemical method (Maxam-Gilbert) and an enzymatic method (Sanger). In the former, chemicals that specifically destroy one of the four bases in the DNA are used to generate a family of DNA fragments of different lengths. These fragments are then separated electrophoretically in a gel strictly according to length, and the nucleotide sequence of the DNA molecule is thus determined.

The enzymatic method, more commonly used than the chemical method nowadays, involves *in vitro* DNA synthesis carried out in the presence of dideoxynucleoside triphosphates (ddNTPs). These modified nucleotides are missing the deoxyribose 3'-OH group present in normal nucleotides. In DNA synthesis, the DNA chain elongates in a 5' to 3' direction—the incoming deoxynucleotide is added to the 3'-OH of the polynucleotide chain. The ddNTPs molecules can be incorporated normally into a growing DNA chain through their 5' triphosphate groups. However, they cannot form phosphodiester bonds with the next incoming deoxynucleotide triphosphates (dNTPs) because of their missing 3'-OH group, and thus they terminate the elongation. For example, when a small amount of ddATP is included along with the four dNTPs, DNA synthesis will stop at a randomly selected *A* in the sequence and generate a series of chains that are specifically terminated at the *A* residue. These chains are then separated and identified using electrophoresis according to their length. To determine the sequence of a DNA molecule, four different chain-terminating nucleoside triphosphates are used in separate DNA synthesis reactions on the same primed single-stranded DNA template. When the products of these four reactions are analyzed by electrophoresis in four parallel lanes of a polyacrylamide gel, the DNA sequence can be directly read from the gel. Figure 7–3 shows an example of a DNA sequencing process using the enzymatic method.

In addition to those described above, other DNA analysis techniques, such as nucleic acid hybridization, DNA microarray, and mass spectroscopy, can also be used in molecular epidemiological studies. DNA microarray technology represents an exciting step toward cost-efficient analysis of genetic materials. Currently, this technology is usually used to analyze gene expression in study samples. A microarray usually contains thousands of cDNA clone inserts that are robotically printed onto the surface of a slide or other substrate. The microarray slides are then hybridized with fluorescently labeled probes that are generated after isolating mRNA from study samples. Because a microarray slide can be designed to contain unique sequences of thousands of genes, the expression status of these genes in a study sample can be determined in a single experiment. With improvement, microarray technology could make the detection of mutations and genotypes in molecular epidemiological studies readily achievable.

EPIDEMIOLOGICAL APPROACHES TO THE STUDY OF CANCER-RELATED GENETIC FACTORS

Various approaches and types of studies can be used to investigate genetic factors and their potential interaction with environmental exposures in the etiology of cancer.[5,30] Two of the most common are family studies and genetic biomarker studies. Family studies are typically conducted within families and use information on the families' histories of disease. The initial evidence for a potential genetic involvement in cancer etiology usually comes from studies using family history as the variable of interest. Both case-

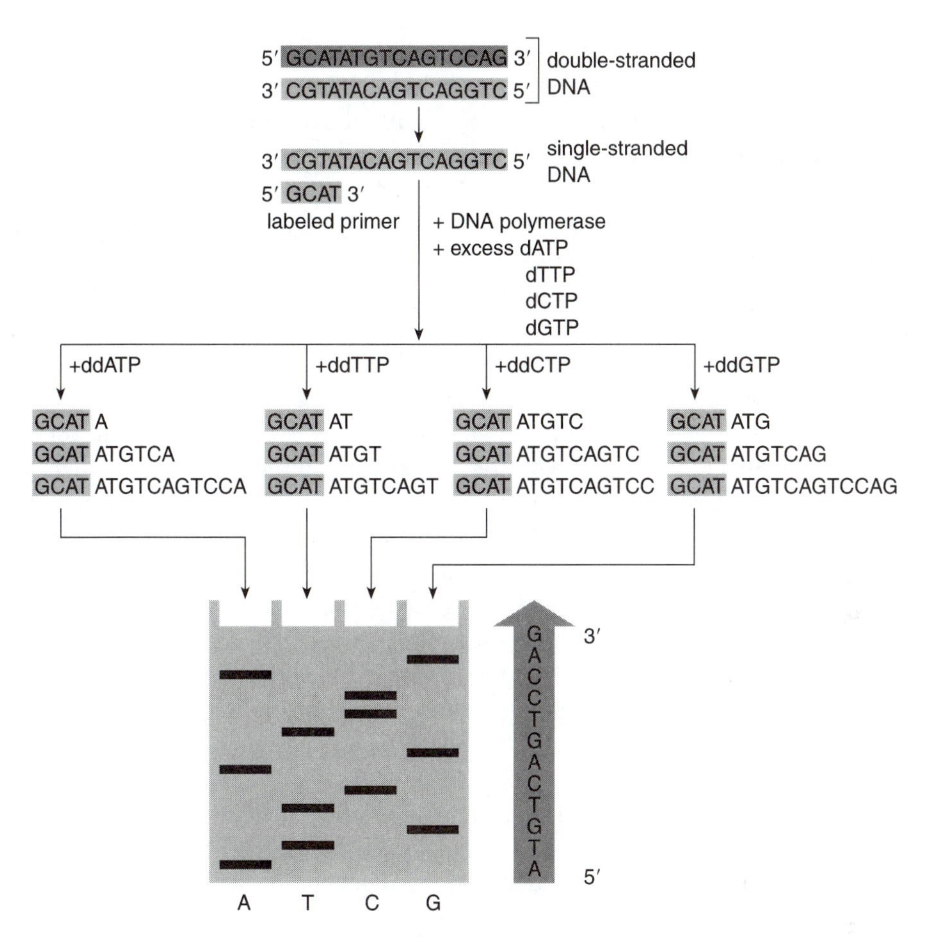

Figure 7–3 The enzymatic method for sequencing DNA. Four different chain-terminating nucleoside triphosphates (ddNTPs) are used in separate DNA synthesis reactions on the same primed single-stranded DNA template. The products of these four reactions are analyzed electrophoretically in four parallel lanes of a polyacrylamide gel, and the DNA sequence can be read directly from the gel. *Source:* Copyright 1994 from *Molecular Biology of the Cell, 3rd Edition* by B. Alberts, et al., eds. Reproduced by permission of Taylor & Francis, Inc., http://www.routledge-ny.com.

---

control and cohort studies can be used to investigate the association between familial cancer history and cancer risk. In studies of the former kind, cancer case and control subjects are compared to examine whether a higher percentage of persons with cancer have a family history of cancer than persons in the control group, while in studies of the latter kind, persons with a family history of cancer are compared with persons without such a history regarding their future risk of cancer occurrence. A notable association between cancer risk and familial cancer history, particularly if cancer has been diagnosed among multiple family members at a young age, would suggest a possible genetic component in the etiology of the cancer. Although epidemiological studies of familial cancer history are an important starting point for genetic epidemiology, data from these studies can be difficult to interpret. Some important environmental factors are also "familial." For example, certain lifestyle factors, such as cigarette smoking and dietary habits, tend to be prevalent among family members, and these factors are known to be associated with the risk of cancer.[31] Therefore, familial cancer aggregation could be a result of genetic factors or shared environmental factors or both.

Segregation analysis can be considered an extension of the traditional epidemiological studies of family history. Segregation analyses are used to determine whether a particular disease or trait is inherited in one of the Mendelian ways described previously. Family data collected from cancer patients (probands) are modeled to identify the most likely disease transmission pattern in families. The specific patterns of transmission within families may vary according to whether the genes are dominant or recessive, autosomal or X-linked, polygenic or multifactorial . The analytic strategy is to fit the study data to various predefined genetic models (null hypotheses) and select the model that best explains the data. As with traditional epidemiological studies, there are some potential biases associated with segregation analysis. Of note is ascertainment bias, which occurs when families with certain genotypic or phenotypic characteristics are more or less likely to be included in the study sample. Misclassification bias could occur when information related to the disease status of relatives or their relationship with the proband is incorrect. Environmental factors, measured or unmeasured, could also affect the parameter estimates in segregation analysis. Because of these limitations, an adequate fit to a genetic model of inheritance does not constitute proof that the model truly explicates the cancer under study, although it may suggest strongly that genetic factors may be involved in the etiology of the cancer.

Twin studies are a special type of family study that includes only monozygotic twins (who are genetically identical) and dizygotic twins (who share, on average, 50% of their genes). A useful statistic for determining if genetic factors are involved in the etiology of a disease is the concordance rate, which is calculated by dividing the number of twin pairs who both have the disease under study by the number of twin pairs in which at least one has the disease. If genetic factors do contribute to the etiology, the concordance rate for monozygotic twins should be significantly greater than that for dizygotic twins. Although twins, regardless of whether mono- or dizygotic, share a similar environment, particularly in their early life, monozygotic twins may be subject to environmental factors that are subtly different from those that dizygotic twins are subject to. For example, the intrauterine environment may be more similar for monozygotic twins than for dizygotic twins. Therefore, the potential influence of environmental factors that covary with zygosity should be considered in twin studies. Population-based twin studies are difficult to apply to the study of cancer occurrence because the low incidence of cancer in the general population makes the estimate of concordance rates difficult. These studies are more useful for investigating quantitative traits, such as mammographic density, an established risk factor for breast cancer.[32,33]

Genetic biomarker studies are used to investigate the links between specific genetic markers and cancer risks and to provide direct evidence for or against the involvement of genetic factors in the etiology of cancer. The two basic kinds are linkage studies and molecular epidemiological association studies. Linkage studies are conducted to evaluate whether a disease is inherited together with a genetic marker in a family (ie, whether the unknown disease gene and a usually well characterized genetic marker are passed as a single unit from parent to child). Linkage studies are based on the fact that two loci physically near one another on the same chromosome are likely to be transmitted to offspring together. During meiosis (the formation of gametes), homologous pairs of chromosomes from parents can undergo recombination through crossing over of the DNA strands. Because of this, the order of genetic markers on the disease-carrying chromosome differs from the order on the chromosome of either parent. The recombination occurs more frequently for genes that are far apart on the chromosome than for those that are close together. A recombination fraction (θ) is estimated in linkage analysis to measure the probability of crossing over of the disease locus and the marker locus (the fraction is a function of the distance between these two loci). Recombination fractions range from .0 to .5; the former indicates complete coinheritance of alleles at the two loci (nonrecombinant) and the latter indicates independent inheritance (recombinant). For example, if one of the five children in a family is a recombinant, the recombination fraction is calculated as 20%.

Whether a disease locus and a marker locus are linked is judged by comparing the likelihood of the inheritance pattern within study families under linkage at the observed recombination fraction to that under the null hypothesis of no linkage ($\theta = 0.5$). In linkage analysis, the logarithm of these odds is referred to as a *log-odds (LOD) score.* An LOD score is computed to measure the likelihood of the data under linkage at some specific recombination fraction. A score of 3.0 or more has been traditionally considered strong evidence of linkage. This score corresponds to an odds of 1,000 to 1 for linkage at a specified recombination fraction. Linkage studies are conducted within families and require data and DNA collected from informative multigeneration families or siblings. Because of a late onset of cancer, historical family data and archived biospecimens are often needed to reconstruct a suitable multigeneration family for linkage studies. The rarity of cancer in the general population makes it impractical for linkage studies to evaluate low-penetrance genes. Therefore, linkage studies are usually used to identify possible loci for high-penetrance mutant genes. Once a gene is mapped to a specific locus, positional cloning can be used to locate and clone the gene.

Association studies are generally conducted in unrelated individuals selected from the general population and are used to evaluate the potential role of candidate genes and their interactions with environmental factors or other genes in the etiology of cancer. Although any traditional epidemiological study design could be used for an association study, the case-control design is most commonly used, because of the cost of bioassays and the rarity of cancer. Therefore, association studies usually focus on common genes, such as polymorphic genes (the frequencies of variant alleles for these genes are much higher in the general population than those for mutant genes).

As with any traditional case-control study, care must be taken in molecular epidemiological association studies to ensure comparability between case and control groups as regards potential confounding variables. Of note is the potential confounding effect of ethnicity. Because there may exist considerable variation in the allele frequencies of a given gene among ethnic groups, difference in ethnicity between cases and controls could potentially lead to bias. One way to eliminate this bias is to collect family-based controls and use transmission disequilibrium test (TDT) statistics. Spielman et al[34] developed the TDT to evaluate whether a given allele is preferentially transmitted from heterozygous parents to affected children. When parents are unavailable, discordant sibpairs can be used along with the sib-TDT statistic to test for associations.[35] Careful attention should also be paid to obtaining relevant exposure information, since many of the polymorphic genes are related to the risk of cancer through their interactions with environmental factors. The design of association studies is simpler than that of linkage studies. With the recent development of sensitive, reliable, and cost-efficient DNA analysis techniques, association studies have been increasingly used for investigating genetic susceptibility factors and their potential interactions with environment and other genes in the etiology of cancer. Table 7–3 compares selected characteristics of linkage studies and association studies.

One of the most common purposes of biomarker association studies is to investigate gene-environment interaction in the etiology of cancer. Most environmental carcinogens are biologically inactive and thus called *procarcinogens*. After absorption, procarcinogens usually undergo two phases of metabolism as part of the cellular detoxification process. The first step is catalyzed by phase I enzymes, primarily cytochrome P-450 enzymes (CYPs), which usually convert inactive, nonpolar compounds to reactive (electrophilic) intermediates. These reactive metabolites are good substrates for phase II enzymes, such as glutathione *S*-transferases, which add conjugating molecules to the reactive intermediates to form excretable hydrophilic complexes. Many of the electrophilic metabolites created by phase I enzymes can covalently bind to DNA and form carcinogen-DNA adducts. DNA damage in critical genes, such as the *p53* gene, if not repaired, could initiate a carcinogenic process. The balance between the metabolic activation and detoxification of carcinogens, as well as the efficiency of DNA repair, determines individual susceptibility to carcinogens. Figure 7–4 illustrates the role of both carcinogenic-metabolic and DNA-repairing enzymes in the etiology of cancer.

Many epidemiological studies have evaluated potential interaction between polycyclic aromatic hydrocarbons (PAHs) and genetic factors in the etiology of lung cancer. PAHs, such as those found in tobacco smoke, have been established as carcinogens in animals and humans. Several enzymes, including aryl hydrocarbon hydroxylase (AHH)

Table 7–3 Comparison of Linkage and Association Studies

	Linkage Studies	*Association Studies*
Usual study setting	Family	Unrelated individuals
Study objective	Identify potential loci for disease genes	Evaluate potential association of specific alleles with a disease
Candidate genes	High-penetrance mutant genes	Low-penetrance polymorphic genes
Study scenario	Prior evidence of Mendelian patterns of inheritance	Biological evidence for a potential link between candidate gene and cancer risk
Other applications	Limited	Evaluation of gene-gene and gene-environment interaction

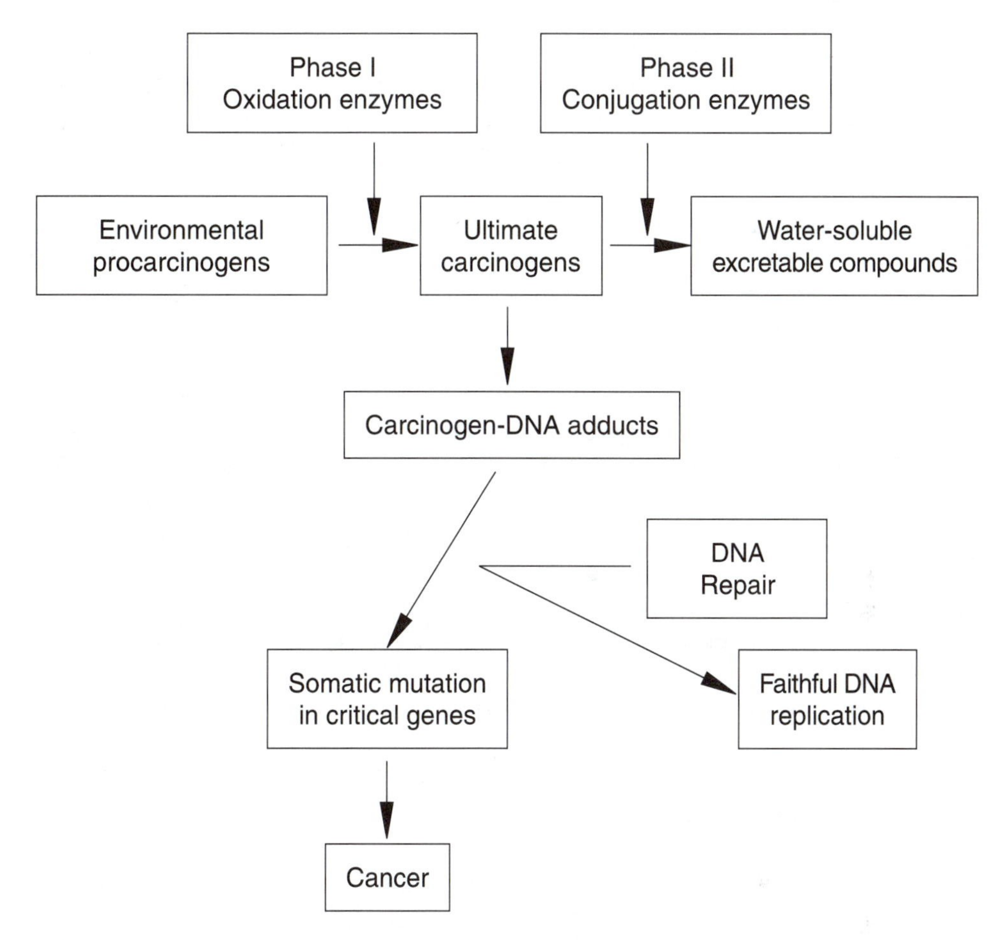

Figure 7–4 Role of carcinogen-metabolic and DNA-repair enzymes in the etiology of cancer.

---

and glutathione *S*-transferases (GSTs), are involved in the metabolism of PAHs, such as benzo[*a*]pyrene. AHH catalyses the oxidation of PAHs to electrophilic metabolites, which are further catalyzed by GSTs to form water-soluble conjugates that are readily excreted from cells. In one of the earliest epidemiological studies to investigate genetic susceptibility factors for cancer, Kellerman et al[36] reported that AHH inducibility in lymphocytes from peripheral blood was trimodally distributed and that the risk of lung cancer was increased substantially with the increased inducibility of this enzyme. Because AHH is highly inducible by PAHs and other compounds, and because lung cancer patients often change their smoking habits after lung cancer diagnosis, the level of AHH measured in blood collected after cancer diagnosis may not reflect the usual level of this enzyme in cancer patients. AHH is encoded by the *CYP1A1* gene. Several genetic polymorphisms of the *CYP1A1* gene have been described.[37] Because the genotype of the *CYP1A1* gene is more easily determined than the inducibility of AHH in epidemiological studies, most recent studies have focused on the investigation of *CYP1A1* genotypes in relation to lung cancer risk.[37] A polymorphism caused by isoleucine to valine substitution in exon 7 of the *CYP1A1* gene has been extensively investigated,[37–41] and the *Val/Val* genotype was associated with a two- to threefold elevated risk of lung cancer, particularly among smokers. This finding is biologically plausible, since this polymorphism has been related to both an increased expression of the gene and an increased activity of the enzyme.[42,43]

As mentioned earlier, the phase II enzymes GSTs play an important role in the detoxification of reactive PAH metabolites. The *GSTM1* gene is absent in about 50% of Asian, European, and North American populations, and deficiency of this gene has been associated with an increased risk of lung cancer.[22] In a recent meta-analysis of 12 case-control studies, McWilliams reported a 41% (95% CI = 1.23–1.61) elevated risk of lung cancer associated with the *GSTM1* null (*GSTM1*0*) genotype.[26] Stratification by race showed that the positive association was stronger in Japanese populations (OR = 1.65, 95% CI = 1.25–2.13) than that found in Caucasian populations (OR = 1.17, 95% CI = 0.98–1.40). Among smokers, *GSTM1* deficiency confers an even greater risk of lung cancer, suggesting this gene may interact with smoking in lung carcinogenesis.[26]

The relative activity level of the bioactivating phase I and inactivating phase II carcinogen-metabolizing enzymes may be an important factor in determining the susceptibility to carcinogens. In the case of tobacco-related cancer, individuals with the combined genotype of *CYP1A1 Val/Val* and *GSTM1*0* may have a greater risk of lung cancer than those who have only one of these two genotypes. In a case-control study conducted in Japan, the combined genotype of *CYP1A1 Val/Val* and *GSTM1*0* was found to be associated with a 5.8-fold elevated risk (95% CI = 2.3–13.3) of lung cancer.[44] The risk was even higher for squamous cell carcinoma (OR = 9.1, 95% CI = 3.4–24.4), the type of lung cancer more closely related to cigarette smoking than adenocarcinoma (OR = 3.5, 95% CI = 1.1–10.8). These findings support the hypothesis of gene-gene and gene-environment interaction in the etiology of lung cancer.

SUMMARY

The aim of genetic epidemiology is to identify inherited susceptibility factors for primary, secondary, and tertiary prevention of diseases. Cumulative evidence indicates that genetic factors contribute to the development of most cancer cases, including those without a clear familial aggregation.

Most hereditary cancer syndromes are caused by the mutation or deletion of a single gene, and the inheritance patterns for some of these syndromes often follow Mendelian transmission models within a family. The genes implicated in hereditary cancer syndromes are usually involved in the critical functions of cells, and defects in these genes may "predetermine" the risk of cancer among carriers. Because germ-line mutations of major cancer genes are rare in the general population, hereditary cancer syndromes explain only a small fraction of cancer cases in humans. On the other hand, polymorphic genes, although each carries a relatively small risk, may contribute to the occurrence of many cancer cases, given their high prevalence in the general population. These genes often interact with environmental agents to increase the risk of cancer.

Epidemiological studies investigating genetic factors can generally be classified as either family studies or genetic biomarker studies. Family studies, including case-control and cohort studies of family history, segregation studies, and twin studies, provide general information on the role and/or inheritance patterns of genetic factors in the etiology of cancer. Biomarker studies, on the other hand, can pinpoint specific genetic factors responsible for the pathogenesis of cancer. Linkage analyses, which make up one of the two major categories of biomarker studies, are generally used to identify possible loci for high-penetrance mutant genes. They are conducted within families. Biomarker association studies, which typically include unrelated individuals in the study population, are used to evaluate common polymorphic genes and their interaction with environmental factors in the etiology of cancer.

Various epidemiological study designs can be used to investigate genetic factors for cancer. The choice of a particular study design depends on the frequency of the disease and the frequency of the genetic factors as well as the mechanism of genetic influence on the disease. Both linkage and association studies are useful in evaluating whether genetic factors influence cancer risk. Linkage studies are more appropriate than association studies for identifying genes for cancer with clear Mendelian patterns of inheritance. Association studies, on the other hand, are often used to evaluate genes that confer only a modest risk or genes that interact with environmental factors to increase the risk of cancer.

The last ten years has seen substantial progress in the field of genetic epidemiology of cancer. Much of the progress is attributable to the remarkable advances in DNA recombinant technology, particularly the application of PCR and related techniques in molecular epidemiological studies. These techniques are, in general, reliable and highly efficient and require only a small amount of DNA. Assuming the current rate of progress in molecular biology is roughly maintained, our understanding of the genetic basis of cancer will continue to develop and will likely help us to design even more effective strategies for cancer prevention.

Discussion Questions

1. Using lung cancer as an example, discuss the notion that many cancers are caused by the interaction of genetic susceptibility factors and environmental exposure.
2. Many genetic factors are likely to be involved in the etiology of breast cancer, including low-penetrance genes such as those encoding estrogen metabolic enzymes. Develop a study design to evaluate the association of these genetic factors with breast cancer, and discuss the limitations and strengths of your study.
3. Discuss the need to identify high-penetrance genes as well as logistical and ethical issues related to the screening of germ-line mutations of these genes in the general population.

References

1. Doll R, Peto R. The causes of cancer. *J Natl Cancer Inst.* 1981;66:1101–1308.
2. Knudson AG Jr. Hereditary predisposition to cancer. *Ann NY Acad Sci.* 1997;833:58–67.
3. Strong LC, Amos CI. Inherited susceptibility. In: Schottenfeld D, Fraumeni JF Jr, eds. *Cancer Epidemiology and Prevention.* 2nd ed. New York: Oxford University Press, 1996:559–583.

4. Caporaso N, Goldstein A. Issues involving biomarkers in the study of the genetics of human cancer. In: Toniolo P, Boffetta P, Shuler DEG, Rothman N, Hulka B, Pearce N., eds. *Application of Biomarkers in Cancer Epidemiology.* Lyon, France: International Agency for Research on Cancer; 1997:237–250. IARC Scientific Publications, No. 142.
5. Khoury MJ, Beaty TM, Cohen BH. *Fundamentals of Genetic Epidemiology.* New York: Oxford University Press; 1993.
6. Adamson RH. Mutagens and carcinogens formed during cooking of foods and methods to minimize their formation. In: DeVita VT Jr, Hellman S, Rosenberg SA, eds. *Cancer Prevention.* Philadelphia: JB Lippincott Co: 1990:1–7.
7. Vatsis KP, Weber WW, Bell DA, et al. Nomenclature for *N*-acetyltransferases. *Pharmacogenetics.* 1995;5:1–17.
8. Hein DW, Doll MA, Fretland AJ, et al. Molecular genetics and epidemiology of the *NAT1* and *NAT2* acetylation polymorphisms: a review. *Cancer Epidemiol Biomarker Prev.* 2000;9:29–42.
9. Deitz AC, Zheng W, Leff MA, et al. *N*-acetyltransferase-2 (*NAT2*) genetic polymorphism, well-done meat intake, and breast cancer risk among post-menopausal women. *Cancer Epidemiol Biomarker Prev.* 2000;9:905–910.
10. Knudson AG Jr. Mutation and cancer: a statistical study of retinoblastoma. *Proc Natl Acad Sci USA.* 1971;68:820–823.
11. Friend SH, Bernards R, Rogelj S, et al. A human DNA segment with properties of the gene that predisposes to retinoblastoma and osteosarcoma. *Nature.* 1986;323:643–646.
12. Bishop DT. Genetic predisposition to cancer: an introduction. In: Eeles RA, Ponder BAJ, Easton DF, Horwich A, eds. *Genetic Predisposition to Cancer.* London: Chapman & Hall Medical, 1996:3–15.
13. Strong LC, Williams WR, Tainsky MA. The Li-Fraumeni syndrome: from clinical epidemiology to molecular genetics. *Am J Epidemiol.* 1992;135:190–199.
14. DeMichele A, Weber BL. Recent advances in breast cancer biology. *Curr Opin Oncol.* 1997;9:499–504.
15. Lindor NM, Greene MH. The concise handbook of family cancer syndromes. Mayo Familial Cancer Program. *J Natl Cancer Inst.* 1998;90:1039–1071.
16. Caporaso N, Goldstein A. Cancer genes: single and susceptibility: exposing the difference. *Pharmacogenetics.* 1995;5:59–63.
17. Lachman HM, Papolos DF, Saito T, Yu YM, Szumlanski CL, Weinshilboum RM. Human catechol-*O*-methyltransferase pharmacogenetics: description of a functional polymorphism and its potential application to neuropsychiatric disorders. *Pharmacogenetics.* 1996;6:243–250.
18. Lavigne JA, Helzlsouer KJ, Huang HY, et al. An association between the allele coding for a low activity variant of catechol-*O*-methyltransferase and the risk for breast cancer. *Cancer Res.* 1997;57:5493–5497.
19. Thompson PA, Shields PG, Freudenheim JL, et al. Genetic polymorphisms in catechol-*O*-methyltransferase, menopausal status, and breast cancer risk. *Cancer Res.* 1998;58:2107–2110.
20. Xie DW, Dai Q, Yager JD, et al. Genetic polymorphisms of catechol-*O*-methyltransferase and the risk of breast cancer: The Shanghai Breast Cancer Study. Presented at the 90th Annual Meeting of the American Association for Cancer Research; April 1999; Philadelphia.
21. Schipper DL, Wagenmans MJH, Wagener DJT, Peters WHM. Glutathione *S*-transferases and cancer. *Intl J Oncol.* 1997;10:1261–1264. Review.
22. Rebbeck TR. Molecular epidemiology of the human glutathione *S*-transferase genotypes *GSTM1* and *GSTT1* in cancer susceptibility. *Cancer Epidemiol Biomarkers Prev.* 1997;6:733–743. Review.
23. Pemble S, Schroeder KR, Spencer SR, et al. Human glutathione *S*-transferase theta (GSTT1): cDNA cloning and the characterization of a genetic polymorphism. *Biochem J.* 1994;300:271–276.
24. Helzlsouer KJ, Selmin O, Huang HY, et al. Association between glutathione *S*-transferase *M1, P1,* and *T1* genetic polymorphisms and development of breast cancer. *J Natl Cancer Inst.* 1998;90:512–518.
25. Zheng W, Xie DW, Heimel AY, et al. *GSTM1* and *GSTT1* polymorphisms, well-done meat intake, cigarette smoking, and breast cancer risk. Presented at the 2000 Keystone Symposia: Molecular Epidemiology: A New Tool in Cancer Prevention; February 2000; Taos, NM.
26. McWilliams JE, Sanderson BJS, Harris EL, Richert-Boe KE, Henner WD. Glutathione *S*-transferase *M1 (GSTM1)* deficiency and lung cancer risk. *Cancer Epidemiol Biomarkers Prev.* 1995;4:589–594.
27. Alberts B, Bray D, Lewis J, Raff M, Roberts K, Watson JD, eds. *Molecular Biology of the Cell.* 3rd ed. New York: Garland Publishing; 1994.
28. Watson JD, Gilman M, Witkowski J, Zoller M, eds. *Recombinant DNA.* 2nd ed. New York: Scientific American Books; 1992.
29. Zheng W, Xie DW, Jin F, et al. Genetic polymorphism of cytochrome P450-1B1 and risk of breast cancer. *Cancer Epidemiol Biomarkers Prev.* 2000;9:147–150.

30. Zhao LP, Hsu L, Davidov O, Potter J, Elston RC, Prentice RL. Population-based family study designs: an interdisciplinary research framework for genetic epidemiology. *Genet Epidemiol.* 1997;14:365–388.
31. Vachon CM, Sellers TA, Kushi LH, Folsom AR. Familial correlation of dietary intakes among post-menopausal women. *Genet Epidemiol.* 1998;15:533–563.
32. Kaprio J, Alanko A, Kivisaari L. Mammographic patterns in twin pairs discordant for breast cancer. *Br J Radiol.* 1987;60:459–462.
33. Oza AM, Boyd NF. Mammographic parenchymal patterns: a marker of breast cancer risk. *Epidemiol Rev.* 1993;15:196–208.
34. Spielman RS, McGinnis RE, Ewens WJ. Transmission test for linkage disequilibrium: the insulin gene region and insulin-dependent diabetes mellitus (IDDM). *Am J Hum Genet.* 1993;52:506–516.
35. Spielman RS, Ewens WJ. A sibship test for linkage in the presence of association: the sib transmission/disequilibrium test. *Am J Hum Genet.* 1998;62:450–458.
36. Kellerman G, Shaw CR, Luyten-Kellerman M. Aryl hydrocarbon hydroxylase inducibility and bronchogenic carcinoma. *N Engl J Med.* 1973;189;934–937.
37. Spivack SD, Fasco MJ, Walker VE, Kaminsky LS. The molecular epidemiology of lung cancer. *Crit Rev Toxicol.* 1997;27:319–365.
38. Kawajiri K, Nakachi K, Imai K, Watanabe J, Hayashi S. The *CYP1A1* gene and cancer susceptibility. *Crit Rev Oncol Hematol.* 1993;14:77–87.
39. Hirvonen A, Husgafvel-Pursiainen K, Karjalainen A, Anttila S, Vainio H. Point-mutational *Mspl* and *Ile-Val* polymorphisms closely linked in the *CYP1A1* gene: lack of association with susceptibility to lung cancer in a Finnish study population. *Cancer Epidemiol Biomarkers Prev.* 1992;1:485–489.
40. Hamada GS, Sugimura H, Suzuki I, et al. The heme-binding region polymorphism of cytochrome P450IA1 (CypIA1), rather than the RsaI polymorphism of IIE1 (CypIIE1), is associated with lung cancer in Rio de Janeiro. *Cancer Epidemiol Biomarkers Prev.* 1995;4:63–67.
41. Drakoulis N, Cascorbi I, Brockmoller J, Gross CR, Roots I. Polymorphisms in the human *CYP1A1* gene as a susceptibility factor for lung cancer. *Clin Invest Med.* 1994;72:240–248.
42. Crofts F, Taioli E, Trachman J, et al. Functional significance of different human *CYP1A1* genotypes. *Carcinogenesis.* 1994;15:2961–2963.
43. Kawamoto T, Koga M, Murata K, Matsuda S, Kodama Y. Effects of *ALDH1, CYP1A1,* and *CYP2E1* genetic polymorphisms and smoking and drinking habits on toluene metabolism in humans. *Toxicol Appl Pharmacol.* 1995;133:295–304.
44. Hayashi SI, Watanabe J, Kawajiri K. High susceptibility to lung cancer analyzed in terms of combined genotypes of P4501A1 and mu-class glutathione *S*-transferase genes. *Jpn J Cancer Res.* 1992;83:866–870.

Chapter 8

Occupation and Cancer

Harris Pastides

There is a long history of scientific research into the possibility that workplace exposures, especially workplace chemicals used in manufacturing, may increase the risk of cancer for employees. Epidemiological studies of workplace exposures have the advantage that employee records are routinely kept and these typically identify employees from the past and present and describe their exposures and work responsibilities. Another advantage is that exposure levels are usually higher in workplace settings. Associations found and confirmed in the workplace can then act as an alert that these same chemicals pose a risk in the nonoccupational environment. The International Agency for Research on Cancer (IARC) is an authoritative source of information about the potential carcinogenicity of factors found in the workplace and in the broader environment.

Fewer than 10% of the agents studied by IARC have been determined to be carcinogenic based on a sufficient body of evidence, although limited evidence of carcinogenicity exists for many others. Cohort and case control studies have been used effectively to study occupational cancer, but the most practical design is the retrospective cohort study. Standardized mortality ratios are derived by comparing the observed number of cases of cancer in an occupational population to the number expected based on a larger comparison population. Recently, advances in the use of cumulative exposure matrices and biological monitoring have enhanced the ability of investigators to measure a worker's former and current exposure and uptake of the agents being studied.

Epidemiological approaches to the study of the occupational causes of cancer are important for several reasons. First, an immense number of individuals spend large amounts of time at their jobs, and a large and expanding group of chemical and physical factors are found in the diverse workplaces of today. Second, workers are generally exposed to much higher levels of potentially hazardous chemical and physical factors than individuals exposed to similar hazards in the ambient environment or in other nonoccupational settings. Therefore, observations of an elevation in the cancer rate in an occupational group should serve as a warning that a widespread community risk may exist. Thirdly, cancer resulting from occupational exposures should be thought of as preventable. Confirmed information about causal cancer agents should lead to removal of the agents or adequate protection of potentially exposed workers.

Unfortunately, the vast majority of chemicals in use in modern workplaces have not been fully tested to determine their potential carcinogenicity. Even so, it is estimated that over seven million workers in the United States alone may be regularly exposed to established carcinogens, while new technologies and industries continue to proliferate. As an example, consider the impact of the advances in microelectronics that have been realized in the recent past. Notebook computers, portable telephones, and compact disc players have all been made possible by remarkably rapid research and engineering advances. In addition to the impact on the consumer, these advances have been accompanied by revolutionary changes in workplace practices and the introduction of new chemicals with unknown health consequences. In comparison with jobs in mining, agriculture, and transportation, jobs in the electronics industry would appear cleaner and safer. Yet workers employed in manufacturing electronic goods are exposed to a wide variety of solvents, acids, lighting conditions, and other environmental characteristics, some of which have not been adequately studied with respect to their potential effects on health. It is wise to assume that neither a high degree of danger nor a high degree of safety exists in workplaces in which new technologies have been implemented. The accelerating pace of technological advances requires systematic investigation of new chemical and physical factors in the workplace as well as of those not thoroughly investigated in the past.

LANDMARKS IN OCCUPATIONAL CANCER RESEARCH

The first recorded studies of occupational illness did not appear until the early 18th century, when Bernardino Ramazzini published a comprehensive treatise on occupational diseases. In this remarkable volume, Ramazzini offered numerous insights. Students of history will not be surprised to learn that most of his assertions were not fully accepted until the 20th century. Ramazzini was especially interested in the effects of metals on human health. For example, he commented on the ill effects of mercury as encountered by miners ("It is from mercury mines that there issues the most cruel bane of all that deals death and destruction to miners"), goldsmiths (". . . and when they later drive off the mercury by fire they cannot avoid receiving the poisonous fumes into their mouths, even though they turn away their faces. Hence craftsmen of this sort very soon become subject to vertigo, asthma and paralysis. Very few of them reach old age"), and surgeons who gave their patients mercury for syphilis (" . . . though they wear a glove when so engaged, it is impossible for them to prevent the mercurial atoms from penetrating the leather and so reaching the hand of him who applies the ointment").[1] Even though we do not have a clear record of how his research and theories were received by medical authorities of the day, they were probably disparaged, given that they were ignored for two hundred years.

Percival Pott is usually credited as being the first to demonstrate that a specific occupational exposure could cause cancer. In 1775, Pott noticed and reported that the boys and young men who swept London's chimneys were dying of cancer of the scrotum at a suspiciously high rate. Without knowing the specific carcinogenic agent or mechanism involved (later shown to be dermal exposure to polycyclic aromatic hydrocarbons found in coal tar), Pott made a simple but poignant connection that was convincing enough for informed prevention strategies to be initiated—not unlike the observation, long before vitamin C deficiency was discovered to be the cause of scurvy, that carrying citrus fruits on long oceanic voyages could prevent the disease in sailors.

More recently, Irving Selikoff and coworkers, using the tools and methods of modern epidemiology, reported the cancer-causing effects of asbestos exposure among insulation workers.[2] While scientists continue to argue about the range of cancers attributable to asbestos exposure and about the specific asbestos fiber types that lead to them, the finding that inhalation of asbestos fibers causes malignant mesothelioma may be legitimately regarded as the most convincingly demonstrated discovery of occupational carcinogenesis known today.

It is worth noting that the successful detection of occupational causes of cancer is not always the result of applying traditional epidemiological methods. In 1974, occupational physicians in the B.F. Goodrich plant in Louisville, Kentucky, observed three cases of angiosarcoma of the liver, a highly lethal cancer affecting the blood vessels of the liver, over a two-year period in factory employees.[3] Knowing how rare this type of cancer is, the physicians took careful histories, and it was discovered that all men had worked continuously for at least 14 years in the section that produced polyvinyl chloride, a widely used plastic resin, using vinyl chloride monomer (VCM).[4] One had been responsible for cleaning out the vats used in polymerization. Follow-up epidemiological studies among VCM workers internationally confirmed that the association between vinyl chloride monomer and angiosarcoma of the liver was causal.[5]

THE MAGNITUDE OF THE PROBLEM OF OCCUPATIONAL CARCINOGENESIS

In a landmark study of the proportional causes of cancer in modern society, Doll and Peto (1981) estimated that 2% to 4% of cancer deaths are attributable to workplace exposures[6]; other estimates have been as high as 20%.[7] The estimate made by Landrigan and Markowitz, that at least 10% of cancer deaths in the United States each year are due to occupational exposures, is a step forward, as the authors tried to account for interactions between occupational factors and nonoccupational factors such as smoking.

The proportion and absolute number of job-related cancers are undoubtedly significant, but it is important to underscore that a potentially large proportion of these cases are avoidable. Through a multifaceted approach involving research epidemiologists, occupational physicians and nurses, industrial hygienists and engineers, and government and industry safety and health officials, the incidence and mortality rates of occupational cancers can be reduced. The best approach would be to combine primary and secondary preventive measures and to tailor these measures to the specific risks in individual workplaces. While not inexpensive or uncomplicated, effective preventive programs are well within the means of the current public health system. In any event, the opportunities for diminishing the impact of occupational cancer are far greater than the opportunities for diminishing the impact of cancers that are inherited or caused by medical treatment, where cancer control is much more difficult.

SOURCES OF INFORMATION ABOUT OCCUPATIONAL CANCER RISKS

The International Agency for Research on Cancer (IARC) is among the most comprehensive programs for evaluating the potential carcinogenicity of specific chemical and physical agents. IARC is an arm of the World Health Organization, and is headquartered in Lyon, France. IARC conducts and promotes epidemiological and laboratory-based research and training, but it is most famous for its series Monographs on the Evaluation of Carcinogenic Risks to Humans. Students of cancer epidemiology should become familiar with these orange-covered monographs, each of which is the product of intensive review of a specific agent (or a related class of agents) conducted by a working group of experts in face-to-face meetings that often last for a week or more. The fields of the experts brought together by IARC vary depending on the material being considered, but they usually include epidemiology, toxicology, genetics, and other scientific fields. The experts are asked to critically assess the pertinent evidence from human studies, animal studies, and metabolic and mechanistic experiments. Although a fundamental decision that an agent is a direct cause of cancer is extremely unlikely to change over time, determinations that are less than totally conclusive because of incomplete or conflicting information are periodically updated by IARC. The result is that the IARC monographs represent a relatively up-to-date summary of occupational and nonoccupational factors that are known or hypothesized to cause cancer.

Other agencies that provide periodic summaries of occupational cancer risk factors are the National Institute for Occupational Safety and Health and the National Toxicology Program. Students should be aware that the classification schemes for designating the strength of the information about a potential occupational carcinogen differ between agencies.

THE IARC CLASSIFICATION SCHEME

Table 8–1 shows the five choices that IARC experts are given for classifying a chemical agent under review. Agents placed in Group 1 are determined to be carcinogenic based on "sufficient" evidence from epidemiological and related studies. Those in Group 2 are deemed to be probably or possibly carcinogenic based on the existence of a "limited" degree of epidemiological evidence relative to the total body of evidence. The carcinogenicity of agents in Group 3 is held to be indeterminate owing to "insufficient" data. Agents belonging to Group 4 are determined to be probably noncarcinogenic. Owing to the impossibility of "proving a negative" in epidemiological studies, IARC cannot state definitively that any agent is absolutely noncarcinogenic. As seen in Table 8–1, there are a large number of agents for which only limited evidence of carcinogenicity

Table 8–1 International Agency for Research on Cancer (IARC) Assessments of Chemical Carcinogenicity

Category	*Carcinogenicity*	*Number of Agents or Exposure Situations (1972–1995)*
Group 1	Carcinogenic to humans	66
Group 2A	Probably carcinogenic to humans	51
Group 2B	Possibly carcinogenic to humans	210
Group 3	Data insufficient to decide carcinogenicity	454
Group 4	Probably not carcinogenic to humans	1
Total evaluated		782

Source: Reprinted with permission from J.M. Stellman and S.D. Stellman, Cancer and the Workplace, *CA - A Cancer Journal for Clinicians*, Vol. 46, pp. 70–92, © 1996, Lippincott-Raven Publishers.

exists. An agent of this type confronts occupational health professionals and regulators with the thankless task of deciding on permissible exposure levels before science has marched forward enough to provide substantial relevant information.

Recently, it has been pointed out that the IARC criteria for "limited" evidence and "inadequate" evidence overlap, creating the potential for confusion.[8] Consider, for example, a positive association that has been observed in one or more credible studies. If the association is based on a small number of cases, or if there are inconsistencies between studies, the overall appraisal may be both limited and inadequate. This could pose a major practical problem for public health officials responsible for regulating a workplace environment. Weiss has suggested replacing the "limited" designation with two categories: "strongly suggestive" and "weakly suggestive." He also suggests using the designation "inadequate" only when an evaluation cannot be made.

Table 8–1 shows that of the 782 chemical agents considered by IARC through 1995, 454 (nearly 60%) remained in class 3 owing to the paucity of relevant published information.

Exhibit 8–1 summarizes a classification of occupations by IARC based on whether the occupational activities involve exposure to chemical agents in Groups 1, 2A, or 2B. An occupation may have been given its particular rating by virtue of worker exposure to a single agent or to several. For example, carpentry and joinery are given a Group 1 rating based on what the working group considered to be sufficient evidence that workers exposed primarily to hardwood dust are at high risk for nasal adenocarcinoma. Studies examining the risk of other cancers among woodworkers, including cancers of the nasopharynx, larynx, lung, gastrointestinal system, and hematopoietic system, provided either limited or inadequate evidence. It should therefore be understood that the overall IARC assessment may appear to establish a general causal relationship between an agent and cancer but is usually based on evidence of a more specific association between an exposure and one or more subcategories of cancer, such as a specific organ, tissue, or cell type. While this may make it difficult to establish whether an occupational exposure caused cancer in an individual worker who developed cancer in an organ not designated as primary, it presents no problem for regulating the workplace. Workers must be protected from all substances that can cause cancer at any site.

THE USE OF EPIDEMIOLOGY IN IDENTIFYING OCCUPATIONAL CANCER RISKS

The occupational physicians who discovered the link between liver angiosarcoma and acute exposure to vinyl chloride monomer were alerted to the link by what is sometimes referred to as a *sentinel event.* This term was coined by Rutstein et al[9] to mean an observed occurrence that serves to warn of a hazardous situation. In reality, most occupational cancer risks manifest their effects more subtly, making it much more difficult to uncover an association between a type of exposure and a type of cancer.

Analytic epidemiology studies, including cross-sectional, cohort, and case-control studies, can of course be applied to investigations of occupation-related cancers. Population-based case-control studies are not considered in this chapter because they are rarely undertaken in order to research associations between occupational exposures and cancer

Exhibit 8–1 Occupational Exposures with Cancer Risks as Determined by the International Agency for Research on Cancer

Known Human Carcinogens—Group 1 Ratings
Aluminum production
Auramine, manufacture of
Boot and shoe manufacture and repair
Coal gasification
Coke production
Furniture and cabinet making
Carpentry and joinery
Hematite mining
Iron and steel founding
Isopropanol manufacture (strong-acid process)
Magenta, manufacture of
Painter
Rubber industry
Strong-inorganic-acid mists containing sulfuric acid

Probable Human Carcinogens—Group 2A Ratings
Hairdresser or barber
Manufacture of art glass, glass containers, and pressed glassware
Spraying and application of nonarsenical insecticides
Petroleum refining

Possible Human Carcinogens—Group 2B Ratings
Textile manufacturing industry

Source: Reprinted with permission from J.M. Stellman and S.D. Stellman, Cancer and the Workplace, *CA - A Cancer Journal for Clinicians*, Vol. 46, pp. 70–92, © 1996, Lippincott-Raven Publishers.

(apart from when done within the base of an occupational cohort). The reason for their rarity is that few geographical areas have a large enough proportion of the population employed in a single industry or even in related industries to satisfy the "exposure-opportunity" requirement of a case-control study (ie, the requirement that a meaningful proportion of subjects would be expected to have at least some exposure).

Cohort studies of occupational cancer can be either prospective or retrospective in design. Prospective cohort studies of occupational cancers are uncommon, primarily because of the long latency period for most cancers (which likewise obstructs prospective research on nonoccupational cancers). In addition, relatively large numbers of exposed workers are required by cohort studies, and there is a pressing "need to know" about alleged workplace cancer risks so that changes can be implemented without delay. Nevertheless, certain exposure-cancer associations may be amenable to prospective epidemiological research methods. For example, if an association between chalk dust exposure and respiratory cancer were hypothesized, a prospective cohort study of teachers might be proposed. Owing to the many thousands of potential participants, the well-organized professional associations and labor unions that exist, and the fact that teachers could be expected to keep accurate and regular records of approximate chalk dust exposure, many of the requirements of a prospective cohort study could be satisfied. The main advantage over a retrospective cohort study of teachers' exposure to chalk dust would be the far better and more detailed cumulative estimates of individual exposure, estimates that could even take into account variability over time, ventilation and other physical characteristics of the classrooms, and other potentially useful information.

In the hypothetical example above, a retrospective cohort study might also be considered. Such studies are identical to their prospective counterparts in fundamental design. The major difference is that the "follow-up" period for the exposed workers and their nonexposed or low-exposed counterparts has already elapsed by the time the study is initiated. This allows the epidemiologists to benefit from a long-term follow-up of employed populations without needing to monitor the target population and expend the money and effort demanded by monitoring.

Retrospective cohort studies begin by identifying an occupational population whose exposure started sometime in the past. Workers are often grouped by exposure level or duration, job title, work area, or some other distinguishing feature of their workplace exposure without regard to disease endpoint. Unfortunately, detailed quantitative records that reflect the exposure experience of individual workers are almost always incomplete and sometimes totally unavailable. In these cases, epidemiologists must rely on whatever records exist, coupled with interviews of industrial hygienists, former employees, plant or area managers or supervisors, and any other sources that may aid in a qualitative exposure reconstruction. Use of an exposure matrix, in which available data from a variety of sources are combined to estimate individual historical exposures, is on the rise. In a study of chromate chemical workers, for example, each member of the cohort was assigned a cumulative exposure value based on records of where in the facility he or she worked in each year of employment. The information was obtained from a comprehensive review of all available personal and area sampling data. The risk of lung cancer was then evaluated by calculating the workers' cumulative exposures to chromate chemicals.[10]

Even when occupational records of general or personal exposure levels exist, rarely do they encompass information required for body burden or dose estimates. A body burden estimate is arrived at by aggregating estimates of entry of the chemical agent through all routes into the body as well as estimates of individual (or average) metabolic rates. For example, a worker employed in the manufacture of chlorine might encounter chlorine and some of its compounds in solid, liquid, and gaseous form. Since the physical states would involve different pathways, an exposure classification scheme based on only one or even two of the states might systematically over- or underestimate the biologically relevant doses for an individual worker, depending on the job and area worked in. A related employee record deficiency is the typical unavailability of information that would allow a qualitative or quantitative appraisal of possible confounders, such as information about past cigarette smoking by individual workers.

Whether prospective or retrospective, cohort studies of occupational cancer frequently rely on general population rates of cancer incidence or mortality in order to determine whether the estimated magnitude of cancer in a workplace is higher, lower, or about the same as "expected." Whereas cancer cohort studies done in the community usually can find numerous groups of nonexposed individuals available for recruitment and study, occupational epidemiologists investigating a cancer hazard in a workplace often do not have the option of selecting nonexposed workers from the same workplace. This is because many chemical agents and physical factors present in a workplace are not restricted to small areas within the occupational environment. Even though the magnitude of exposure may vary between departments or locations within a factory, there may be no area that is absolutely free from exposure. Furthermore, even when a chemical agent is limited to one area or job type, it may be difficult to find a large enough group of "comparison workers" without any current or former exposure to the agent of interest. For example, an epidemiologist may be concerned about the cancer risk among workers who package pesticides (as opposed to those who manufacture them) because of exposure patterns that take place in the packaging department. In this case, the epidemiologist would want to ensure that workers from other departments who make up the comparison group have not been employed in the packaging department, and ensuring this may not be practical. One approach might be to use multiple comparison groups even if members of one or more groups cannot convincingly be assumed to be completely unexposed. Alternatively, a cumulative exposure matrix might be developed for assigning an individual cohort member a total exposure level or score based on his or her job title or work area for each year that he or she was potentially exposed to the suspect chemical. Finally, the epidemiologist would have to confirm that there is no plausible cancer risk posed by the chemicals to which the comparison group is exposed to; otherwise the results could by biased in such a way that a true cancer risk would escape detection.

Another required task of an occupational cohort study is cohort follow-up, which is done to determine the presence or absence of the cancers being studied and other diseases or causes of death. The biasing of results is likely when the proportion of the study's subjects lost to follow-up is reasonably large. In clinical trials of the therapeutic efficacy of a new drug, the loss to follow-up is usually very small owing to the special interest subjects have in discovering the immediate outcomes to their health. In occupational research, however, follow-up activities are generally passive. That is, they often consist of matching the name, date of birth, and social security number (or comparable identifying information in international studies) with the computerized files of local, state, and national agencies that maintain records of disease or death, including local and state vital registry departments. At the national level, two particularly useful sources of data for performing mortality follow-up are the National Death Index of the National Center for Health Statistics and the Master Beneficiary Record of the Social Security Administration. Numerous other large reliable databases appropriate for monitoring cancer incidence or cancer deaths exist, such as the Beneficiary Identification and Records Locator Subsystem (BIRLS) of the Department of Veterans Affairs, which is a fairly complete source for tracking the vital status of US veterans.[11]

In occupational cohort studies in which observed cancer incidence or mortality patterns among a group of workers are compared to the experience of some larger community, it is common to calculate a standardized incidence ratio (SIR) or standardized mortality ratio (SMR). Initially, cancer excesses and deficits can be examined as a way to screen for unanticipated associations that would need further study and possibly more refined information from the literature and from related fields such as toxicology. Alternatively, when a specific hypothesis exists, SIRs and SMRs can help confirm the absence or presence of a cancer risk, especially if carefully selected subgroup analyses are performed (eg, analyses by duration of employment, job type, assumed latency period, and so on).

The SIR and SMR are calculated by first stratifying the cohort by gender, age, calendar year, and other variables of interest. Next, the number of cases or deaths in all of the strata are added to obtain the numerator. The denominator is obtained by multiplying the rates in comparable strata from the comparison population (eg, US black or white, female or male) by the corresponding numbers of person-years in the cohort to estimate the expected number of cases.[12] The denominator of the SIR or SMR may be considered to be the number of cases that would have been expected to occur in the cohort had the population illness rates been experienced. Person-years represent the total number of years that a cohort has been followed since the members' first relevant exposure to the factor being studied. Person-years for the follow-up period are terminated upon death, upon diagnosis of the disease being studied, or at some other endpoint that represents the particular analytic interest of the researcher. Person-years are estimated for each member of the cohort and then summed to estimate the total number for the cohort.

Table 8–2 demonstrates the importance of choosing an appropriate standard population for deriving the expected number of deaths. Substantial differences in the estimated cancer SMR and the standardized proportional mortality ratio (SPMR) can be expected. The SPMR for a given cancer site depends not only on the cancer mortality experience but also on the proportion of deaths from other causes in the standard population. Numerous examples of these studies can be found by perusing issues of journals specializing in occupational health.

Table 8–2 Sample Comparisons of Standardized Mortality Ratio (SMR) and Standardized Proportional Mortality Ratio (SPMR)

	Study Population	*Standard Populations*			
		A	*B*	*C*	*D*
Total population	10,000	100,000	100,000	100,000	100,000
Total deaths	100	1,000	1,000	1,500	1,200
Cancer deaths	20	200	300	300	200
CHD deaths	40	300	400	450	500
Other deaths	40	500	300	750	500
Death rate (all causes)	0.01	0.01	0.01	0.015	0.012
Cancer death rate	0.002	0.002	0.003	0.003	0.002
CHD death rate	0.004	0.003	0.004	0.005	0.005
Cancer PMR	0.20	0.20	0.30	0.20	0.17
Standardized rates for study population using as standard:					
Cancer SMR		1.00	0.67	0.67	1.00
Cancer SPMR		1.00	0.67	1.00	1.18

Nested case-control studies compare the occupational exposure histories of individuals who developed cancer or another disease being researched (case subjects) to a sample of individuals who remained disease free and are matched to the case subjects. Once the subjects have been identified and the relevant information on relevant exposures and confounders has been collected, the information is analyzed in the same way as in population-based case-control studies. One variant of the case-control study is termed *a case-cohort study.*[13] In this latter type of study, the control subjects are not matched to the case subjects but constitute a random sample of all of the cohort members who remained disease free. More detailed descriptions of these types of comparisons are available in occupational epidemiology textbooks.[12]

BIOLOGICAL MONITORING

Biological monitoring (or biomonitoring) may be defined as the measurement of chemical markers present in the human body that result from exposure to physical or chemical agents or their metabolites. It can be used to help estimate acute or cumulative exposures of interest in individual workers or commonly exposed groups of workers, to help evaluate the subclinical effects or anticipated effects of exposures on workers, and as a tool in occupational surveillance.

Traditional methods for estimating human exposures to occupational hazards have included monitoring the ambient air or the dust on surfaces within a workplace. However, because of different work habits; different work activities; and different genetic, physical, and physiologic characteristics among individuals, environmental measures often lack direct correlation with biologic measures of exposure. In addition, environmental measures generally gauge the amount of entry of a chemical agent only for a single route. Biologic measures provide a mechanism for estimating the amount of agent absorbed regardless of the route.[14] Biomarkers, therefore, allow more direct and accurate estimates of the body burden associated with occupational exposures to hazardous materials. Occupational biomarkers are typically derived from the analysis of blood, urine, or exhaled breath, and they may include chemicals and their biologic metabolites, biochemical conjugates or adducts formed as a result of exposure, and endogenous enzymes.[15]

Often there are several available biomarkers that can be used in an epidemiological study of an occupational cancer issue. The best choice (or choices) usually represents a compromise between accuracy, feasibility, and ethical considerations. The range of potential markers is indicated in a study by Pan et al.[16] In evaluating the association between leukemia and polycyclic aromatic hydrocarbons (PAHs), these authors employed several kinds of biomarkers: 1-hydroxypyrene (internal dose), leukocyte aromatic DNA adducts (biologically effective dose), serum p53 proteins (response), and genetic polymorphisms of cytochrome P-450 (genetic susceptibility). Consider how much more sensitive this approach would be for estimating the exposures of interest than relying on industrial hygiene measurements of the work environment or on self-reported information.

Biological markers are now largely considered to be complementary to traditional environmental measures of occupational hazards, and data from biomonitoring may be used to estimate exposure levels in epidemiological studies. Biomonitoring should not replace rigorous environmental surveillance, however, because, like any measure, biomarkers themselves are subject to variation (owing to homeostatic mechanisms, the bioavailability of specific chemicals, and varying chemical half-lives).[17] The possible causes of biomarker variability must be carefully considered in any occupational epidemiological study that uses biomarkers. Biomarkers of exposure are generally most appropriate for longitudinal and cross-sectional studies of exposures for which the latency period is relatively short.

Despite the work done to establish the applicability of biochemical markers to help measure exposure in epidemiological studies, little attention has been focused on measuring the biological effects of exposure to hazardous materials. Though markers of internal dose may deliver more accurate estimates of actual exposure to environmental carcinogens, individual responses to exposure are known to vary greatly. As a result, markers of internal dose may not correlate well with measures of biologically effective dose or actual biological effect. Unfortunately, the biological effect is thought to be the most relevant for the assessment of cancer risks.[18] Common markers for biologically effective dose include sister chromatid exchanges and DNA adducts, and markers of biological effect include gene mutations, chromosomal aberrations, and micronuclei.[19] These cytogenic compounds have been the focus of recent studies of occupational cancer,[20] but results thus far have been mixed. A large European study of several occupational cancers revealed a predictive value of chromosomal aberrations for occupational cancer risk but found no such value for sister chromatid exchanges or micronuclei.[21] Similar positive results for chromosomal aberrations and negative results for sister chromatid exchanges have been reported for workers exposed to chromium (VI).[22] Positive associations with DNA adducts have been reported for occupational exposure to styrene[23] and for exposure to polycyclic aromatic hydrocarbons,[24] as has an association between chromosomal aberrations and hospital workers exposed to ionizing radiation.[25]

Because biomonitoring can be expensive and invasive, it may not be appropriate for some occupational surveillance situations. In general, the use of biomonitoring is recommended when routes of exposure other than inhalation are important, when unanticipated exposures occur, or when it is required or strongly recommended by regulators (eg, to gauge blood lead levels). Biomonitoring has obvious advantages as a supplement to environmental surveillance, as it creates an index of directly measured exposure for each toxic substance of interest, and, in areas where reporting is mandated by a state agency, it may facilitate the wide dissemination of surveillance data. Note that biologic assays do not exist for all hazardous substances. Also, they may be prohibitively expensive for small businesses, and quality control programs for biomarker analyses are limited.[26] Furthermore, biomarkers may provide direct evidence of biologic effects of carcinogens or serve as early endpoints for the onset of cancer. Consequently, biomarkers offer a mechanism for the prevention and early identification and treatment of occupational cancers. As more epidemiological studies provide evidence for or against the relationship between particular biomarkers and cancer, the role of biomonitoring in occupational cancer surveillance will become more appropriately defined.

MEDICAL SURVEILLANCE

As with any program intended to identify cancer in asymptomatic individuals, medical screening or surveillance programs in the workplace should be instituted only for cancers for which treatment can alter the patient's prognosis. For example, there is some evidence that workers who are at increased risk for bladder cancer as a result of exposure to aromatic amines used in dyes can benefit from early detection by means of urine testing and cytoscopy. On the other hand, there is little evidence that screening for asbestos-associated bronchogenic carcinoma would alter an individual's life expectancy.[27] The Occupational Safety and Health Administration (OSHA) requires medical surveillance for a large number of workplace chemicals (Exhibit 8–2). The list is not cancer-based but includes chemicals believed to have a significant effect on health. Obviously, the chemicals listed make up only a very small percentage of the extraordinary range of chemicals in widespread use. It should be remembered that the carcinogenicity of many chemicals has not been thoroughly evaluated.

OCCUPATIONAL CARCINOGENESIS IN DEVELOPING COUNTRIES

The burden of occupation-related cancers worldwide falls disproportionately on developing countries. While about 80% of the world's people live in these countries, more than this percentage of occupational health problems are estimated to occur in them.[28] Furthermore, tightening industrial regulations and increasing labor costs in developed countries are causing the transfer of certain hazardous industries, such as asbestos brake lining manufacture, from developed countries to developing ones. Another aspect of the problem is that, in developing countries, occupational activity takes place in relatively small shops and factories, making inspection and enforcement of rules regarding the use of protective clothing, respirators, and other safety devices especially difficult. Finally, there are relatively few epidemiological studies of occupational cancer risks performed in developing countries, mainly because numerous acute health prob-

---

Exhibit 8–2 Carcinogens for Which OSHA Requires Medical Surveillance by the Employer

2-Acetylaminofluorene
Acrylonitrile
4-Aminodiphenyl
Arsenic (inorganic)
Asbestos
Benzidine (and its salts)
Bis-chloromethyl ether
Coke oven emissions
1,2-Dibromo-3-chloropropane
3,3'-Dichlorobenzidine (and its salts)
Ethylenimine
Ethylene dibromide
Ethylene oxide
4,4'-Methyelenebis (2-chloroaniline)
Methyl chloromethyl ether
α-Naphthylamine
β-Naphthylamine
4-Nitrobiphenyl
N-Nitrosodimethylamine
β-Propiolactone
Vinyl Chloride

Source: Copyright © 2000, State of California, reprinted with permission of the State of California. Any reproduction in whole or in part by any means is expressly prohibited without written permission of the State of California.

lems, often infectious in nature, compete with occupational disease and take up the immediate attention of the public health and scientific communities in these countries. Unfortunately, lack of direct evidence of a cancer risk in a local population, coupled with the potential for adverse economic consequences related to environmental workplace controls and other interventions, may make lawmakers reluctant to legislate regulatory standards or to better enforce existing laws.

Quantifying the occupational cancer risks in developing countries in a detailed manner is very difficult due to the lack of reliable data. Nevertheless, specific associations of importance have been identified. These include mesothelioma and lung cancer from asbestos mining (South Africa and China); lung cancer among gold miners (South Africa), tin miners (China), and hematite miners (China); and lung cancer among copper- and arsenic-smelting workers (China).[29]

SUMMARY

When cancer results from a person's occupational activities, it must be viewed as a public health failure. Except for some predictable number of cancers that will be induced as a result of former exposures to carcinogenic substances (eg, asbestos exposure), current technology and regulations should suffice to prevent occupation-related cancers in developed nations. In developing nations, on the other hand, the educational programs and government regulations will need to be improved and economic barriers will need to be addressed if meaningful reductions in the incidence of occupation-related cancers are to occur. Epidemiological studies of occupation-related cancers face many methodological challenges and are not easy to execute. When designed and performed carefully, as many have been, meaningful information can be generated and guide the implementation of primary and secondary prevention activities. Given the proliferation of new chemicals introduced into the workplace annually, public health scientists will continue to face the challenge of researching the potential carcinogenicity of substances that people are exposed to in their occupations.

Discussion Questions

1. Compare the relative difficulty of conducting cancer epidemiology studies of workplace exposures and studies of broader environmental exposures. Develop a hypothesis about one potential occupational carcinogen and one potential environmental carcinogen and describe several available sources of exposure data, at the individual or group level, that may assist the study.
2. Assume that two epidemiological studies are conducted, one of the potential role of coal dust in the development of lung cancer in miners, and another of the potential role of radiation in the development of leukemia in lab workers. For each study, identify the major potential confounding variables that you would hope to control for. Next, assume that an SMR (retrospective cohort) study is conducted and comment on the researchers' likely ability to acquire information on the confounders. Finally, assume that a cohort study having an internal control group and using personal interviews is conducted, and comment on the same issue.

3. Try to design a survey that can be used to assess an individual's lifetime occupational history, focusing on the nature of the person's work, the duration of employment in each job, and the major exposures he or she might have experienced in each job. Try administering the survey to several individuals. What are the relative advantages of a self-administered questionnaire versus an interviewer-administered questionnaire?

References

1. Ramazzini B; Wright WC, trans. *Diseases of Workers.* New York: Hafner; 1964.
2. Selikoff IJ, Churg J, Hammond EC. Asbestos exposure and neoplasia. *JAMA.* 1964;188:22–26.
3. Creech JL Jr, Johnson MN. Angiosarcoma of the liver in the manufacture of polyvinyl chloride. *J Occup Med.* 1974;16:150–151.
4. Centers for Disease Control and Prevention. Angiosarcoma of the liver among polyvinyl chloride workers—Kentucky. *MMWR.* 1997;46:97–101.
5. Tabershaw IR, Gaffey WR. Mortality study of workers in the manufacture of vinyl chloride and its polymers. *J Occup Med.* 1974;16;509–518.
6. Doll R, Peto R. The causes of cancer: quantitative estimates of avoidable risks of cancer in the United States today. *J Natl Cancer Inst.* 1981;66:1191–1308.
7. Fox AJ, Adelstein AM. Occupational mortality: work or way of life? *J Epidemiol Community Health.* 1978;32:73–78.
8. Weiss NS. Ambiguities in the IARC criteria for evaluation of carcinogenic risks to humans, and a recommendation. *Epidemiology.* 1995;7:105–106.
9. Rutstein DD, Mullan RJ, Frazier TM, et al. Sentinel health events (occupational): a basis for physician recognition and public health surveillance. *Am J Public Health.* 1983;73:1054–1062.
10. Pastides H, Austin R, Lemeshow S, Klar J, Mundt KA. A retrospective-cohort study of occupational exposure to hexavalent chromium. *Am J Indust Med.* 1994;25:663–675.
11. Page WF, Mahan CM, Kang HK. Vital status ascertainment through the files of the Department of Veterans Affairs and the Social Security Administration. *Ann Epidemiol.* 1996;6:102–109.
12. Checkoway H, Pearce NE, Crawford-Brown DJ. *Research Methods in Occupational Epidemiology.* New York: Oxford University Press; 1989.
13. Prentice RL. A case-cohort design for epidemiologic cohort and disease prevention trials. *Biometrika.* 1986;73:1–9.
14. Rempel DM, Rosenberg J, Harrison RJ. Biologic monitoring. In: LaDou J, ed. *Occupational Medicine.* Norwalk, CT: Appleton & Lange; 1990:459–466.
15. Templeton DJ, Weinberg RA. Principles of cancer biology. In: Murphy GP, Lawrence W Jr, Lenhard RE, eds. *American Cancer Society Textbook of Clinical Oncology.* 2nd ed. Atlanta, GA: American Cancer Society; 1995:164–177.
16. Pan G, Hanaoka T, Yamano Y, et al. A study of multiple biomarkers in coke oven workers: a cross-sectional study in China. *Carcinogenesis.* 1998;19:1963–1968.
17. Perera FP. Molecular epidemiology in cancer prevention. In: Schottenfeld D, Fraumeni JF, eds. *Cancer Epidemiology and Prevention.* 2nd ed. New York: Oxford University Press; 1996:101–115.
18. van Delft JHM, Baan RA, Roza L. Biological effect markers for exposure to carcinogenic compounds and their relevance for risk assessment. *Crit Rev Toxicol.* 1998;28:477–510.
19. Hagmar L, Bonassi S, Stromberg U, et al. Cancer predictive value of cytogenetic markers used in occupational health surveillance programs: a report from an ongoing study by the European Study Group on cytogenetic biomarkers and health. *Mutat Res.* 1998;405:171–178.
20. Vainio H. Use of biomarkers: new frontiers in occupational toxicology and epidemiology. *Toxicol Lett.* 1998;103:581–589.
21. Hagmar L, Bonassi S, Stromberg U, et al. Chromosomal aberrations in lymphocytes predict human cancer: a report from the European Study Group on Cytogenetic Biomarkers and Health (ESCH). *Cancer Res.* 1998;58:4117–4121.

22. Kortenkamp A. Problems in the biological monitoring of chromium (VI) exposed individuals. *Biomarkers.* 1997;2:73–79.
23. Rappaport SM, Yeowell-O'Connell K, Bodell W, Yager JW, Symanski E. An investigation of multiple biomarkers among workers exposed to styrene and styrene-7,8-oxide. *Cancer Res.* 1996;56:5410–5416.
24. Tang DL, Santella RM, Blackwood AM, et al. A molecular epidemiologic case-control study of lung-cancer. *Cancer Epidemiol Biomarkers Prev.* 1995;4:341–346.
25. Bonassi S, Forni A, Bigatti P, et al. Chromosome aberrations in hospital workers: evidence from surveillance studies in Italy (1963–1993). *Am J Ind Med.* 1997;31:353–360.
26. Baker EL, Matte TP. Surveillance for occupational hazards and disease. In: Rosenstock L, Cullen MR, eds. *Textbook of Clinical Occupational and Environmental Medicine.* Philadelphia: WB Saunders Co; 1994:61–67.
27. Fischman ML, Cadman EC, Desmond S. Occupational cancer. In Ladou, ed. *Occupational Medicine.* Norwalk, CT: Appleton & Lange; 1990:182–208.
28. Pearce N, Matos E, Boffetta P, et al. Occupational exposures to carcinogens in developing countries. *Ann Acad Med Singapore.* 1994;23:684–689.
29. Pearce N, Matos E, Vainio H, Boffetta P, Kogevinas M. *Occupational Cancer in Developing Countries.* Lyon, France: International Agency for Research on Cancer; 1994. IARC Scientific Publications No. 129.

Chapter 9

Tobacco and Cancer

Philip C. Nasca

Etiological relationships between exposures to various tobacco products and various forms of cancer are well established in the literature. The goal of this chapter is to provide an historical framework for this large body of research. The chapter provides an overview of tobacco use patterns from 1880 to the present, the health and economic impacts of tobacco use, and the biological basis for considering tobacco smoke to be an important source of carcinogenic agents. The chapter also includes a review of the studies that led to the establishment of clear etiological relationships between tobacco smoke and upper respiratory and bladder cancers, among others, and the methodological issues involved in measuring human exposure to tobacco products are discussed within the context of this historical account. In addition, the chapter covers current thinking regarding possible relationships between the use of tobacco products and cancers in other sites, such as leukemias and cancers of the breast and reproductive organs; the etiologic role of smokeless tobacco and cancer of the oral cavity; and methodological issues involved in studies of environmental tobacco smoke and lung cancer and interactions between tobacco smoke and other environmental exposures. Given recent advances in molecular genetics, the established etiological relationship between cigarette smoking and lung cancer provides an excellent opportunity to study gene-environment interactions for a major cancer site, and examples of studies of gene-environment interactions are presented at the end of the chapter.

Perhaps the most extensively studied etiologic relation between an environmental exposure and a specific site of cancer is cigarette smoking and lung cancer. In 1964, the Report of the US Surgeon General[1] identified cigarette smoking as the probable cause of the worldwide epidemic of lung cancer that started after World War I. The report also presented evidence linking cigarette smoking and other forms of tobacco use to other types of cancer. Research done in the three decades since the release of the surgeon general's report has served to solidify the scientific consensus that cigarette smoking and other tobacco exposures represent a major source of human carcinogenic exposure. The present chapter provides an overview of secular trends in tobacco use patterns in the United States, respiratory cancer incidence and mortality trends, and estimates of the impact of tobacco use on mortality from cancer and other diseases. Also described are epidemiological studies that define the etiologic relation between tobacco use and cancer, interactions between tobacco exposures and other environmental exposures, the relation between environmental or "passive" smoking and cancer risk, and the role of smokeless tobacco in the etiology of oral cancers.

TOBACCO USE IN THE UNITED STATES FROM 1880 TO 1995

During this period, tobacco was used mainly in the form of cigarettes, cigars, pipe and roll-your-own loose-leaf tobacco, chewing tobacco, and snuff. Long-term trends in the per capita consumption of these various types of tobacco are shown in Figure 9–1. From 1880 until just after World War I, commercially produced cigarettes represented a small proportion of overall tobacco consumption in the United States. Cigars, roll-your-owns, pipes, and chewing tobacco accounted for most tobacco use during this period. Per capita consumption of commercially produced cigarettes rose dramatically from 1920 to 1945, and commercially produced cigarettes became the dominant form of tobacco use among Americans. Cigarette consumption leveled off between 1945 and 1965 and then declined dramatically between 1965 and 1995.

The relation between trends in adult per capita consumption of cigarettes and major historical events is shown in Figure 9–2. The graph shows there was a steady increase in cigarette consumption from 1915 until 1955, with short-term decreases in use during the early years of the great depression and at the end of World War II. Since 1950, scientific reports linking cigarette smoking with various forms of cancer and other chronic diseases, bans on TV and radio advertising, the growth of the nonsmokers rights movement, and a dramatic increase in federal and state cigarette taxes have combined to reduce the public demand for cigarettes. The per capita consumption of other forms of tobacco use has shown similar patterns of decline over this same period.

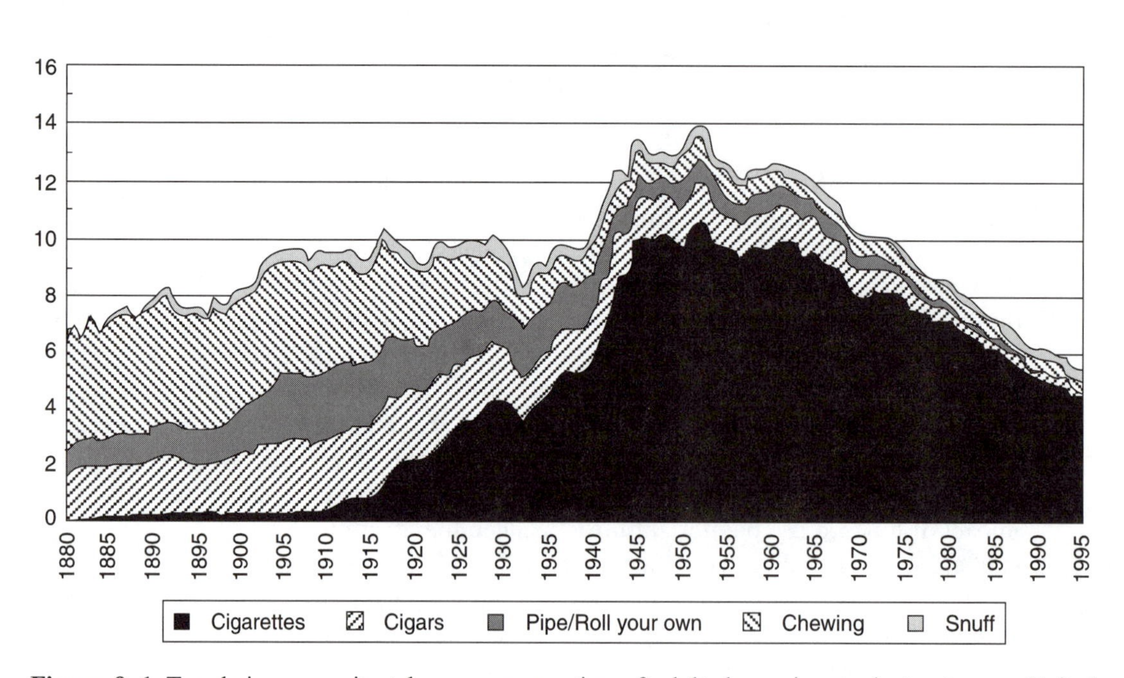

Figure 9–1 Trends in per capita tobacco consumption of adults by major product category, United States, 1880–1995. *Note:* Adults are persons aged 18 and over. The 1979 and 1980 data for snuff and chewing tobacco are estimated. *Source:* Reprinted from *Tobacco Situation and Outlook Report*, 1997, U.S. Department of Agriculture, Commodity Economics Division, Economic Research Service.

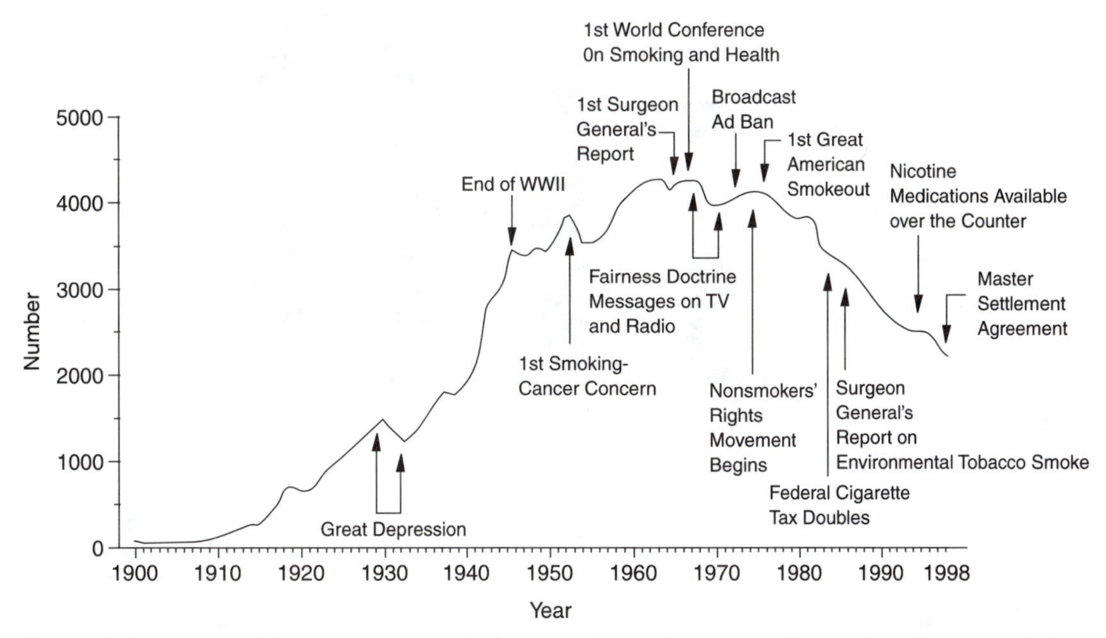

Figure 9–2 Annual adult per capita cigarette consumption and major smoking and health events, United States, 1900–1998. *Source:* Reprinted from *Reducing the Health Consequences of Smoking: 25 Years of Progress: A Report of the Surgeon General,* 1989, U.S. Department of Health and Human Services, the Centers for Disease Control and Prevention, National Center for Chronic Disease Prevention, and Health Promotion Office on Smoking and Health.

Data from the National Household Survey on Drug Abuse[2] show that, among persons who ever smoked, most began smoking on a daily basis by the time they reached 18 years of age. Data from the Youth Risk Behavior Surveillance System provide insights into some disturbing recent trends in cigarette smoking among adolescents. The data presented in Figure 9–3 show significant increases in smoking rates for students in grades 9–12 between 1991 and 1997.

HEALTH AND ECONOMIC IMPACTS OF CIGARETTE SMOKING

Cigarette smoking is a major contributor to mortality in the United States. Cigarette smoking was responsible for an estimated 430,000 deaths (20% of all deaths) among Americans each year from 1990 to 1994 (Figure 9–4).[3] The majority of these premature deaths are attributed to lung cancer and ischemic heart disease. In addition, over 100,000 premature deaths a year from chronic lung disease, stroke, and other cancers are attributed to cigarette smoking. Annual deaths attributed to cigarette smoking far exceed the number of deaths attributed to other causes, including AIDS, alcohol, motor vehicle injuries, and illicit drug use (Figure 9–5). Another approach to measuring the impact of cigarette smoking on health is to calculate the years of potential life lost (YPLL) as a result of dying prematurely from a smoking-related disease. This is accomplished by subtracting the age at which each individual dies from a smoking-related disease from age 65 or from the current gender-specific life expectancy. In 1990, cigarette smoking was responsible for 1,152,635 YPLL to age 65 and 5,048,740 YPLL to current life expectancy.[3]

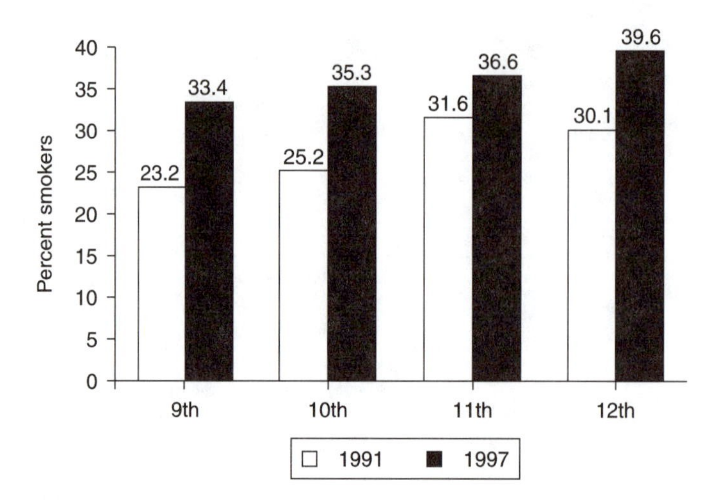

Figure 9–3 Cigarette smoking (one or more cigarettes) anytime in the past 30 days by school grade, United States, 1991 and 1997. *Source:* Reprinted from Youth Risk Behavior Surveillance System, the Centers for Disease Control and Prevention.

Smoking has been shown to have a major impact on medical care expenditures. In 1993, the University of California and the Centers for Disease Control utilized data from the National Medical Expenditures Survey and the Health Care Financing Administration to estimate the smoking-attributable costs for direct medical care expenditures. These expenditures included prescription drugs, hospitalizations, physician care, home health care, and nursing home care.[4] Models developed for estimating these costs in-

---

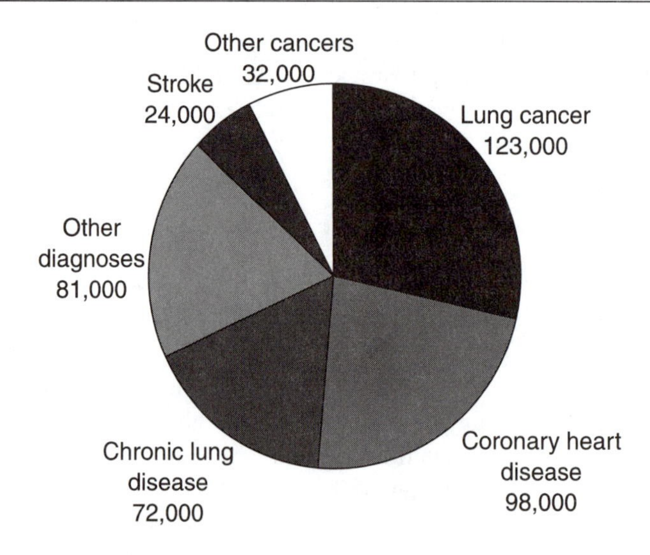

Figure 9–4 Average annual number of deaths attributed to cigarette smoking, United States, 1990–1994. *Source:* Reprinted from Smoking-Attributable Mortality and Years of Potential Life Lost—United States, 1984, *Morbidity and Mortality Weekly Report,* Vol. 46, pp. 444–451, 1997, the Centers for Disease Control and Prevention.

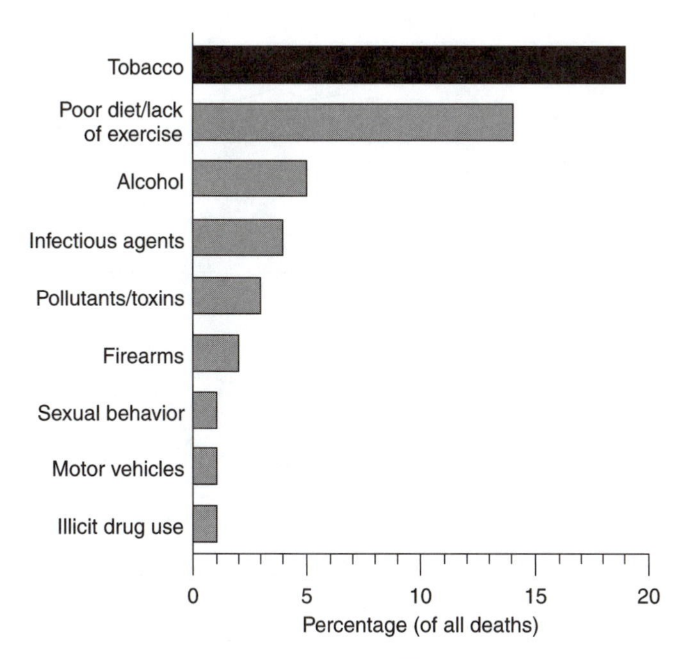

Figure 9–5 Actual causes of death, United States, 1990. The percentages are composite approximations derived from published scientific studies that attributed deaths to these causes. *Source:* Reprinted from J.M. McGinnis and W.H. Foege, Actual Causes of Death in the United States, *Journal of the American Medical Association*, Vol. 270, pp. 2207–2212, 1997, American Medical Association.

cluded a number of potentially confounding variables, such as age, race/ethnicity, poverty status, marital status, education, medical insurance status, region of residence, safety belt nonuse, and obesity. Direct medical care costs attributed to smoking were estimated to be $50 billion in 1993. Smoking-attributable costs represented approximately 7% of total medical care costs in the United States in 1993, with public funding covering 43.3% of the smoking-related expenditures. Among persons aged 65 and older, the public's share of smoking-related direct medical expenditures was estimated to be 61%. In addition to direct costs, smoking-related cancers also produce indirect costs, such as time lost from work, housekeeping expenses, and lost income.[5] These indirect morbidity and mortality costs represent 75% of the total costs associated with cancer (10% morbidity costs, 65% mortality costs). In 1990, respiratory cancers alone accounted for $17.123 billion in mortality costs.

Secular trends for cancers of the lung and bronchus among males and females in the United States are an excellent reflection of the relation between cigarette smoking prevalence and the health consequences of smoking. The data in Figure 9–6 show that lung cancer incidence rates began to level off after 50 years of steady increase that started, in males, after World War II and that continued until the beginning of the 1980s. The lung cancer incidence rates then leveled off and began to decline during the 1980s and the early 1990s. The change in the cancer incidence rates among males is a direct result of the dramatic decrease in smoking prevalence that occurred among males during the 1960s and 1970s, following the first surgeon general's report on the health consequences

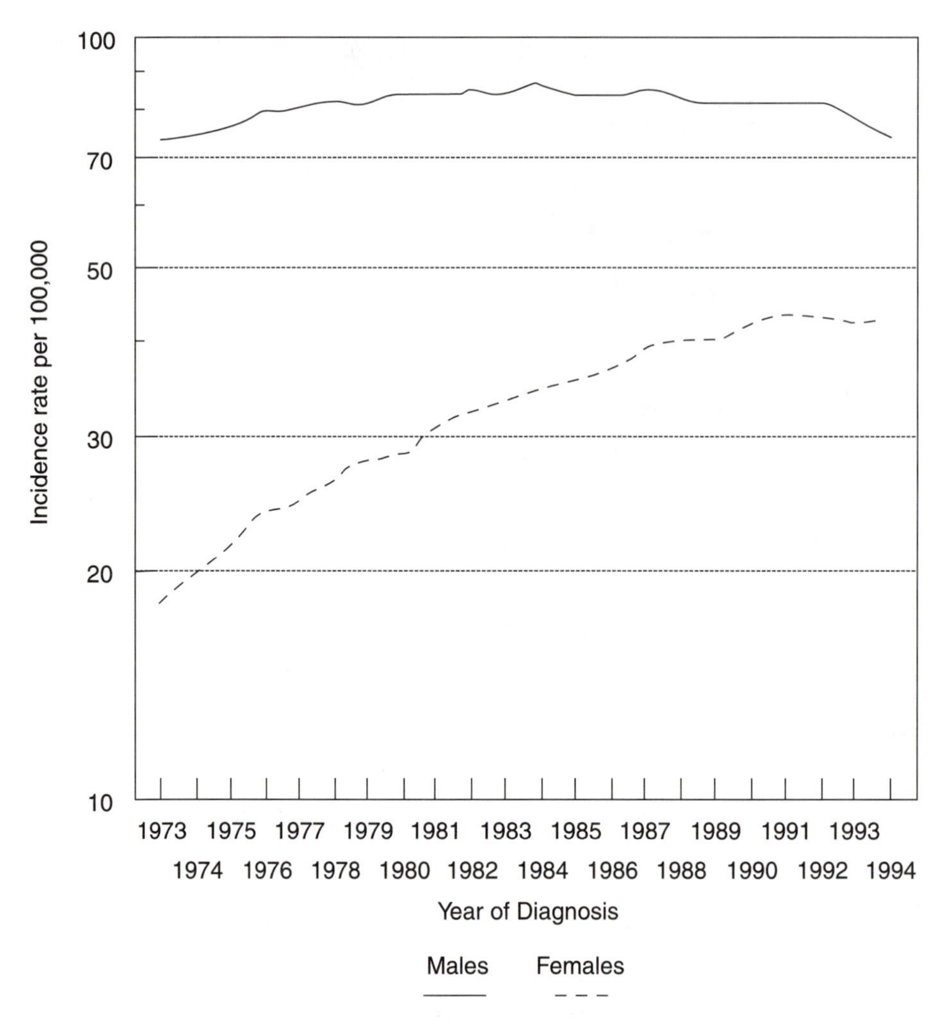

Figure 9–6 Age-adjusted incidence rates per 100,000, cancers of the lung and bronchus, 1973–1994. *Source:* Data from Surveillance, Epidemiology and End-Results Program, National Cancer Institute.

of cigarette smoking. The rise in lung cancer incidence rates observed among women during the 1970s and early 1980s ended in the early 1990s, when the rates leveled off, again as a result of a decline in smoking prevalence among women.

MUTAGENS AND CARCINOGENS IN TOBACCO SMOKE

A burning cigarette produces both mainstream and sidestream smoke. Mainstream smoke is drawn from the burning end of the cigarette through the tobacco directly into the smoker's mouth. Sidestream smoke is produced at the burning end of the cigarette during the intervals when the smoker is not actively drawing smoke through the cigarette.[6] Laboratory experiments have used smoking machines and chambers to identify the chemical constituents of both mainstream and sidestream tobacco smoke. Although these controlled laboratory experiments do not totally reflect variations in human smoking patterns,[7] the data do provide reasonable insights into the potential for human exposure to mutagenic and carcinogenic chemicals present in tobacco smoke.

A wide variety of chemicals have been detected in both mainstream and sidestream smoke, including carbon monoxide, benzene, *N*-nitroso compounds, and formaldehyde. Concentrations of various chemicals in mainstream smoke in both vapor and particulate form are shown in Table 9–1. Also shown in this table is the ratio of each chemical

Table 9–1 Concentrations of Selected Compounds in Nonfilter Cigarette Mainstream Smoke and Ratio of Relative Distribution in Sidestream Smoke

Compound	*Mainstream Smoke*	*Sidestream Smoke: Mainstream Smoke*
Vapor phase		
Carbon monoxide	10–23 mg	2.5–4.7
Carbon dioxide	20–60 mg	8–11
Carbonyl sulphide	18–42 μg	0.03–0.13
Benzene	12–48 μg	10
Toluene	160 μg	6–8
Formaldehyde	70–100 μg	0.1 ≃ 50
Acrolein	60–100 μg	8–15
Acetone	100–250 μg	2–5
Pyridine	16–40 μg	7–20
3-Vinylpyridine	15–30 μg	20–40
Hydrogen cyanide	400–500 μg	0.1–0.25
Hydrazine	32 ng	3.0
Ammonia	50–150 μg	40–170
Methylamine	17.5–28.7 μg	4.2–6.4
Dimethylamine	7.8–10 μg	3.7–5.1
Nitrogen oxides	100–600 μg	4–10
N-Nitrosodimethylamine	10–40 ng	20–100
N-Nitrosopyrrolidine	6–30 ng	6–30
Formic acid	210–478 μg	1.4–1.6
Acetic acid	330–810 μg	1.9–3.9
Particulate phase		
Particulate matter	15–40 mg	1.3–1.9
Nicotine	1.7–3.3 mg	1.8–3.3
Anatabine	2.4–20.1 μg	0.1–0.5
Phenol	60–140 μg	1.6–3.0
Catechol	100–360 μg	0.6–0.9
Hydroquinone	110–300 μg	0.7–0.9
Aniline	360 ng	30
ortho-Toluidine	160 ng	19
2-Naphthylamine	1.7 ng	30
4-Aminobiphenyl	4.6 ng	31
Benz[*a*]anthracene	20–70 ng	2.2–4
Benzo[*a*]pyrene	20–40 ng	2.5–3.5
Cholesterol	14.2 μg	0.9

continues

Table 9–1 continued

Compound	*Mainstream Smoke*	*Sidestream Smoke: Mainstream Smoke*
γ-Butyrolactone	10–22 μg	3.6–5.0
Quinoline	0.5–2 μg	8–11
Harman	1.7–3.1 μg	0.7–1.9
N'-Nitrosonornicotine	200–3000 ng	0.5–3
4-(Methylnitrosamino)-1-(3-pyridyl)-1-butanone	100–1000 ng	1–4
N-Nitrosodiethanolamine	20–70 ng	1.2
Cadmium	100 ng	3.6–7.2
Nickel	20–80 ng	0.2–30
Zinc	60 ng	0.2–6.7
Polonium-210	0.03–0.5 pCi*	1.06–3.7
Benzoic acid	14–28 μg	0.67–0.95
Lactic acid	63–174 μg	0.5–0.7
Glycolic acid	37–126 μg	0.6–0.95
Succinic acid	112–163 μg	0.43–0.62

*0.001–0.019 Bq

Source: Reprinted with permission from R.I. Hernning, et al., Puff Volume Increases When Low-Nicotine Cigarettes are Smoked, *British Medical Journal*, Vol. 283, pp. 187–189, © 1981, BMJ Publishing Group.

concentration in sidestream smoke relative to the amount of chemical detected in mainstream smoke. Some chemicals show higher concentrations in sidestream smoke whereas other chemicals are more heavily concentrated in mainstream smoke. It is clear that individuals can be exposed to a number of potentially harmful substances found in cigarette smoke, either through active smoking or through breathing the ambient air in a smoke-filled room. Environmental studies of indoor spaces such as worksites, restaurants, taverns, and other public gathering places have shown large concentrations of chemical pollutants caused by cigarette smoking (Figure 9–7).

A number of the chemicals detected in mainstream and sidestream smoke are mutagenic in in vitro studies using mammalian and nonmammalian cells.[6] As previously noted, chemicals found to be mutagenic in these test systems are often found to be carcinogenic agents.[8] For many of the chemicals found in mainstream and sidestream smoke, there is already sufficient evidence to classify them as animal or human carcinogens. Many other chemicals show some evidence of carcinogenicity, and many others have not been tested enough to rule out potential carcinogenicity.[6(p389)]

MEASURING HUMAN EXPOSURE TO TOBACCO PRODUCTS

As discussed in the next section, much of the evidence suggesting a causal relation between tobacco use and various forms of cancer is derived from epidemiological research. Epidemiological studies have relied primarily on self-reported smoking histories, and these histories may have been subject to some degree of misclassification. Both the size and direction of the misclassification bias need to be considered. Nondifferential

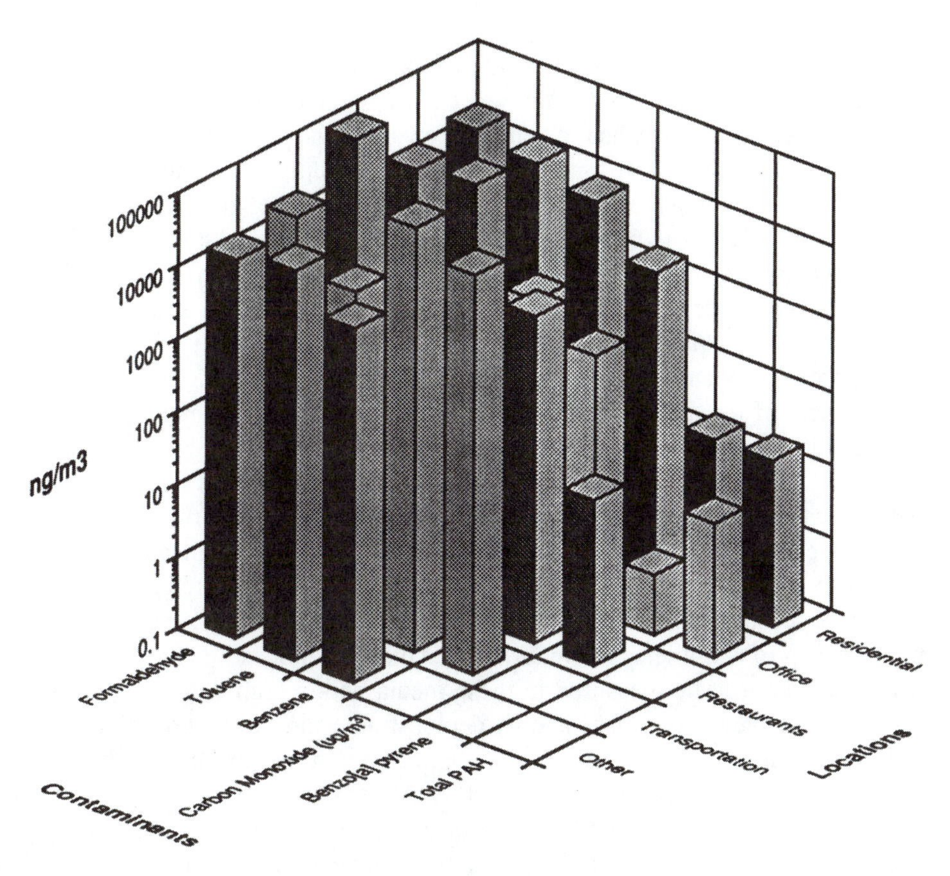

Figure 9–7 Concentrations of indoor chemical pollutants caused by cigarette smoking. Shown are a range of average indoor concentrations for notable ETS contaminants associated with smoking occupancy for different indoor environments. Background levels are subtracted. Maximum recorded values are typically orders of magnitude higher than averages shown. *Source:* Reprinted with permission from R.I. Hernning, et al., Puff Volume Increases When Low-Nicotine Cigarettes are Smoked, *British Medical Journal*, Vol. 283, pp. 187–189, © 1981, BMJ Publishing Group.

---

misclassification of smoking patterns, where the degree of misclassification is similar for cases and controls, is likely to bias the relative risk for smoking toward the null value. The relative risk observed in the study would be an underestimate of the true disease risk associated with the exposure. If the degree of exposure misclassification was significantly different for cases and controls, then the effect might be to bias the relative risk in either direction. Differential misclassification might hide a real association between the exposure and disease or might produce a spurious association where a real association did not in fact exist.[9,10]

Unlike in the case of long-term dietary patterns, subjects participating in epidemiological research studies are unlikely to seriously misreport their smoking habits owing to faulty recall. Studies designed to establish the reliability of smoking histories have been conducted by interviewing subjects many years after they had originally reported their current smoking patterns.[11–13] These studies invariably show that, many years after the original interviews, study subjects tend to recall smoking patterns with a fair degree of accuracy. It should also be noted that the early epidemiological studies were conducted at a time when the public was not generally aware of the potential adverse health effects of tobacco use. Although tobacco use was frowned upon by some religious sects, tobacco use was enjoying the peak of its popularity and was not viewed as socially undesirable, as it is today. It is unlikely that subjects in these early studies would have had sufficient reason to deny tobacco use or to seriously underreport their level of use. Moreover, epidemiological studies conducted after these early reports were published and made known to the public continue to show a strong relation between tobacco use and various forms of cancer. The cohort studies ascertained smoking histories prior to the development of the disease under study, thus minimizing the potential for differential misclassification. Any misclassification bias that existed with regard to measuring tobacco use was likely to be nondifferential and probably tended to underestimate rather than overestimate the association between tobacco and various forms of cancer. If differential misclassification of smoking use did exist, the level of misclassification would have to be large in order to produce the large relative risks reported for lung cancer.

More recently, it has been shown that smoking histories correlate well with the measurement of cotinine in serum, urine, or saliva specimens.[11] Cotinine is a metabolite of nicotine that can be measured in these media with a high degree of sensitivity and specificity. However, this test can only demonstrate exposure to tobacco within the past few days and cannot distinguish levels of exposure to tobacco smoke.[11] It has also been shown that hemoglobin and DNA adducts that are associated with tobacco carcinogens can be detected in the blood of smokers and snuff users and can be related to the level of smoking.[14–16] Finally, metabolites of a known lung carcinogen have been quantified in the urine of cigarette smokers.[17]

EPIDEMIOLOGICAL STUDIES

Lung Cancer

The dramatic rise in lung cancer mortality rates in the 1930s and 1940s (20 years after the rise in popularity of cigarette smoking) aroused the suspicions of medical researchers that a causal relation might exist between tobacco use and respiratory cancer.[18,19] However, some investigators[20,21] argued that the increase in the documented lung cancer rate might be due in large part to improvements in diagnosis and past errors in classifying the cause of death rather than an increase in the actual incidence of the disease.[6]

Investigators also attempted to determine smoking prevalence among cancer patients. Some early studies, while suggestive of an association between cigarette smoking and lung cancer, tended to be plagued by limitations, including small sample sizes, the use of inadequate comparison groups, and crude assessment of smoking patterns in study subjects. Three case-control studies[22–24] reported in 1950 and two cohort studies[25,26] reported in the early 1960s helped to establish a link between cigarette smoking and lung cancer. These studies represent some of the first systematic attempts to utilize epidemiological methods to investigate the etiology of cancer, heart disease, and other chronic diseases.

The first two case-control studies were conducted in the United States by research groups from the New York State Department of Health[22] and the Washington University School of Medicine.[23] The study by Levin et al[22] included 1,045 cancer patients and 605 noncancer patients identified from the medical files of the Roswell Park Memorial Institute (RPMI) in Buffalo, New York. Approximately half the patients entering RPMI were eventually found not to have cancer, thus providing a source of comparison subjects. Beginning in 1938, a questionnaire was administered to all patients entering RPMI for the first time. The questionnaire was designed to collect information in a number of areas, such as previous medical history, occupation, and various lifestyle exposures, including the use of tobacco products. The questionnaire was administered to patients prior to the establishment of a cancer or noncancer diagnosis, greatly reducing the chance that patients would provide biased responses to the smoking questions. This approach to minimizing potential information bias between cancer patients and noncancer comparison patients was a significant methodological improvement over previous retrospective studies. Information on smoking included the age smoking began, duration of smoking, type of smoking, and number of cigarettes smoked per day. Cancer patients and noncancer patients showed significantly different age distributions. Because the risk of lung cancer and the incidence of smoking both increased with age, it was necessary to control for possible confounding by age-adjusting all study findings. The results of this study showed a statistically significant excess amount of cigarette smoking among the lung cancer patients when compared with the patients without cancer. The observation that pipe smoking was found to be associated with lip cancer but that cigar and pipe smoking were not related to lung cancer was cited as evidence for the specificity of the association between cigarette smoking and lung cancer.

The case-control study by Wynder and Graham[23] included 684 lung cancer patients and a comparison group of 780 noncancer patients selected from the surgical and medical wards at four of the participating hospitals. Study results again showed a significantly higher prevalence of cigarette smoking among the lung cancer patients when compared with the patients without cancer. In addition, noncancer patients who smoked tended to be lighter smokers than the lung cancer patients, suggesting a dose-response relationship between the amount of cigarettes smoked per day and the risk of developing lung cancer. This study also demonstrated the specificity of the relationship between cigarette smoking and lung cancer since other forms of tobacco use showed weaker associations with this malignancy.

The third case-control study, conducted by Doll and Hill[24] in Great Britain, included 709 lung cancer patients and an equal number of noncancer patients whose diseases were diagnosed at London area hospitals. A structured questionnaire was used to obtain information on smoking at any time in the patient's life, the patient's ages at starting and stopping smoking, the amount smoked, major changes in smoking patterns over time, the type of tobacco exposure, and whether or not the patient inhaled when smoking. A significantly higher prevalence of cigarette smoking was observed among the lung cancer patients than among the noncancer patients. Lung cancer patients also reported higher amounts of tobacco use than controls, again suggesting a dose-response relation.

In order to overcome concerns about the essentially retrospective nature of these studies, two prospective cohort studies were begun in Great Britain[25] and the United

States.[26] These studies were designed to assemble large numbers of males not previously diagnosed with cancer. Cohort members were classified according to smoking status before the study subjects or the investigators had any knowledge of disease status. The cohort members were then followed for a number of years to determine mortality rates in smokers and nonsmokers. In the United States, Hammond and Horn[26] used American Cancer Society volunteers to assemble a cohort of 187,783 men aged 50–69. The volunteers collected information on lifetime smoking patterns, including the types of tobacco products used, duration of smoking, and usual daily amount smoked. The cohort members were then followed for a period of 44 months, with death certificates obtained for subjects known to have died. Investigators compared the observed number of cancer deaths attributed to lung cancer among the smokers with the "expected" number of lung cancer deaths. The expected number of lung cancer deaths was calculated by applying age-specific death rates for those who did not smoke to the person-years of exposure in the various smoking groups. Separate analyses were conducted for adenocarcinomas and for all other cell types of lung cancer combined.

The results for the adenocarcinomas showed a strong association between cigarette smoking and lung cancer mortality. A total of 26 subjects were found to have died from lung cancer, compared with only 6 expected deaths from bronchogenic cancer, for an observed to expected death ratio of 4.33. The results for other lung cancer cell types were even more striking: a total of 279 smokers died from lung cancer, as compared with only 9 expected deaths, representing a 31-fold excess of lung cancer mortality among smokers over nonsmokers. Also examined was the risk of dying from lung cancer based on the number of cigarettes smoked daily. The data showed that the death rates attributable to lung cancer increased dramatically as the number of cigarettes smoked daily increased. The lung cancer death rate was only 3.4 per 100,000 person-years among nonsmokers but it was 59.3 among men who smoked between a half and a full pack of cigarettes per day and 217.3 among men who smoked two or more packs per day. The investigators nonetheless recognized that lung cancer deaths and cigarette smoking both occurred more frequently in urban than in suburban and rural areas, and that it was therefore possible the observed association between cigarette smoking and lung cancer might be confounded by usual place of residence (ie, the causative agent might be another factor related to urban living, such as air pollution).

In order to take the possibility of confounding by place of residence into account, the investigators did a stratified analysis: they calculated lung cancer death rates for smokers and nonsmokers living within four types of residential areas, ranging from the most urban to the most rural. Within each type of residential area, smokers experienced significantly higher lung cancer death rates than nonsmokers, showing that the association between lung cancer and cigarette smoking was direct and not a result of confounding by place of residence. The Hammond and Horn study also showed higher death rates among smokers for cancers of the oral cavity and pharynx, larynx, esophagus, and genitourinary system as well as excess mortality rates for other pulmonary diseases and cardiovascular disease. Although the relative risk of developing lung cancer is higher than the relative risk observed for heart disease, the absolute difference in disease rates between smokers and nonsmokers is actually higher for heart disease. Of the 2,665 excess deaths observed among smokers, 52.1% were due to heart disease, 13.5% to lung cancer, and 13.5% to cancers in other sites.

The second cohort study by Doll and Hill[26] was designed to study cancer mortality among all physicians in the United Kingdom. A baseline questionnaire was sent to all members of the medical profession in October 1951. It was designed to collect data that could be used to classify each physician as a current smoker, former smoker, or never smoker. Physicians who reported being current or former smokers were asked about the age they started smoking, the method of smoking (cigarette, pipe, cigar, or combination), and the amount they usually smoked each day. The physicians were then followed until March 1956 to determine the number of deaths attributed to lung cancer and other diseases in this cohort. Lung cancer as the primary site of the cancer was established by autopsy, biopsy at the time of operation, bronchoscopy, or radiological examination. A total of 84 males with confirmed lung cancer were included in the study. The analysis was limited to males because only 3 females died from lung cancer during the follow-up period.

Overall, 34,494 males provided 148,686 person-years of risk, which served as the denominator for calculating rates of disease among current smokers, former smokers, and never smokers. The lung cancer mortality rate per year was 0.90 per 1,000 male smokers, which was significantly higher than the rate of 0.07 observed among never smokers. The lung cancer mortality rate was also shown to increase in a steady manner with increasing amounts of average daily smoking. For physicians who smoked 1–14 grams of tobacco per day, the annual lung cancer mortality rate was 0.47 per 1,000. For physicians who smoked 15–24 grams of tobacco per day, the rate doubled to 0.86, and it doubled again, to 1.66, for physicians smoking more than 25 grams of tobacco per day.

The dose-response relation between increasing lung cancer mortality rates and increasing levels of daily cigarette smoking was observed for all age groups, thus eliminating age as a potential confounding factor. The association between tobacco use and lung cancer was restricted to cigarette smokers, and no increased risk was observed among those who smoked pipes or cigars exclusively. Because data on cigarette smoking were available only through the baseline questionnaire, the analysis could not take into account life-time smoking patterns or changes in smoking patterns that might have occurred after the initial smoking data were collected. Doll and Hill indicate that any potential bias created by changes in smoking habits would most likely result in their study underestimating the already strong association between cigarette smoking and lung cancer. The Doll and Hill study also confirmed observations from previous retrospective studies that cigarette smoking appeared to be more strongly associated with epidermoid and anaplastic histologic types of lung cancer than with adenocarcinomas. Additional cohort and case-control studies and ongoing follow-up of the earlier cohort studies confirmed the strong association between cigarette smoking and lung cancer.[6]

These pioneering studies and others that followed formed the basis for official governmental recognition of the role of tobacco in the etiology of cancer and other chronic diseases and helped to stimulate government health agencies to try to reduce tobacco consumption in the population. In 1957, the Medical Research Council of Great Britain[27] published a statement on the relationship between tobacco smoking and cancer of the lung. The council concluded that the strong epidemiological evidence, coupled with the identification of several carcinogens in tobacco smoke, provided support for a direct causal relation between cigarette smoking and lung cancer. In 1964, Luther Terry, the surgeon general of the United States, issued a landmark report[1] that laid out in great detail the relation between tobacco use and cancer, heart disease, and other chronic conditions. The US Surgeon General's Report on Tobacco and Health placed heavy emphasis on the epidemic nature of the 30-year increase in lung cancer mortality and the strong associations between cigarette smoking and lung cancer observed in the case-control and cohort studies. The report utilized the now famous criteria suggested by Sir Bradford Hill[28] for assessing the possible causal nature of epidemiological associations. Application of the Hill criteria to the smoking and lung cancer data can be summarized as follows.

The Consistency of the Association

At the time of the 1964 surgeon general's report, 29 retrospective and 7 prospective studies had all demonstrated an association between cigarette smoking and lung cancer. Similar findings had thus been reported from a large number of studies conducted by independent investigators using different methodological approaches in vastly different populations.

Strength of the Association

The overall association between ever smoking cigarettes and lung cancer risk in men is shown in data from several of the large cohort studies available at the time of the surgeon general's report (Figure 9–8). Relative risks ranged from 3.8 to 14.2, with eight of the nine studies reporting relative risks of 7.0 or greater. Among women, who generally tended to smoke less than men, the relative risks for lung cancer associated with ever smoking cigarettes ranged from 2.0 to 5.0, with three of the four studies reporting relative risks in excess of 3.0. In several studies, men and women who smoked one or more packs of cigarettes per day experienced a 25- to 30-fold increased risk of dying from lung cancer when compared with nonsmokers.

Dose-Response Relationship

The existence of a dose-response relationship between cigarette smoking and lung cancer risk constitutes further evidence of a causal relationship. Data from several major cohort studies showing the relation between daily smoking levels and lung cancer risk are plotted in Figure 9–9. The similarity of the dose-response curves reported by several studies conducted by different investigators in different countries is striking.

Specificity of the Association

The surgeon general's report also acknowledged the growing realization among medical researchers that the etiology of chronic diseases like lung cancer might be related to several causes and that a single agent might be able to cause different forms of cancer. The degree of specificity between lung cancer and cigarette smoking is revealed by calculating an estimate of the attributable risk (ie, the proportion of lung cancer risk in the general population that can be attributed to cigarette smoking). The calculation of the attributable risk takes into account the relative risk associated with exposure to cigarette smoking and the percentage of the population exposed. It has been estimated that 85% to 90% of lung cancer mortality in men is due to cigarette smoking.[6(pp228–235)] The remaining 10% to15% can be attributed to other factors, such as occupational chemical exposures and residential radon exposures. The observation that all smokers do not develop lung

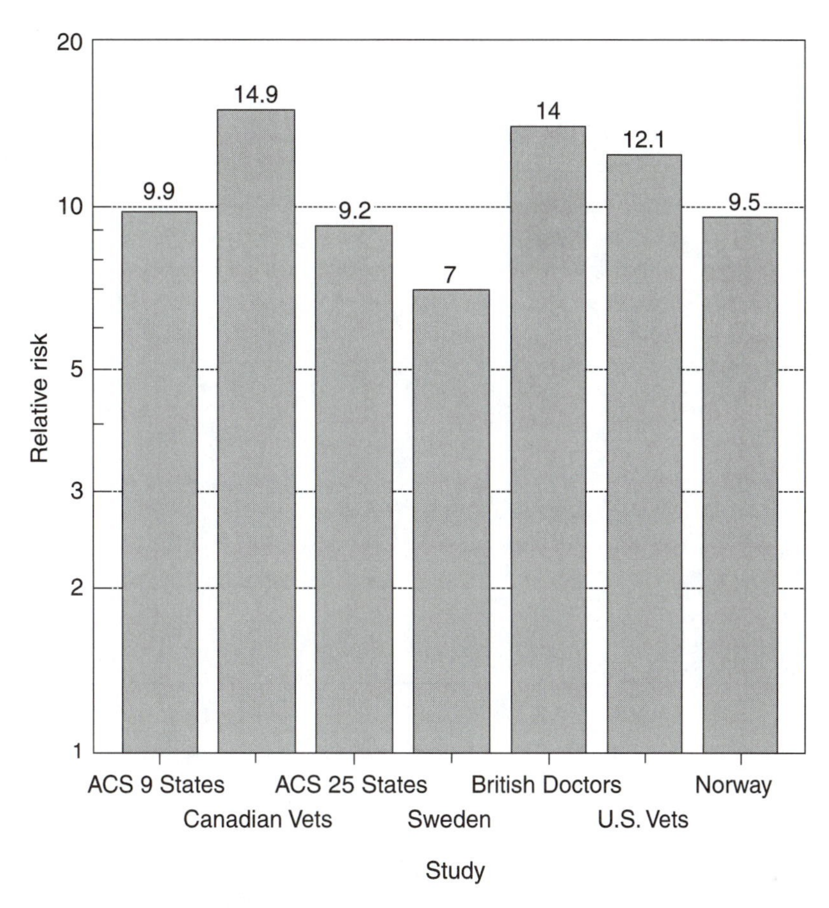

Figure 9–8 Relative risk of lung cancer from current smoking of cigarettes only (versus never smoking). Results from selected studies are shown. *Source:* Adapted with permission from *Tobacco Smoking*, IARC Monographs on the Evaluation of Carcinogenic Risk of Chemicals to Humans, No. 38, p. 205, © 1986, International Agency for Research on Cancer.

---

cancer indicates the influence of factors such as competing causes of death and underlying genetic differences in individuals' metabolism of carcinogenic agents.

Temporal Relationship of Cigarette Smoking and Lung Cancer

The onset of cigarette smoking was observed to occur many years prior to the diagnosis of cancer. The possibility that an undiagnosed lung cancer might exist in a patient prior to the onset of smoking and remain silent for two to three decades has never been adequately supported by actual research data. In addition, studies of chemical carcinogens have made clear that a 20- to 30-year latent period between first exposure to a carcinogen and cancer diagnosis is the rule rather than the exception.

Coherence of the Association

The judgment that there is a causal relation between cigarette smoking and lung cancer also rests on the extent to which the the known distribution of the disease and of

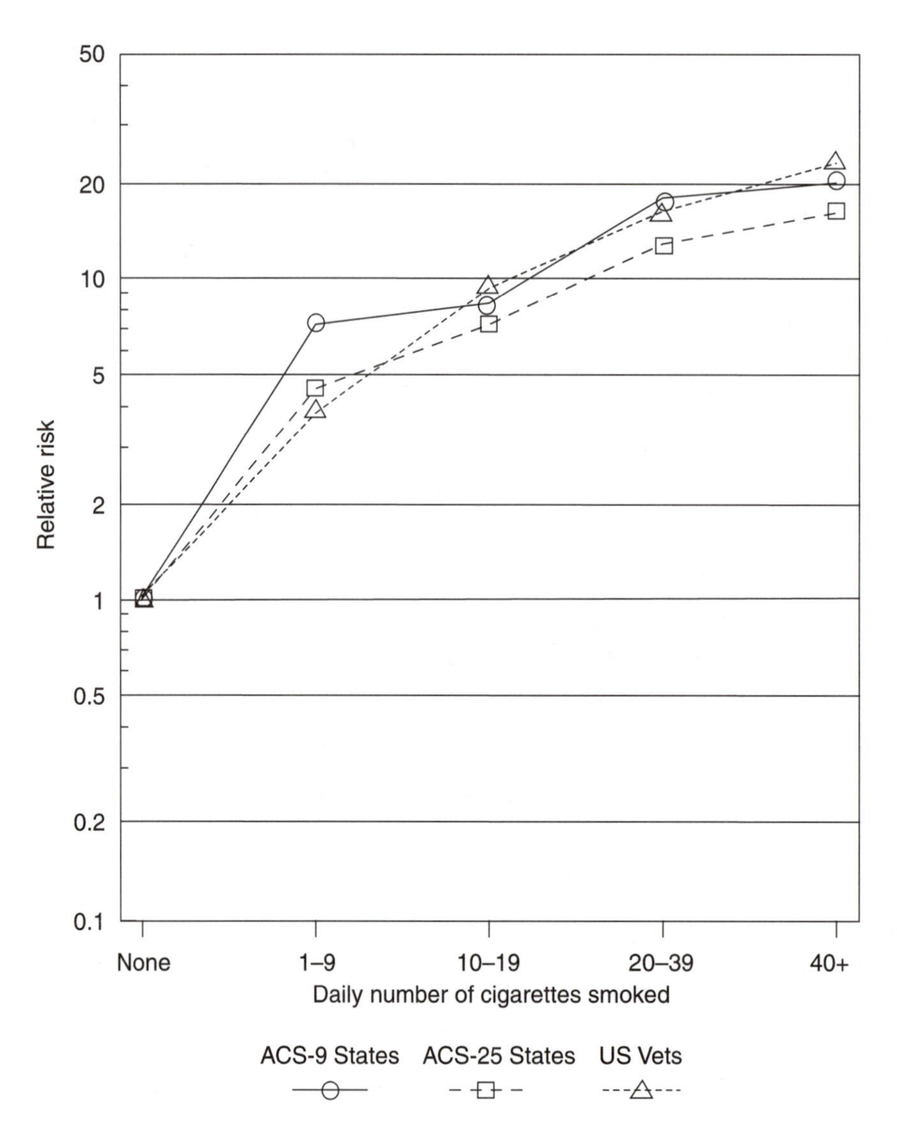

Figure 9–9 Data from three cohort studies showing the relation between lung cancer risk and daily number of cigarettes smoked. *Source:* Adapted with permission from *Tobacco Smoking*, IARC Monographs on the Evaluation of Carcinogenic Risk of Chemicals to Humans, No. 38, pp. 215–216, © 1986, International Agency for Research on Cancer.

cigarette smoking are similar with regard to person, place, and time. The coherence of the association with existing knowledge concerning the natural history and biology of the disease is also notable. The surgeon general's report cited the rapid rise in per capita consumption of cigarettes and the rapid increase in lung cancer mortality that occurred after a suitable period of latency. The distribution of cigarette smoking among the sexes, among rural and urban residents, and among different socioeconomic classes was similar to the distribution of lung cancer among these groups, and this fact was taken as further evidence of a causal connection between cigarette smoking and lung cancer. The existence of a dose-response relation and the decrease in risk observed among those who quit smoking also provided support for a coherent association between cigarette smoking and lung cancer. Data from several studies [26,29–31] show that cessation of smoking for 10 years or more tends to significantly reduce lung cancer risk among former smokers. In addition, a number of studies showed an especially high lung cancer risk associated with inhalation of tobacco smoke and the use of nonfiltered, high-tar cigarettes.[6(pp218–220)] The strong correlation between the type of tobacco used and the anatomic site of the cancer also tended to lend support to the association.

In summary, the association between cigarette smoking and lung cancer was judged to represent a causal relationship. This conclusion was based on the consistency and magnitude of the relative risk, the specificity of the association, the apparent temporal relationship between the exposure and the disease, the coherence of the association with the known descriptive epidemiology of lung cancer, and the agreement between the findings and our understanding of the disease.

Cancers of the Upper Respiratory and Upper Digestive System

Tobacco smoking has also been shown to be associated with head and neck cancers. Cigarette smokers have been shown to be at increased risk for developing cancers of the oral cavity and pharynx, larynx, and esophagus, as compared with nonsmokers, and pipe smokers have been shown to be at increased risk for developing lip cancer.[6] Risk estimates for cigarette smoking and cancers of the upper respiratory and digestive tracts are shown in Figure 9–10. These estimates are for smoking in the absence of alcohol consumption and use of smokeless tobacco, which are other strong risk factors for upper respiratory and digestive tract cancers. The effect of combined exposure to tobacco and alcohol and the impact of smokeless tobacco on the development of these cancers are discussed later in this chapter. The data show significantly elevated relative risks for head and neck cancers among cigarette smokers. They also show a dose-response relation between cancer risk and daily number of cigarettes smoked. The risk of disease among smokers in the highest dose category (relative to the risk for nonsmokers) ranges from 8.0 or 9.0 for cancers of the buccal cavity and esophagus to around 21.0 for cancers of the pharynx and larynx.

Other Digestive System Cancers

A causal relationship has been established between cigarette smoking and cancer of the pancreas. For other digestive organs, including the stomach and liver, an etiologic relationship is less certain. For stomach cancer, the association with cigarette smoking has been weak, and no consistent dose-response relations have been observed.[6] More consistent elevations in risk have been observed in studies of hepatocellular carcinomas.[6] However, these studies have been based on small numbers of cases and have not always adequately controlled for potential confounding by other risk factors, such as alcohol use, hepatitis B infection, or exposure to aflatoxins.[6] Studies of cigarette smoking and pancreatic cancer are stronger, with ecological studies[6] showing correlations be-

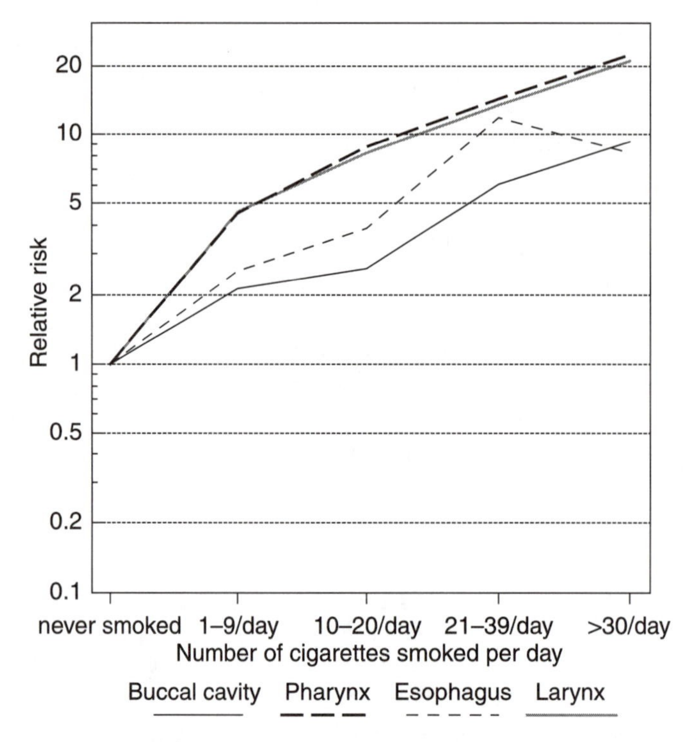

Figure 9–10 Relative risk of cancers of the upper respiratory and digestive tract from current smoking of cigarettes (versus never smoking) in a US prospective study. *Source:* Adapted with permission from *Tobacco Smoking*, IARC Monographs on the Evaluation of Carcinogenic Risk of Chemicals to Humans, No. 38, p. 272, © 1986, International Agency for Research on Cancer.

---

tween geographic distributions of pancreatic cancer and cigarette consumption. Both cohort studies[6]and case-control studies[6] have shown approximately twofold increased risks and suggestions of a dose-response relation between cigarette smoking and pancreatic cancer.

Cancers of the Lower Urinary Tract

Cigarette smoking has been shown to be strongly related to cancers of the lower urinary tract, including the renal pelvis, ureter, bladder, and urethra.[6] Significantly elevated risks have been observed among smokers (relative to nonsmokers), from around 2 to as high as 15 (in the highest daily smoking categories). Both cohort and case-control studies have consistently shown a dose-response relation between risk and amount of cigarettes smoked each day. The association between cigarette smoking and cancers of the lower urinary tract has been observed among both men and women, although the relative risks observed in women have been lower than those observed in men. One study[32] showed higher risks among black male and female cigarette smokers than among whites, but a second study[33]found the opposite. Increased risk has been observed among patients with noninvasive and invasive disease. However, the cigarette smoking effect appears to be stronger in patients in which the disease is at a more advanced clinical stage.[34] The relation between cigarette smoking and cancers of the lower urinary tract was not found to be confounded by other risk factors for these malignancies. Siemiatychi et al[35] showed that the relation between smoking and bladder cancer remained strong even after adjustment for occupational exposures. The risk of developing a cancer of the lower urinary tract also appears to increase with decreasing age at first exposure and increasing duration of exposure. Because age at first exposure is correlated with total duration of exposure, it is difficult to determine the independent effects of these two variables. A causal relation between smoking and bladder cancer is also suggested by the reduction in risk observed among former smokers.[6] Reductions in bladder cancer have been shown to be related to time since quitting. In one study,[36] the bladder cancer risk in subjects who had stopped smoking cigarettes for at least 5 years was less than one-third that of current smokers.

A number of studies also examined the relation of cigarette smoking to urinary cancers with respect to type of tobacco used, use of filtered and unfiltered cigarettes, and the extent of inhalation. In two studies,[36,37] users of both black and blond tobacco experienced an increased risk of bladder cancer. However, the risk was significantly higher in those using black tobacco. Another study[38] showed no significant risk in users of blond tobacco cigarettes, but the number of such users was small. Several studies[38–40] have shown an attenuated risk among users of filtered and low-tar cigarettes, while one study[41] failed to demonstrate a difference in risk between users of filtered and users of unfiltered cigarettes. Higher bladder cancer risk has also been associated with deep inhalation.[38,39,41] The stronger association between bladder cancer and cigarette smoking in those reporting deep inhalation, the use of black tobacco, and the use of unfiltered, high-tar cigarettes suggests that these individuals receive a stronger dose of various carcinogenic agents present in cigarette smoke. These observations, combined with the consistency of the association and the presence of a dose-response relation in most studies, strongly suggest a causal role for cigarette smoking in the development of cancer of the lower urinary tract. Assuming that the association between cigarette smoking and cancer of the lower urinary tract is causal, the population attributable risk (PAR) can be estimated to be in the range of 45% to 55% for men and 33% to 40% for women.[39–44]

Cancers of the Reproductive Organs and Breast

Initial reports[45–48] of an association between cigarette smoking and squamous cell cancer of the uterine cervix were greeted with skepticism. Concerns were raised regarding inadequate control of potential confounding variables and the lack of a biological rationale for the association. A large number of subsequent studies[49–69] have shown a moderate increase in cervical cancer risk among cigarette smokers, with some evidence of a dose-response relation. However, several studies have failed to show this association.[70–73] The more recent studies have included extensive efforts to control for the possible confounding effects of important risk factors, including sexual activity, Pap screening, and infection with various viral agents. Control for human papillomavirus (HPV) infection tends to significantly reduce the risk associated with cigarette smoking.[63,71,73] A recent meta-analysis[74] used sensitivity analysis to estimate pooled relative risks assuming various levels of potential confounding. Under the assumption of no confounding, the sensitivity analysis produced a pooled relative risk estimate of 1.81 for cancer of the uterine cervix among current cigarette smokers. Assuming low (10%) and high (30%) degrees of confounding, the analysis produced relative risks of 1.63 and 1.27, respectively. The exact role of cigarette smoking in the etiology of cancer of the uterine cervix is still unclear. Cigarette smoking may act as a cofactor that enhances the carcinogenic action of the papillomavirus.

Squamous cell carcinomas of the vulva and cervix may share a common etiology. Epidemiological studies have shown cigarette smoking to be associated with an increased vulvar cancer risk. Brinton et al[75] also showed an interesting association between cigarette smoking and a history of venereal warts, a condition caused by human papillomavirus. Their study showed a relative risk of 3.0 for venereal warts in the absence of cigarette smoking and a relative risk of 11.0 in the presence of cigarette smoking. These figures are based on small numbers of case and control subjects and should be interpreted with caution, but they do suggest that cigarette smoking may enhance the carcinogenic effect of HPV.

A biological rationale was proposed by Winkelstein,[76,77] who reported ecological data showing high correlations between areas with high age-adjusted incidence rates for lung cancer in males and high incidence rates for cancer of the uterine cervix. Winkelstein also pointed out that squamous cell carcinomas predominate in the uterine cervix and that cigarette smoking has been most strongly linked with squamous cell carcinomas of the lung. Later studies of adenocarcinomas of the uterine cervix[78–80] showed no clear association between this cell type and cigarette smoking. In addition, no consistent association has been found between cigarette smoking and cancers of the ovary and female breast or cancers of the prostate gland. Winkelstein also provided examples of other cancer sites where multiple risk factors have been identified and cited research showing that chemicals found in cigarette smoke can be absorbed into the bloodstream and transported to other organs. Holly et al[81] tested the cervical fluids of 78 women for mutagenicity using the Ames *Salmonella* microsomal assay. These investigators reported that 39% of cigarette smokers, as compared with only 12% of nonsmokers, tested positive in the Ames test for mutagenicity. In another study,[82] nicotine was detected in the cervical mucus of all smokers tested, while cotinine, a metabolite of nicotine, was detected in 84% of the smokers. The levels of these compounds detected in the cervical mucus were found to be significantly correlated with the subject's usual daily number of cigarettes smoked and the number smoked in the 24 hours prior to testing.

Epidemiological studies have shown a decreased risk for endometrial cancer among cigarette smokers.[83–95] An antiestrogenic effect has been proposed to explain the apparent protection offered by cigarette smoking. However, studies designed to measure estrogen levels in the blood or urine of smokers and nonsmokers have been inconsistent. In a study of 167 premenopausal and 200 postmenopausal women, Key et al[96] found no differences between smokers and nonsmokers with regard to geometric mean excretion of estrone or estradiol in the urine. They did report estriol excretion to be 19% lower in smokers than in nonsmokers. Austin et al[94] found no differences in serum estrone levels between smokers and nonsmokers. They also reported lower serum levels of estradiol and higher serum androstenedione levels in smokers. The study by Khaw et al[97] also showed no differences in the serum levels of estrone, estradiol, or estriol between smokers and nonsmokers. Conversely, this study did show a significant increase in androgen plasma levels in smokers, and a dose-response relation was observed between androgen levels and the amount of cigarettes smoked. These studies do not provide strong support for the hypoestrogenism hypothesis. Additional research is needed to help identify the role androgens may play in the biological mechanism underlying the reduced endometrial cancer risk observed in cigarette smokers.

Epidemiological studies of endometrial cancers and cigarette smoking provide interesting insights into the etiology of these malignancies. However, promotion of cigarette smoking as a preventive for endometrial cancer is not recommended.[87,98] Cancer of the endometrium is much less common than lung cancer and other smoking-related diseases and is usually detected at an early clinical stage, leading to high 5- and 10-year survival rates. Lung cancer is usually detected at a late stage and the survival rates are low. Screening is not capable of detecting lung cancer in an early treatable form, and reduction of smoking is the only effective public health preventive measure.

Leukemia

A large number of epidemiological studies have shown a small to moderate increased leukemia risk associated with cigarette smoking. However, a number of epidemiological studies of both cohort and case-control design have failed to confirm these findings. The excess risk appears to be most strongly associated with myeloid leukemias. Two meta-analyses of epidemiological studies of leukemia risk reported pooled relative risk estimates of 1.51 and 1.40 for myeloid leukemias in the cohort studies. One of these analyses[99] estimated the pooled relative risk in the case-control studies at 1.23 for myeloid leukemias, while the second[100] estimated the pooled relative risk in the case-control studies at 1.3 for leukemias classified as acute nonlymphocytic. The specificity of the findings for myeloid leukemias and the observation of a dose-response relation in the majority of positive studies lend support to the hypothesis that smoking is a cause of these cancers. Cigarette smoke has also been shown to contain compounds that are known leukemogenic agents. Benzene and lead-210, established leukemogenic agents, have both been isolated from cigarette smoke. Wallace[101] reported significantly higher breath concentrations of benzene in smokers than in nonsmokers as well as a dose-response relation between increasing benzene levels and the daily number of cigarettes smoked. Ong et al[102] examined the urine concentrations of three benzene-related compounds in smokers and nonsmokers. The urine concentrations of catechol, hydroquinone, trans, and trans-muconic acid were found to be higher in smokers than in nonsmokers. This same study reported higher levels of cotinine in the smokers than in nonsmokers. Smokers have also shown increased levels of lead-210 in bones and soft tissues.[103,104]

In their review of the literature on smoking and leukemias, Brownson et al[100] cited a number of studies that have shown significantly higher leukocyte counts (of both acute and long-term duration) in smokers than in nonsmokers. A higher likelihood of cytogenetic lesions has also been observed in smokers with leukemias than in nonsmokers with these cancers, and the likelihood of an abnormal karyotype is associated with the number of cigarettes smoked daily.[105] Siegal[99] has reviewed some of the weaknesses of the negative studies reported through 1991, including low follow-up rates in one cohort study and the potential for selection bias in two of the negative case-control studies. Despite the sound arguments in support of a causal relation between cigarette smoking and leukemia, these studies report increased relative risks that are small to moderate in size and might easily be caused by some form of systematic bias. Lack of adequate control of confounding by race, socioeconomic status, and exposure to known leukemogenic agents may have affected study results.

ENVIRONMENTAL TOBACCO SMOKE

The carcinogenic effects of environmental tobacco smoke (ETS) or passive smoking on human lung tissues have been a source of controversy during the past decade.[106–112] ETS consists of sidestream smoke and mainstream smoke exhaled by active smokers. As shown earlier in this chapter, both mainstream and sidestream smoke contain about 40 different chemicals that are suspected or proven carcinogens, and sidestream smoke often contains larger concentrations of these chemicals than mainstream smoke. In 1992, the US Environmental Protection Agency (EPA) published a report[106] that labeled ETS a Group A carcinogen (known human carcinogen). The basic thrust of the evidence provided by the EPA to support this classification included the following:

- the firmly established dose-response relation between active cigarette smoking and lung cancer, which extends down to doses low enough to be roughly equivalent to doses commonly received through ETS
- the results from air sampling and biomarker (nicotine and cotinine) studies, which show widespread distribution of ETS in various locations, such as private homes, work sites, and restaurants
- the presence of known or suspected carcinogens in sidestream smoke in concentrations that often exceed concentrations found in mainstream smoke
- experimental data from animal bioassays and genotoxicity studies demonstrating the carcinogenicity of mainstream and sidestream smoke
- results from a majority of epidemiological studies showing an increased risk of lung cancer in nonsmoking women whose spouses are smokers.

Approximately 90% of the subjects included in the existing epidemiological studies of ETS are women. The case-control studies have consisted of nonsmoking female lung case and control subjects. The majority of these studies have been hospital based rather than population based. Estimates of ETS exposure have been arrived at primarily by determining the smoking habits of the women's spouses. Most investigators have attempted to collect data on spousal smoking habits and potential confounding variables through face-to-face interviews. The high case-fatality rate associated with lung cancer has required the use of next-of-kin interviews for approximately 50% of the subjects included in these studies. Three cohort studies of ETS exposure and lung cancer have also been conducted.[113] One overall estimate of the relative risk associated with ETS based on spousal smoking as the measure of exposure is 1.47 (95% CI = 1.12–1.92).[113] A dose-response relation between spousal smoking and lung cancer risk has been observed in many but not all studies.

Because of the basic design of these studies, certain biases may be responsible for the observed increased lung cancer risk associated with ETS. Many study reports have not provided detailed information on diagnostic criteria and have not included an independent review of pathology slides. The case series also tend to contain mostly adenocarcinomas, which are only weakly associated with active cigarette smoking. Some critics have suggested that these studies may have included many cancers that did not originate in the lung but spread to the lung from another primary site.[111] Selection bias has also been proposed as an alternative explanation for reported findings. Since most studies were hospital based, the hospital-based controls may have exposure distributions dissimilar from the exposure distributions of the underlying population from which the cases were selected.[113] The main source of concern is the potential for information bias. Most studies relied solely on spousal smoking habits for measuring ETS exposure, and the exclusion of occupational, recreational, and childhood exposures may have biased the findings. Several studies[114–117] compared original interview responses with reinterview data for samples of study subjects and used cotinine levels in the urine as a marker of exposure. Although one study suggested that spousal data were unreliable,[118] these studies generally indicated that spousal data are reasonably reliable and valid in identifying nonsmoking women but that misclassification is significantly higher when more complex measures of exposure are used.[113] If the exposure misclassification is nondifferential, then the effect is to dilute the true effect of ETS on lung cancer risk. Differential misclassification of ETS exposure between cases and controls would be more likely to cause a spurious increased risk for lung cancer. High levels of unreported active smoking by lung cancer patients, as compared with controls, and smoking concordance between spouses could produce an inflated relative risk estimate. The extent to which the observed relative risk is adjusted downward depends not only on the statistical model used but also on the estimate of unreported active smoking used in the model. The choice of appropriate models and parameter estimates has been a particularly contentious part of the ETS controversy.[107,119–121] Assuming the relation between ETS and lung cancer is causal, ETS is estimated to be responsible for between 10% and 15% of all lung cancers.[113]

SMOKELESS TOBACCO

Smokeless tobacco includes both chewing tobacco and snuff. The characteristics of the various smokeless tobacco products are shown in Table 9–2. In 1986, a scientific advisory committee[122] to the US surgeon general concluded that a causal relation between the use of snuff and oral cancer has been demonstrated and that a causal relation between chewing tobacco and oral cancer is suggested by the evidence. The expert panel noted the presence of potent carcinogens in smokeless tobacco, including nitrosamines, polycyclic aromatic hydrocarbons, and radiation-emitting polonium. The panel also noted the development of white patches (leukoplakias) in the mouths of smokeless tobacco users. A certain portion of these benign lesions undergo further transformation into malignant lesions. Finally, the presence of nicotine in smokeless tobacco at levels similar to those found in cigarettes supported the hypothesis that tobacco in this form might also be addictive.

Case series and individual case reports have shown that smokeless tobacco is used frequently by patients diagnosed with oral cancer and that oral lesions occur in the areas of the mouth where the tobacco was held between the gum and cheek.[122] In North America and Europe, case-control studies of smokeless tobacco and oral cancer have faced limitations caused by the small number of available subjects and the infrequency

Table 9–2 Characteristics of Smokeless Tobacco Products

Product	*Description*	*How Used*	*Packaging**
Chewing tobacco			
Looseleaf	Made from air-cured, cigar leaf tobaccos of Pennsylvania and Wisconsin. Consists of stripped and processed tobacco leaves. The leaves are stemmed, cut, or granulated and are loosely packed to form small strips of shredded tobacco. Most brands are sweetened and flavored with licorice.	A piece of tobacco, 3/4 to 1 inch in diameter, is tucked between the gum and jaw, usually to the back of the mouth.	Pouch, typically 3 ounces. A few brands market a 1.5-ounce pouch.
Plug	Made from enriched tobacco leaves (Burley and bright tobacco and cigar tobacco) or fragments wrapped in fine tobacco and pressed into bricks. May be firm (less than 15 percent moisture) or moist (15 percent or greater moisture). Most plug tobacco is sweetened and flavored with licorice.	Chewed or held in the cheek or lower lip. May be held in the mouth for several hours.	A compressed brick or flat block wrapped inside natural tobacco leaves. Packaged in clear plastic. Packages range from 7 to 13 ounces. Also sold by the piece.
Twist	Handmade of dark, air-cured leaf tobacco treated with a tarlike tobacco leaf extract and twisted into strands that are dried. Majority is sold without flavoring and sweeteners.	Similar to plug.	A pliable but dry rope. Sold by the piece, packaged in plastic bags. No standard weight. Sold in small (approximately 1–2 ounces) and larger sizes based on the number of leaves in the twist.
Snuff			
Moist	Made from air-cured and fire-cured tobacco. Consists of tobacco stems and leaves that are processed into fine particles or strips. Some products are flavored. Has a moisture content of up to 50 percent.	A small amount ("pinch") is placed between the lip or cheek and gum and is typically held for 30 minutes or longer per pinch.	Cans and plastic containers, typically 1.2 ounces.
Dry	Most dry snuff is made from fire-cured tobaccos of Kentucky and Tennessee. After initial curing, the tobacco is fermented further and processed into a dry powdered form. Products vary in strength and flavoring. Generally has a moisture content of less than 10 percent.	Same as moist snuff. May also be sniffed.	Metal cans or glass containers, vary from 1.15 to 7 ounces per container.

*Product weight (includes moisture).

Source: Reprinted from *The Health Consequences of Using Smokeless Tobacco: A Report of the Advisory Committee to the Surgeon General,* p. 6, 1986, U.S. Department of Health and Human Services, National Institutes of Health.

of smokeless tobacco use in the general population. These studies were conducted prior to the advent of multivariate statistical techniques and relied primarily on stratified analyses to control for potential confounding by cigarette smoking, alcohol, and poor dentition.[122] Despite these limitations, the relative risks observed in these studies have been large (on the order of 6.0 to 12.0), and they have been shown to increase with increasing duration of use. The study by Winn et al[123] involved 255 women with oral and pharyngeal cancers and approximately twice as many control subjects, who were individually matched to the case subjects by age, race, and source of ascertainment. These investigators observed a fourfold increased risk among white women who did not smoke cigarettes. This increased risk was maintained after controlling for cigarette smoking, alcohol consumption, poor dentition, diet, and use of mouthwash.[124] Snuff was used by nearly all patients with cheek and gum tumors, and long-term snuff users experienced a 50-fold increased risk of cancers of the gum and buccal mucosa. The authors also estimated that smokeless tobacco use accounted for approximately 87% of these cancers.

Studies in Asian and African populations have also provided strong support for a causal relation between smokeless tobacco and oral cancers.[122] Most Asian and African countries show oral cancer incidence rates approximately 10 times higher than those seen in Europe and North America. In these countries, smokeless tobacco is usually used in combination with other compounds. One combination popular in India contains tobacco, betel leaf, areca nut, and lime, while other mixtures are used in other countries. Several studies[125–130] included comparisons of patients and controls who used betel quids with and without tobacco. Three studies showed an increased risk in the 2.9–3.6 range for the use betel quids not containing tobacco, while two studies showed no increased risk. An increased relative risk of oral cancers in users of betel quids containing smokeless tobacco was observed in all studies, and the magnitude of the increase, in the 4.3–25 range, was much greater than for betel leaf alone (Figure 9–11). These studies also showed that smokeless tobacco use was reported by nearly all case subjects, thus making this exposure the major source of oral cancers in these populations.[131,132] Most importantly, four of these studies included no cigarette smokers, and the remaining study showed similar elevated risks among smokeless tobacco users after controlling for cigarette smoking. The combined evidence from the case-control studies conducted in several parts of the world clearly supports the view that a causal relation exists between smokeless tobacco use and oral cancers.

Cohort studies[133–137] have been only minimally informative owing to the small number of exposed subjects. An increased risk of death due to cancers of the buccal cavity, pharynx, and esophagus was reported by cohort studies conducted in Norway[135] and one conducted in the United States.[136] The 16-year study of US veterans[136] reported no cases of oral or pharyngeal cancer in a small cohort of 951 users of smokeless tobacco products. Similar negative results were reported by a study of 1,500 patients followed for changes in the oral mucosa.[133,134]

INTERACTIONS BETWEEN TOBACCO AND OTHER ENVIRONMENTAL EXPOSURES

Investigators have also attempted to determine if tobacco interacts with other environmental exposures to greatly increase an individual's risk of developing various forms

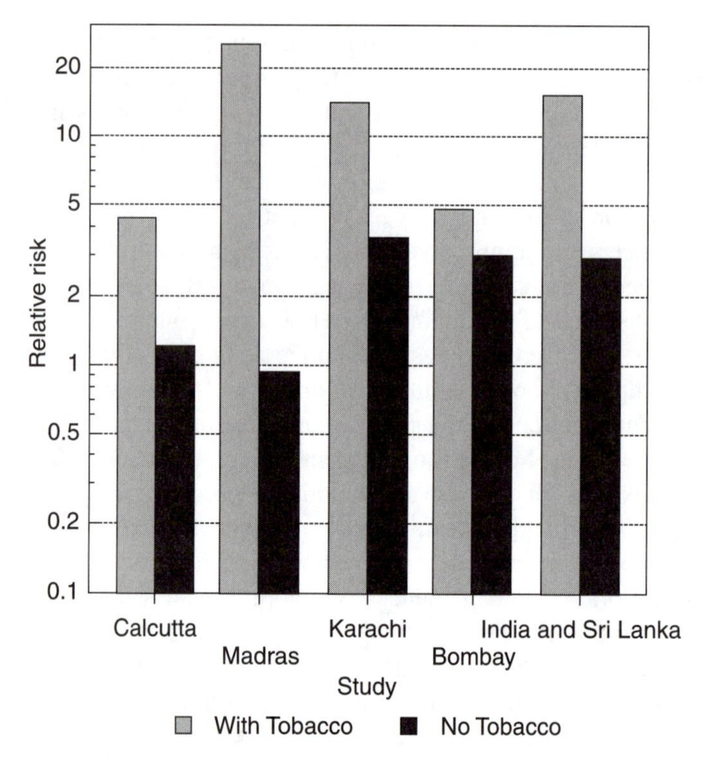

Figure 9–11 Relative risk of oral cancer from chewing betel quids with and without tobacco (versus not chewing betel in any form). Data from selected studies are shown. *Source:* Adapted from *The Health Consequences of Using Smokeless Tobacco: A Report of the Advisory Committee to the Surgeon General,* p. 46, 1986, U.S. Department of Health and Human Services, National Institutes of Health.

---

of cancer. Possible effects of the interaction between cigarette smoking and alcohol abuse on the development of cancers of the mouth, pharynx, larynx, and esophagus[138–141] have received much attention. A detailed discussion of the modeling approaches used to study these interactions can be found in the article by Saracci.[142] Studies of the effects of interaction between cigarette smoking and alcohol on head and neck cancers have produced mixed results, with both additive and multiplicative models fitting the observed data. Similar variations have been observed for cigarette smoking and asbestos, ionizing radiation, and arsenic in relation to lung cancer and for cigarette smoking and aromatic amines in relation to bladder cancer. The failure to identify unequivocal effects of the interaction between cigarette smoking and other environmental exposures may be the result of crude measurement or misclassification of exposures, which might artificially reduce the observed magnitude of the interactions.[142]

GENE-ENVIRONMENTAL INTERACTIONS

Although cigarette smoking is responsible for approximately 80% of all lung cancers, only about 20% of smokers will actually develop this form of cancer.[143] In addition, family studies[144–147] and twin studies[148] have shown that lung cancers can aggregate in families independent of smoking status and occupational exposures.[149] The study findings suggest that inherited susceptibility to chemicals in cigarette smoke is partially responsible for significant interindividual risk for lung cancer. Wei and Spitz[149] published a comprehensive review of two areas of research regarding inherited susceptibility. Below is a brief summary of the issues covered in their review.

Extensive research has been directed toward uncovering the role of mutagenic sensitivity and DNA repair mechanisms in determining susceptibility to lung carcinogens. This research is based on the observation that approximately 80% of all cancers are probably related to environmental carcinogens. These carcinogens are genotoxic, often causing mutations of proto-oncogenes and tumor suppressor genes, which play important roles in regulating the cell cycle and can activate or inhibit cell death (apoptosis).[150–152] Failure to repair mutagenic damage to these important regulatory genes may result in carcinogenesis. Interindividual variation in sensitivity to various mutagens and the ability of the host cells to monitor and repair DNA damage could result in significant variability in susceptibility to carcinogens in tobacco smoke.[149]

A number of laboratory approaches have been developed to measure possible interactions between cigarette smoking and the inherited sensitivity of the host DNA to mutagenic damage. The initial assay developed to measure mutagenic sensitivity involves treating an individual's peripheral blood lymphocytes with the drug bleomycin in cell culture.[153] Mutagenic sensitivity is measured by the number of DNA breaks observed per cell. Sensitivity has been generally defined as one or more breaks per cell examined. The assay is based on the assumption that peripheral lymphocytes can serve as a useful surrogate for lung tissue, where the carcinogenic process actually takes place.[149] The assay has high reliability. In one statistical analysis,[154] the correlation coefficient between the first and second reading by the same reader was 0.72. Sensitivity and specificity were also estimated at 75% and 95%, respectively.

This assay has been used in case-control studies of lung and head and neck cancers.[155,156] In general, these studies show a dose-response relationship between the number of breaks per cell and lung cancer risk. In one study,[155] a 4.80 relative risk was observed in the highest quartile of mutagen sensitivity. In addition, the combined relative risk for high mutagen sensitivity and ever smoking was 28.07, compared with a relative risk of 8.07 for smoking only and 4.68 for mutagen sensitivity alone. The combination of high sensitivity to mutagens and cigarette smoking confers a relative risk that exceeds the additive effects of the two risk factors. Similar results were reported by Cloos et al.[156] The bleomycin assay was extended by utilizing benzo[*a*]pyrene diol epoxide (BPDE) as the mutagenic agent. This chemical is a known genotoxic carcinogen found in cigarette smoke.[157] The use of this form of the assay in a case-control design again showed a dose-response relation between the various levels of mutagenic sensitivity and lung cancer risk after adjustment for age, sex, ethnicity, and smoking status.

The goal of the second phase of the research is to demonstrate the existence of a relation between lung cancer risk and a measure of DNA repair capacity (DRC). An assay that measures expression of damaged reporter genes has been developed. The assay is very useful in population studies because of its efficiency (in terms of time and cost) and its repeatability.[149] In a case-control study by Wei et al,[158] mean DRC levels were lower in case subjects than in control subjects, and case subjects were five times more likely than control subjects to have DRC levels below the median (OR = 5.7; 95% CI = 2.1–15.7). Also, higher risk was associated with cigarette smoking and young age at onset of lung cancer, and a dose-response relationship was observed between reduced DRC levels and increased lung cancer risk.

Studies have also been conducted to show a relationship between environmental exposures and inherited ability to repair DNA damage. DNA adduct levels in cells treated with known carcinogens are thought to reflect the balance between the damage caused by the environmental exposure and the extent of DNA repair.[149] Adduct levels are used as a marker of the effectiveness of DNA repair mechanisms and metabolic protection. The ^{32}P-postlabeling assay is the most sensitive test available for quantifying DNA adducts.[159,160] Studies designed to detect differences in the levels of DNA adducts between smokers and nonsmokers have produced inconsistent results. The inconsistency may be due to measurement error or to the effects of polymorphisms that have not been characterized.[149]

A number of metabolic polymorphisms have also been identified that affect carcinogen absorption, distribution, and accumulation[149] (see Chapters 6 and 7 for further discussion of this topic). Phase I enzymes are responsible for converting relatively inactive chemicals into active compounds that can react with and damage cellular DNA. The cytochrome P-450 (CYP) family of enzymes play a major role in carcinogen activation. These enzymes use an oxidative process to create highly reactive intermediates, which are more reactive than the chemicals from which they are derived. These active intermediates can bind covalently with DNA to form adducts.[158] The phase II enzymes form new inactivate compounds from active carcinogens by a process called conjugation. These new compounds are more easily excreted than the more active carcinogens.[158] Genotyping has been used to identify cytochrome P-450 genes that code for a number of phenotypes that have been evaluated with respect to lung cancer risk. Results from these studies have been inconsistent, possibly owing to misclassification of the genotypes. For example, Wu et al[161] conducted a case-control study that examined P-450E1 (CYP2E1), which is involved in the activation of *N*-nitrosamines, known carcinogenic agents found in tobacco smoke. The genotype was found to be associated with a 14-fold increase in lung cancer risk in Mexican Americans, but no increased risk was observed in African Americans. In addition these authors reported a 9.9-fold increase in risk in Mexican Americans who were former smokers but not in nonsmokers or current smokers. These authors also reported a 15-fold increase in risk in Mexican American males with the genotype but not in females.

Examples of phase II enzyme systems include the glutathione *S*-transferases (GSTs), which conjugate a number of highly reactive compounds, and the *N*-acetylation polymorphism, which separates individuals into fast, intermediate, and slow excreters of carcinogenic substances. Study results on the relationship between these enzyme systems and lung cancer risk have been inconsistent. The actions of these enzymes systems are apparently complex. A highly reactive compound can be converted to a less reactive compound but the new compound can in turn serve as a precursor for conversion to another highly reactive compound.[149] The relation between inherited susceptibility and lung cancer is a new and exciting area of research, and the relation between inherited susceptibility and other forms of cancer is also starting to be investigated. Research goals include improving assay methods and obtaining further insights into how various metabolic pathways influence the carcinogenic process.

SUMMARY

Various forms of tobacco use have been shown to be causally related to a number of cancers. Cigarette smoking is the major cause of the respiratory cancer epidemic that occurred in developed countries in the past century. Tobacco-associated diseases, including cancers, have a major impact on morbidity and mortality and are major contributors to health care costs. Although the relation between active cigarette smoking and lung cancer is well established, the relation between environmental tobacco smoke and lung cancer is still being debated. The data are, however, strongly suggestive, making it reasonable to enact laws designed to limit the public's exposure to the carcinogenic chemicals present in sidestream smoke. Finally, smokeless tobacco products, particularly snuff, can lead to the development of cancers of the oral cavity.

Potential interactions between cigarette smoking and other environmental exposures have been observed in some but not all studies. Recent advances in molecular genetics and the established etiological relationship between cigarette smoking and lung cancer provide an excellent opportunity to study gene-environmental interactions for a major cancer site. Given the clear etiologic relations between various chemical agents and various forms of cancer and the possibility of significant interactions, it seems prudent to develop public health interventions intended to eliminate or reduce exposure to both cigarette smoking and other sources of environmental carcinogens. A recent report from the National Cancer Institute[162] presents data from long-term follow-up of subjects enrolled in the early American Cancer Society's cancer prevention studies I and II, the US veterans study, and the more recent Kaiser Permanente and Nurses' Health studies. These data add to the substantial weight of evidence causally linking cigarette smoking with many chronic diseases.

Discussion Questions

1. Discuss the scientific evidence that supports a causal relationship between cigarette smoking and lung cancer in light of Bradford Hill's guidelines for assessing causality in epidemiological research.
2. Discuss concerns about information bias arising from the methods used in epidemiological studies to measure human exposure to tobacco smoke.
3. Discuss the various epidemiological design and measurement issues of concern that arise in studies of environmental tobacco smoke and lung cancer.
4. Discuss the methods used to measure genetic susceptibility to tobacco smoke in gene-environmental interaction studies of lung cancer.
5. Discuss the biological mechanism through which cigarette smoking might be related to cancer of the uterine cervix.
6. Discuss the epidemiological and experimental evidence linking smokeless tobacco use with cancers of the oral cavity.

References

1. US Surgeon General's Advisory Committee on Smoking and Health. *Smoking and Health.* Washington, DC: US Government Printing Office; 1964.USDHEW publication No. 1103.
2. US Department of Health and Human Services. *The Prevalence and Correlates of Treatment for Drug Problems.* Rockville, MD: Substance Abuse and Mental Health Administration, Office of Applied Studies; April 1997.
3. Public Health Practice Program Office, Epidemiology Branch, Office on Smoking and Health; Centers for Disease Control, National Center for Chronic Disease Prevention and Health Promotion. Cigarette smoking: attributable mortality and years of potential life lost—United States, 1990. *MMWR.* 1993;42:645–649.
4. Bartlett JC, Miller LS, Rice DP, Max WB. Medical-care expenditures attributable to cigarette smoking—United States, 1993. *MMWR* 1994;43:469–472.
5. Brown ML, Hodgson TA, Rice DA. Economic impact of cancer in the United States. In: Schohenfield D, Fraumeni JF Jr, eds. *Cancer Epidemiology and Prevention.* 2nd ed. New York: Oxford University Press; 1996:255–266.
6. International Agency for Research on Cancer. *Tobacco Smoking.* Lyon, France: World Health Organization; 1986:83–126. IARC Monographs on the Evaluation of the Carcinogenic Risk of Chemicals to Humans, No. 38.
7. Hernning RI, Jones RT, Bachman J, Mines AH. Puff volume increases when low-nicotine cigarettes are smoked. *BMJ.* 1981;283:187–189.
8. Ames, BN, Lee FD, Durston WE. An improved bacterial test system for the detection and classification of mutagens and carcinogens. *Proc Natl Acad Sci USA.* 1973;70:782–786.
9. Rothman KJ. *Modern Epidemiology.* Boston: Little, Brown & Co; 1986:84–85.
10. Kleinbaum DG, Kupper LL, Morgenstern H. *Epidemiologic Research: Principles and Quantitative Methods.* Belmont, CA: Lifetime Learning Publications; 1982:226–227.
11. US Department of Health and Human Services. *The Health Benefits of Smoking Cessation: A Report of the Surgeon General.* Rockville, MD: US Department of Health and Human Resources, Public Health Service, Centers for Disease Prevention and Health Promotion, Office on Smoking and Health; 1990. UDHHS (PHS) publication No. 90–8416.
12. Kroll EA, Valadian I, Dwyer JT, Gardner J. Accuracy of recalled smoking data. *Am J Public Health.* 1989;79:200–206.
13. Coultas DB, Peake GT, Samot JM. Questionnaire assessment of lifetime and recent exposure to environmental tobacco smoke. *Am J Epidemiol.* 1989;130:338–347.
14. Perera FP, Santella RM, Brenner D, et al. DNA adducts, protein adducts, and sister chromatid exchange in cigarette smokers and non-smokers. *J Natl Cancer Inst.* 1987;79:449–456.
15. Carmella SG, Kagan SS, Kagan M, et al. Mass spectometric analysis of tobacco-specific nitrosamine hemoglobin adducts in snuff dippers, smokers and non-smokers. *Cancer Res.* 1990:50:5438–5445.
16. Foiles PG, Akerkar SA, Carmella SG, Kagan M, et al. Mass spectometric analysis of tobacco-specific nitrosamine DNA adducts in smokers and non-smokers. *Chem Res Toxicol.* 1991;4:364–368.
17. Carmella SG, Akerkars S, Hecht SS. Metabolites of the tobacco-specific nitrosamine 4-(methylnitrosamineo)-1-(3-pyridyl)-butanone in smoker's urine. *Cancer Res.* 1993;53:721–724.
18. Stocks P. *Regional and Local Differences in Cancer Death Rates.* London: His Majesty's Stationery Office; 1947. Studies on Medical and Population Subjects, No. 1.
19. Kennaway EL, Kennaway NM. A further study of the incidence of cancer of the lung and larynx. *Br J Cancer.* 1947;1:260–298.
20. Clemmesen J, Busk T. On the apparent increase in the incidence of lung cancer in Denmark, 1931–1945. *Br J Cancer.* 1947;1:253–259.
21. Steiner PE. Incidence of primary carcinoma of the lung with special reference to its increase. *Arch Path.* 1944;37:185–195.
22. Levin ML, Goldstein H, Gerhardt PR. Cancer and tobacco smoking: a preliminary report. *JAMA.* 1950;143:336–338.
23. Wynder EL, Graham EA. Tobacco smoking as a possible etiologic factor in bronchiogenic carcinoma: a study of six hundred and eighty-four proved cases. *JAMA.* 1950;143:329–336.
24. Doll R, Hill AB. Smoking and carcinoma of the lung: preliminary report. *BMJ.* 1950;2:739–748.
25. Doll R, Hill AB. Lung cancer and other causes of death in relation to smoking: a second report of the mortality of British doctors. *BMJ.* 1956;2:1072–1081.

26. Hammond EC, Horn D. Smoking and death notes: report on forty-four months of follow-up of 187,783 men, II: death rates by cause. *JAMA.* 1958;166:1294–1308.
27. Medical Research Council. Tobacco smoking and cancer of the lung: statement of the Medical Research Council. *BMJ.* 1957;1:1523–1524.
28. Hill AB. The environment and disease: association or causation? *Proc R Soc Med.* 1965;58:295–300.
29. Hirayama T. Smoking in Relation to the Death Rates of 265,118 Men and Women in Japan. Tokyo: National Cancer Center Research Institute; 1967.
30. Cederlöf R, Friberg L, Hrubec Z, Lorich U. *The Relationship of Smoking and Some Social Co-variables to Mortality and Cancer Morbidity: A Ten Year Follow-up in a Probability Sample of 55,000 Swedish Subjects, Aged 18–69.* Parts 1, 2. Stockholm: Karolinska Institute, Department of Environmental Hygiene; 1975.
31. Rogot E, Murray JL. Smoking and causes of death among US veterans: 16 years of observation. *Publ Health Rep.* 1980;95:213–222.
32. Burns PB, Swanson GM. Risk of urinary bladder cancer among blacks and whites: the role of cigarette use and occupation. *Cancer Causes Control.* 1991;2:371–379.
33. Harris RE, Chen-Backlund JY, Wynder EL. Cancer of the urinary bladder in blacks and whites: a case-control study. *Cancer.* 1990;66:2673–2680.
34. Sturgeon SR, Hartge P, Silverman DT, et al. Associations between bladder cancer risk factors and tumor stage and grade at diagnosis. *Epidemiology.* 1994;5:218–225.
35. Siemiatycki J, Dewar R, Krewski D, Désy M, Richardson L, Franco E. Are the apparent effects of cigarette smoking on lung and bladder cancers due to uncontrolled confounding by occupational exposures? *Epidemiology.* 1994;5:57–65.
36. Iscovich J, Castelletto R, Estéve J, et al. Tobacco smoking, occupation exposure and bladder cancer in Argentina. *Int J Cancer.* 1987;40:734–740.
37. D'Avanzo B, Negri E, LaVecchia C, et al. Cigarette smoking and bladder cancer. *Eur J Cancer.* 1990;26:714–718.
38. López-Abente G, González CA, Errezola M, et al. Tobacco smoke inhalation pattern, tobacco type, and bladder cancer in Spain. *Am J Epidemiol.* 1991;134:830–839.
39. Jensen OM, Knudsen JB, McLaughlin JK, Strensen BL. The Copenhagen case-control study of renal pelvis and ureter cancer: role of smoking and occupational exposures. *Int J Cancer.* 1988;41:557–561.
40. Hartge P, Silverman D, Hoover R, et al. Changing cigarette habits and bladder cancer risk: a case-control study. *J Natl Cancer Inst.* 1987;78:1119–1125.
41. Burch JD, Rohan TE, Howe GR, et al. Risk of bladder cancer by source and type of tobacco exposure: a case-control study. *Int J Cancer.* 1989;44:622–628.
42. Slattery ML, Schumacher MC, West DW, Robison LM. Smoking and bladder cancer: the modifying effect of cigarettes on other factors. *Cancer.* 1988;61:402–408.
43. Sorahan T, Lancashire RJ, Sole G. Urothelial cancer and cigarette smoking: findings from a regional case-controlled study. *Br J Urol.* 1994;74:753–756.
44. Chyou PH, Nomura AM, Stemmermann GN. A prospective study of the attributable risk of cancer due to cigarette smoking. *Am J Public Health.* 1992;82:37–40.
45. Naguib SM, Landin FE Jr, Davis HJ. Relation of various epidemiologic factors to cervical cancer as determined by a screening program. *Obstet Gynecol.* 1966;28:451–459.
46. Thomas DB. An epidemiologic study of carcinoma in-situ and squamous dysplasia of the uterine cervix. *Am J Epidemiol.* 1973;98:10–28.
47. Cederlöf R, Friberg L, Hrubec Z, Lorich U. *The Relationship of Smoking and Some Social Co-variables to Mortality and Cancer Morbidity: A Ten Year Follow-up in a Probability Sample of 55,000 Swedish Subjects, Aged 18–69.* Parts 1, 2. Stockholm: Karolinska Institute, Department of Environmental Hygiene; 1975.
48. Williams RR, Horm JW. Association of cancer sites with tobacco and alcohol consumption and socioeconomic status of patients: interview study from the Third National Cancer Survey. *J Natl Cancer Inst.* 1977;58:525–547.
49. Wright NH, Vessey MP, Kenward B, et al. Neoplasia and dysplasia of the cervix uteri and contraception: a possible protective of the diaphragm. *Br J Cancer.* 1978;38:273–279.
50. Wigle DT, Mao Y, Grace M. Re: Smoking and cancer of the uterine cervix: hypothesis. *Am J Epidemiol.* 1980;111:125–127.
51. Stellman SD, Austin H, Wynder EL. Cervix cancer and cigarette smoking: a case-control study. *Am J Epidemiol.* 1980;111:383–388.

52. Clark EA, Morgan RW, Newman AM. Smoking as a risk factor in cancer of the uterine cervix: additional evidence from a case-control study. *Am J Epidemiol.* 1982;115:59–66.

53. Marshall JR, Graham S, Byers T, et al. Diet and smoking in the epidemiology of cancer of the cervix. *J Natl Cancer Inst.* 1983;70:847–851.

54. Trevathan E, Layde P, Webster LA, et al. Cigarette smoking and dysplasia and carcinoma in situ of the uterine cervix. *JAMA.* 1983;250:499–502.

55. Lyon JL, Gardner JW, West DW, et al. Smoking and carcinoma in situ of the uterine cervix. *Am J Public Health.* 1983;73:558–562.

56. LaVecchia C, Franceschi S, DeCarli A, et al. Cigarette smoking and the risk of cervical neoplasia. *Am J Epidemiol.* 1986;123:22–29.

57. Brinton LA, Schairer C, Haenszel W, et al. Cigarette smoking and invasive cervical cancer. *JAMA.* 1986;255:3265–3269.

58. Peters RK, Thomas D, Hagan DG, et al. Risk factors for invasive cervical cancer among Latinas and non-Latinas in Los Angeles County. *J Natl Cancer Inst.* 1986;77:1063–1077.

59. Nischan P, Ebeling K, Schindler C. Smoking and invasive cervical cancer risk: results from a case-control study. *Am J Epidemiol.* 1988;128:74–77.

60. Brisson J, Roy M, Fortier M, et al. Condyloma and intraepithelial neoplasia of the uterine cervix: a case-control study. *Am J Epidemiol.* 1988;128:337–342.

61. Licciardone JC, Wilkins JR III, Brownson RC, Chang JC. Cigarette smoking and alcohol consumption in the aetiology of uterine cervical cancer. *Int J Epidemiol.* 1989;18:533–537.

62. Brock KE, MacLennan R, Brinton LA, et al. Smoking and infectious agents and risk of in situ cervical cancer in Sidney, Australia. *Cancer Res.* 1989;49:4925–4928.

63. Herrero R, Brinton LA, Reeves WC, et al. Invasive cervical cancer and smoking in Latin America. *J Natl Cancer Inst.* 1989;81:205–211.

64. Cuzick J, Singer A, DeStavola BL, Chomet J. Case-control study of risk factors for CIN in young women. *Eur J Cancer.* 1990;76:684–690.

65. Jones CJ, Brinton LA, Hamman RF, et al. Risk factors for in situ cervical cancer: results from a case-control study. *Cancer Res.* 1990;50:3657–3662.

66. Daling JR, Sherman KJ, Hislop TG, et al. Cigarette smoking and the risk of anogenital cancer. *Am J Epidemiol.* 1992;135:180–189.

67. Becker TM, Wheeler CM, McGough NS, et al. Cigarette smoking and other risk factors for cervical dysplasia in southwestern Hispanic and non-Hispanic white women. *Cancer Epidemiol Biomarkers Prev.* 1994;3:113–119.

68. Kjaer SK, Van den Brule AJC, Bock JE, et al. Human papilloma virus—the most significant risk determinant for cervical intraepithelial neoplasia: a population-based prospective cohort study from Copenhagen. *Int J Cancer.* 1996;65:601–606.

69. Kjaer SK, Engholm G, Dahl C, Bock JE. Case-control study of risk factors for cervical squamous cell neoplasia in Denmark, IV: role of smoking habits. *Eur J Cancer Prev.* 1996;5:359–365.

70. Peng H, Liu S, Mann V, et al. Human papilloma virus types 16 and 33, herpes simplex virus type 2 and other risk factors for cervical cancer in Sichuan Province, China. *Int J Cancer.* 1991;47:711–716.

71. Bosch FX, Munoz N, DeSanjose S, et al. Risk factors for cervical cancer in Columbia and Spain. *Int J Cancer.* 1992;52:750–758.

72. Coker AL, Jenkins GR, Busnardo MS, et al. Human papilloma virus and cervical neoplasia in South Carolina. *Cancer Epidemiol Biomarkers Prev.* 1993;2:207–212.

73. Schiffman MH, Bauer HM, Hoover RN, et al. Epidemiologic evidence showing that human papilloma virus infection causes most cervical intraepithelial neoplasia. *J Natl Cancer Inst.* 1993;85:958–964.

74. Licciardone JC, Brownson RC, Chang JC, Wilkins JR III. Uterine cervical cancer risk in cigarette smokers: a meta-analytic study. *Am J Prev Med.* 1990;6:274–281.

75. Brinton LA, Nasca PC, Mallin K, et al. Case-control study of cancer of the vulva. *Obstet Gynecol.* 1990;75:859–866.

76. Winkelstein W. Smoking and cancer of the uterine cervix: hypothesis. *Am J Epidemiol.* 1977;106:257–259.

77. Winkelstein W, Shillitoe EJ, Brand R, Johnson KK. Further comments on cancer of the uterine cervix, smoking, and herpes virus infection. *Am J Epidemiol.* 1984;119:1–8.

78. Brinton LA, Tashima KT, Lehman HF, et al. Epidemiology of cervical cancer by cell type. *Cancer Res.* 1987;47:1706–1711.

79. Silcocks PBS, Thornton-Jones H, Murphy M. Squamous and adenocarcinoma of the uterine cervix: a comparison using routine data. *Br J Cancer.* 1987;55:321–325.

80. Parazzini F, La Vecchia C, Negri F, et al. Risk factors for adenocarcinoma of the cervix: a case-control study. *Br J Cancer.* 1988;57:201–204.

81. Holly EA, Petrakis NL, Friend NF, et al. Mutagenic mucus in the cervix of smokers. *J Natl Cancer Inst.* 1986;76:983–986.

82. McCann MF, Irwin DE, Walton LA, et al. Nicotine and cotinine in the cervical mucus of smokers, passive smokers, and non-smokers. *Cancer Epidemiol Biomarkers Prev.* 1992;1:125–129.

83. Smith EM, Sowers MF, Burn TL. Effects of smoking on the development of female reproductive cancers. *J Natl Cancer Inst.* 1984;73:371–376.

84. Lesko SM, Rosenberg L, Kaufman DW, et al. Cigarette smoking and the risk of endometrial cancer. *N Engl J Med.* 1985;313:593–596.

85. Baron JA, Byers T, Greenberg ER, et al. Cigarette smoking in women with cancers of the breast and reproductive organs. *J Natl Cancer Inst.* 1986;77:677–680.

86. Franks AL, Kendrick JS, Tyler CW Jr. Postmenopausal smoking, estrogen replacement therapy, and the risk of endometrial cancer. *Am J Obstet Gynecol.* 1987;156:20–23.

87. Lawrence C, Tessaro I, Durgerian S, et al. Smoking, body weight, and early-stage endometrial cancer. *Cancer.* 1987;59:1665–1669.

88. Stockwell HG, Lyman GH. Cigarette smoking and the risk of female reproductive cancer. *Am J Obstet Gynecol.* 1987;157:35–40.

89. Levi F, LaVecchia C, DeCarli A. Cigarette smoking and the risk of endometrial cancer. *Eur J Cancer Clin Oncol.* 1987;23:1025–1029.

90. Paganini-Hill A, Boss RK, Henderson BE. Endometrial cancer and patterns of use of oestrogen replacement therapy: a cohort study. *Br J Cancer.* 1989;59:445–447.

91. Koumantaki Y, Tzonou A, Koumantakis E, et al. A case-control study of cancer of endometrium in Athens. *Int J Cancer.* 1989;43:795–799.

92. Dahlgren E, Friberg LG, Johansson S, et al. Endometrial carcinoma; ovarian dysfunction: a risk factor in young women. *Eur J Obstet Gynecol Reprod Biol.* 1991;41:143–150.

93. Brinton LA, Barrett RJ, Berman ML, et al. Cigarette smoking and the risk of endometrial cancer. *Am J Epidemiol.* 1993;137:281–291.

94. Austin H, Drews C, Partridge EE. A case-control study of endometrial cancer in relation to cigarette smoking, serum estrogen levels and alcohol use. *Am J Obstet Gynecol.* 1993;169:1086–1091.

95. Parazzini F, LaVecchia C, Negri E, et al. Smoking and risk of endometrial cancer: results from an Italian case-control study. *Gynecol Oncol.* 1995;56:195–199.

96. Key TJ, Pike MC, Brown JB, et al. Cigarette smoking and urinary estrogen excretion in pre-menopausal and post-menopausal women. *Br J Cancer.* 1996;74:1313–1316.

97. Khaw KT, Tazuke S, Barrett-Connor E. Cigarette smoking and levels of adrenal androgens in post-menopausal women. *N Engl J Med.* 1988;318:1705–1709.

98. Baron JA. Beneficial effects of cigarette smoking: the real, the possible, and the spurious. *Br Med Bull.* 1996;52:58–73.

99. Siegel M. Smoking and leukemia: evaluation of a causal hypothesis. *Am J Epidemiol.* 1993;138:1–9.

100. Brownson RC, Novotny TE, Perry MC. Cigarette smoking and adult leukemia: a meta-analysis. *Arch Intern Med.* 1993;153:469–475.

101. Wallace L, Pellizzari E, Hartwell TD, et al. Exposures to benzene and other volatile compounds from active and passive smoking. *Environ Health.* 1987;42:272–279.

102. Ong CN, Lee BL, Shi CY, et al. Elevated levels of benzene related compounds in the urine of cigarette smokers. *Int J Cancer.* 1994;59:177–180.

103. Holtzman RB, Ilcewica FH. Lead-210 and polonium-210 in tissues of cigarette smokers. *Science.* 1966;153:1259–1260.

104. Blanchard RL. Concentrations of 210 P_b and 210 P_o in human soft tissues. *Health Phys.* 1967;13:625–632.

105. Crane MM, Keating MJ, Trujillo JM, et al. Environmental exposures in cytogenetically defined subsets of acute non-lymphocytic leukemia. *JAMA.* 1989;262:634–639.

106. National Research Council. *Environmental Tobacco Smoke: Measuring Exposures and Assessing Health Effects.* Washington DC: National Academy Press;1986.

107. US Environmental Protection Agency. *Respiratory Health Effects of Passive Smoking: Lung Cancer and Other Disorders.* Washington, DC: US Environmental Protection Agency; 1992. EPA/6001 6-901006F.

108. Gori GB. Sciences, policy, and ethics: the case of environmental tobacco smoke. *J Clin Epidemiol.* 1994;47:325–334.

109. Farland W, Bayard S, Jinot J. Environmental tobacco smoke: a public health conspiracy? A dissenting view. *J Clin Epidemiol.* 1994;47:335–337.

110. Jinot J, Bayard S. Respiratory health effects of passive smoking: EPA's weight-of-evidence analysis. *J Clin Epidemiol.* 1994;47:339–349.

111. Gross AJ. The risk of lung cancer in nonsmokers in the United States and its reported association with environmental tobacco smoke. *J Clin Epidemiol.* 1995;48:587–598.

112. VanLeeuwen FE. The risk of lung cancer in nonsmokers in the United States: a causal association with environmental tobacco smoke. *J Clin Epidemiol.* 1995;48:599–601.

113. Pershagen G. Passive smoking and lung cancer. In: Samet J, ed. *Epidemiology of Lung Cancer.* New York: Dekker; 1994:109–130.

114. Kabat GC, Stellman SD, Wynder EL. Relation between exposure to environmental tobacco smoke and lung cancer in lifetime nonsmokers. *Am J Epidemiol.* 1995;142:141–148.

115. Brownson RC, Alavanja MC, Hock ET. Reliability of passive smoke exposure histories in a case-control study of lung cancer. *Int J Epidemiol.* 1993;22:804–808.

116. Becher H, Zatonski W, Jockel KH. Passive smoking in Germany and Poland: comparison of exposure levels, sources of exposure, validity, and perception. *Epidemiology.* 1992;3:509–514.

117. Riboli E, Haley NJ, Tredaniel J, et al. Misclassification of smoking status among women in relation to exposure to environmental tobacco smoke. *Eur Respir J.* 1995;8:285–290.

118. Ogden MW, Morgan WT, Heavner DL, et al. National incidence of smoking and misclassification among the US married female population. *J Clin Epidemiol.* 1997;50:253–263.

119. Tweedie RL, Mengersen KL. Meta-analytic approaches to dose-response relationships, with application in studies of lung cancer and exposure to environmental tobacco smoke. *Stat Med.* 1995;14:545–569.

120. Lee PN, Forgey BA. Misclassification of smoking habits as a source of bias in the study of environmental tobacco smoke and lung cancer. *Stat Med.* 1996;15:581–605.

121. Barry D. Differential recall bias and spurious associations in case-control studies. *Stat Med.* 1996;15:2603–2616.

122. US Department of Health and Human Services. *The Health Consequences of Using Smokeless Tobacco: A Report of the Advisory Committee to the Surgeon General, 1986.* Bethesda, MD: National Institutes of Health; 1986. NIH publication No. 86-2874.

123. Winn DM, Blot WJ, Shy CM, et al. Snuff dipping and oral cancer among women in the southern United States. *N Engl J Med.* 1981;304:745–749.

124. Winn DM. Smokeless tobacco and oral-pharynx cancer: the role of cofactors. In: Hoffman D, Harris CC, eds. *Mechanism in Tobacco Carcinogenesis.* Cold Spring Harbor, NY: Cold Spring Harbor Laboratory; 1986. Banbury Report No. 23.

125. Orr IM. Oral cancer in betel nut chewers in Travancore. *Lancet.* 1933;2:575–580.

126. Shanta V, Krishnamurthi S. A study of aetiological factors in oral squamous cell carcinoma. *Br J Cancer.* 1959;13:381.

127. Chandra A. Different habits and their relation with cheek cancer. *Bulletin Cancer Hospital National Cancer Research Center.* 1962;1:33.

128. Wahi PN. The epidemiology of oral and oropharyngeal cancer. *Bull World Health Organ.* 1968;38:495–521.

129. Jussawala DJ, Deshpande VA. Evaluation of cancer risk in tobacco chewers and smokers: an epidemiologic assessment. *Cancer.* 1971;28:244–252.

130. Jafary NA, Zaidi SH. Carcinoma of the oral cavity in Karachi, Pakistan: an appraisal. *Trop Doct.* 1976;6:63.

131. Gupta PC, Pindborg JJ, Mehta FS. Comparison of carcinogenicity of betel quid with and without tobacco: an epidemiological review. *Ecol Dis.* 1982;1:213–219.

132. Jayant K, Balakrishnan V Sanghvi LD, Jussawalla DJ. Quantification of the role of smoking and chewing tobacco in oral, pharyngeal, and esophageal cancers. *Br J Cancer.* 1977;35:232–235.

133. Smith JF, Mincer HA, Hopins KP, Bell J. Snuff-dippers lesion: a cytological and pathological study in a large population. *Arch Otolaryngol.* 1970;92:450–456.

134. Smith JF. Snuff dippers lesion: a ten-year follow-up. *Arch Otolaryngol.* 1975;101:2767–277.

135. Bjelke E, Schuman LM. Chewing tobacco and use of snuff: relationships to cancer of the pancreas and other sites in two prospective studies. In: Proceedings of the 13th International Congress on Cancer; September 1982; Seattle, WA.

136. Winn DM, Walrath J, Blot W, Rogot E. Chewing tobacco and snuff in relation to cause of death in a large prospective cohort. *Am J Epidemiol.* 1982;116:567.

137. International Agency for Research on Cancer. *Tobacco Habits Other Than Smoking: Betel-Quid and Areca-Nut Chewing and Some Related Nitrosamines.* Lyon, France: World Health Organization; 1985:103–104. IARC Monographs on the Evaluation of the Carcinogenic Risk of Chemicals to Humans, No. 37.

138. Schwartz D, Denoix PF, Anquerra G. Recherche des localisations du cancer associées aux facteurs tabac et alcool chez L'homme. *Bulletin Association Etude Cancer.* 1957;44:336–361.

139. Wynder EL, Bross IG, Feldman RM. A study of etiological factors in cancer of the mouth. *Cancer.* 1957;10:1300–1322.

140. Keller AZ, Terris M. The association of alcohol and tobacco with cancer of the mouth and pharynx. *Am J Public Health.* 1965;55:1578–1585.

141. Rothman K, Keller A. The effect of joint exposure to alcohol and tobacco on risk of cancer of the mouth and pharynx. *J Chronic Dis.* 1972;25:711–716.

142. Saraccci R. The interactions of tobacco smoking and other agents in etiology. *Epidemiology Rev.* 1987;9:175–193.

143. Shopland DR, Eyre HJ, Pechacek TF. Smoking-attributable cancer mortality in 1991: is lung cancer now the leading cause of death among smokers in the United States? *J Natl Cancer Institute.* 1991;83:1142–1148.

144. Tokuhata GK, Lilienfeld AM. Familial aggregation of lung cancer in humans. *J Natl Cancer Inst.* 1963;30:289–312.

145. Ooi WL, Elston RC, Chen VW, et al. Increased familial risk for lung cancer. *J Natl Cancer Inst.* 1986;76:217–222.

146. Sellers TA, Elston RC, Rothchild H. Familial risk of cancer among randomly selected probands. *Genet Epidemiol.* 1988;5:381–392.

147. Sellers TA, Baily-Wilson JE, Elston RC, et al. Evidence for Mendelian inheritance in the pathogenesis of lung cancer? *J Natl Cancer Inst.* 1990;82:1272–1279.

148. Carmelli D, Swan GE, Robinerre D, Fabsitz R. Genetic influence on smoking: a study of male twins. *N Engl J Med.* 1992;327:829–833.

149. Wei Q, Spitz MR. The role of DNA repair capacity in susceptibility to lung cancer: a review. *Cancer Metastasis Rev.* 1997;16:295–307.

150. Bishop JM. Molecular themes in oncogenesis. *Cell.* 1991;64:235–248.

151. Levine AJ. The tumor suppressor genes. *Annu Rev Biochem.* 1993;62:623–651.

152. Sherr CJ. Cancer cell cycles. *Science.* 1996;274:1672–1677.

153. Hsu TC, Johnston DA, Cherry LM, et al. Sensitivity to genotoxic events of bleomycin in humans: possible relationship to environmental carcinogens. *Int J Cancer.* 1989;43:403–409.

154. Lee JJ, Trizna Z, Hsu TC, et al. A statistical analysis of the reliability and classification error in application of the mutagen sensitivity assay. *Cancer Epidemiol Biomarkers Prev.* 1996;5:191–197.

155. Spitz MR, Hsu TC, Wu X, et al. Mutagen sensitivity as a biomarker of lung cancer risk in African Americans. *Cancer Epidemiol Biomarkers Prev.* 1995;4:99–103.

156. Cloos J, Spitz MR, Schantz SP, et al. Genetic susceptibility to head and neck squamous cell carcinoma. *J Natl Cancer Inst.* 1996;88:530–535.

157. Wei Q, Gu J, Cheng L, et al. Benzo[*a*]pyrene diol epoxide induced chromosomal aberrations in normal human lymphocytes. *Cancer Res.* 1996;56:3975–3979.

158. Wei Q, Cheng L, Hong WK, Spitz MR. Reduced DNA repair capacity in lung cancer patients. *Cancer Res.* 56:4103–4107.

159. Reddy MV, Randerath K. Nuclease P1-mediated enhancement of sensitivity of ^{32}P-postlabeling test for structurally diverse DNA adducts. *Carcinogenesis.* 1986;7:1543–1551.

160. Watson WP. Postradiolabeling for detection of DNA damage. *Mutagenesis.* 1987;2:319–331.

161. Wu X, Shi H, Jiang H, et al. Associations between cytochrome P-4502E1 genotype, mutagen sensitivity, cigarette smoking and susceptibility to lung cancer. *Carcinogenesis.* 1997;18:967–973.

162. National Cancer Institute. Changes in cigarette-related disease risks and their implication for prevention and control. Washington, DC: National Institutes of Health; 1997. NIH publication No. 97-4213.

Chapter 10

Alcohol and Cancer

Philip C. Nasca

The chapter begins by providing an overview of alcohol consumption patterns in the United States over the past 60 years and by discussing the enormous economic impact of alcohol abuse on our society, including both medical and nonmedical costs. It then reviews the scientific evidence supporting the existence of a causal relationship between excess alcohol consumption and cancers of the upper aerodigestive tract, bladder, and liver. It first focuses on experimental studies and discusses their strengths and weaknesses in light of the general principles of good laboratory practice (see Chapter 5). Next it examines descriptive epidemiological studies of concomitant variations between alcohol consumption patterns and cancer incidence and mortality patterns, including the role of these studies in generating hypotheses and in providing findings to confirm or disconfirm the results derived from analytic epidemiological studies. The chapter also provides a detailed review of methodological studies designed to assess the reliability and validity of alcohol intake measurement in epidemiological studies. Finally, it looks at the large number of studies that have investigated the relationship between alcohol consumption and breast cancer risk. Particular emphasis is placed on assessing the extent to which existing data support a causal relationship between alcohol consumption and breast cancer.

Alcohol has been shown to be causally related to cancers of the oral cavity and pharynx, esophagus, and larynx. Associations have also been reported for alcohol and cancers of the bladder and liver and female breast, although the nature of the relation between these cancers and alcohol consumption has not been fully elucidated. This chapter examines the experimental and epidemiological data that support a causal relation between alcohol consumption and cancers of the upper respiratory and digestive tract. It also describes the current state of our knowledge about alcohol and other cancers, including gaps in the existing research, and discusses the validity of alcohol consumption data derived from epidemiological studies.

ALCOHOL CONSUMPTION PATTERNS AND THE ECONOMIC COSTS OF ALCOHOL ABUSE

Alcohol use patterns can be tracked over time by means of a number of approaches. In a recent report for the National Institute of Alcohol Abuse and Alcoholism (NIAAA), Williams et al[1] presented time trends for US per capita consumption for the years 1935–1994 (Figure 10–1). These consumption estimates are based on sales of alcoholic beverages, state tax receipts, and shipment figures provided by major industry sources. An estimate of the average ethanol content of each beverage is used to convert gallons of

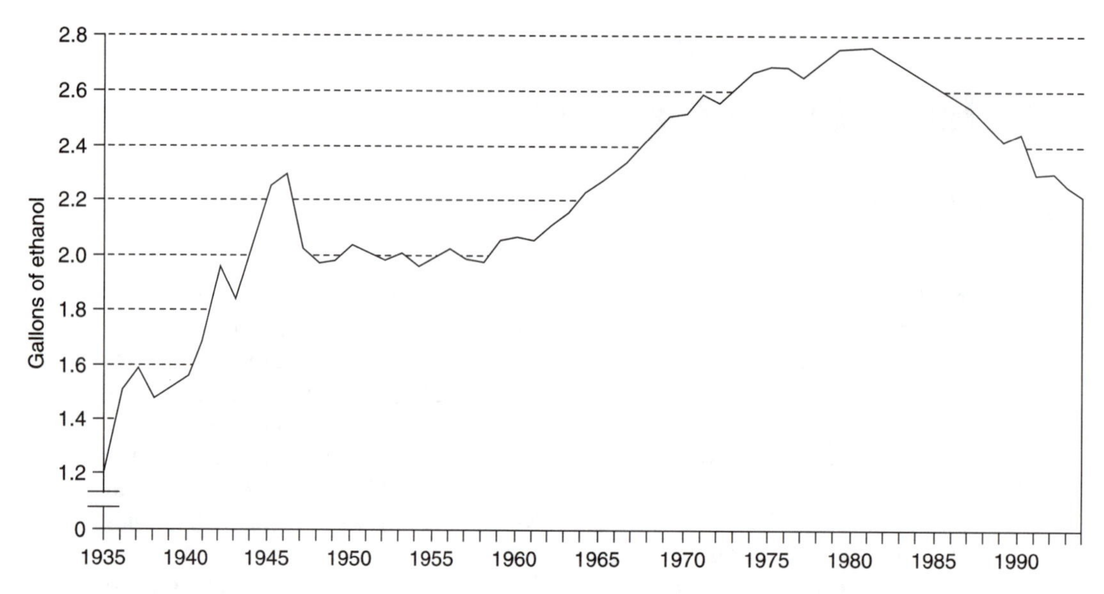

Figure 10–1 Total per capita ethanol consumption, United States, 1935–94. *Source:* Adapted from G.D. Williams, et al., *Apparent Per Capita Alcohol Consumption: National, State, and Regional Trends, 1977–1994*, Surveillance Report No. 39, pp. 1–37, 1996, National Institute on Alcohol Abuse and Alcoholism.

sold or shipped beverages into gallons of ethanol prior to calculating per capita consumption. The data show large increases in per capita ethanol consumption from 1935 through the end of World War II. The consumption level remained fairly stable from 1946 until the end of the 1950s but increased again between 1960 and 1980. Beginning in the early 1980s, consumption began to decrease dramatically, declining from just under 2.8 gallons per capita to just over 2.2 gallons per capita in 1994. The declines have been most prominent for spirits (so-called hard liquor) and wine, with beer consumption remaining somewhat stable over time.

A second approach to measuring trends in alcohol consumption involves the use of population-based surveys designed to measure health-related behaviors. In 1995, Bray et al[2] reported alcohol use patterns for active-duty military personnel. These data cover six selected years between 1980 and 1995. The percentage of respondents reporting heavy or moderate to heavy alcohol use declined significantly over time. In 1980, 53.2% of those interviewed reported heavy or moderate to heavy use. By 1990, the percentage of respondents reporting these levels of drinking had declined to 41.3%. The percentage reporting negative effects from alcohol consumption, including productivity loss or dependence, declined from 52% to 29.6%. Another source of data on alcohol consumption patterns is the Behavioral Risk Factor Surveillance System (BRFSS), which is designed to collect risk factor data from a random sample of the population residing in each of the 50 states. According to 1995 BRFSS data,[3] 21.3% of men and 6.9% of women reported binge drinking, which was defined as drinking five or more alcoholic beverages on at least one occasion during the previous month. The data also show higher rates of chronic drinking among men (4.8%) than among women (0.7%). Chronic or type II drinking is defined as consumption of 60 or more alcoholic beverages during the previous month.

A third approach to estimating changes in drinking patterns over time is to track mortality rates for diseases in which alcohol abuse is an established contributing cause. It has been estimated that between 41% and 95% of all cirrhosis deaths may be attributable to alcohol abuse.[4] DeBakey et al[5] reported age-adjusted death rates for liver cirrhosis in the United States by sex for the years 1933–1993 (Figure 10–2). After 1914, the overall rate of death attributed to cirrhosis declined dramatically, reaching an all-time low in 1932 of 8.0 per 100,000 population. The rate remained fairly constant throughout the 1930s and 1940s but then began to increase steadily, reaching a peak in 1973 of 14.9 per 100,000. Since 1973, it has again shown declining trends, reaching a low of 7.9 per 100,000 in 1993. Throughout the period 1910–1993, the male cirrhosis death rate has been significantly higher than the rate for females, but the time trends have been quite similar for both genders.

Alcohol consumption patterns have been shown to vary significantly by gender. Table 10–1 shows that men are significantly more likely than women to be classified as current drinkers. Indicators of alcohol abuse are also more prevalent among men than women. Men are more likely than women to engage in binge drinking and driving while intoxicated and to be classified as chronic drinkers.

In addition to the human costs of alcohol, the economic costs of alcohol abuse are enormous and pose a serious challenge for public health policy in the United States and other countries throughout the world. Total costs include direct health care and indirect morbidity and mortality costs and non-health-sector expenditures associated with alcohol abuse.[6,7] Two studies have estimated the total societal losses due to alcohol abuse in the United States to be between $70.3 billion and $116 billion per annum. The difference in the estimates results from the use of different methodologies and sources of data. However, even assuming the lower estimate, alcohol abuse clearly represents a significant financial burden for the nation.

SCIENTIFIC EVIDENCE LINKING ALCOHOL AND SELECTED CANCERS

Experimental Studies

Alcohol beverages consist primarily of ethanol, water, and volatile and nonvolatile compounds that contribute to flavor and are derived from the raw materials, the fermentation process, or the wooden casks in which the beverages are aged. The type and amount of each compound vary by beverage type. Numerous additives are also used in the production of alcoholic beverages, such as hops, synthetic flavor enhancers, preservatives, and trace elements. In addition, a number of contaminants have been detected in alcoholic beverages, including compounds with proven mutagenic or carcinogenic properties. These include *N*-nitrosamines, mycotoxins (eg, aflatoxin), urethane, asbestos, arsenic compounds, and pesticides—all substances known or strongly suspected to be carcinogenic agents in various animal models or in humans.[8]

The characteristics of experimental studies designed to examine the potential carcinogenicity of alcohol or its metabolites are summarized in Exhibit 10–1. Experiments have been conducted that involve the direct feeding of alcohol beverages or ethanol to various rodent species, the application of ethanol to the skin of these animals, or the

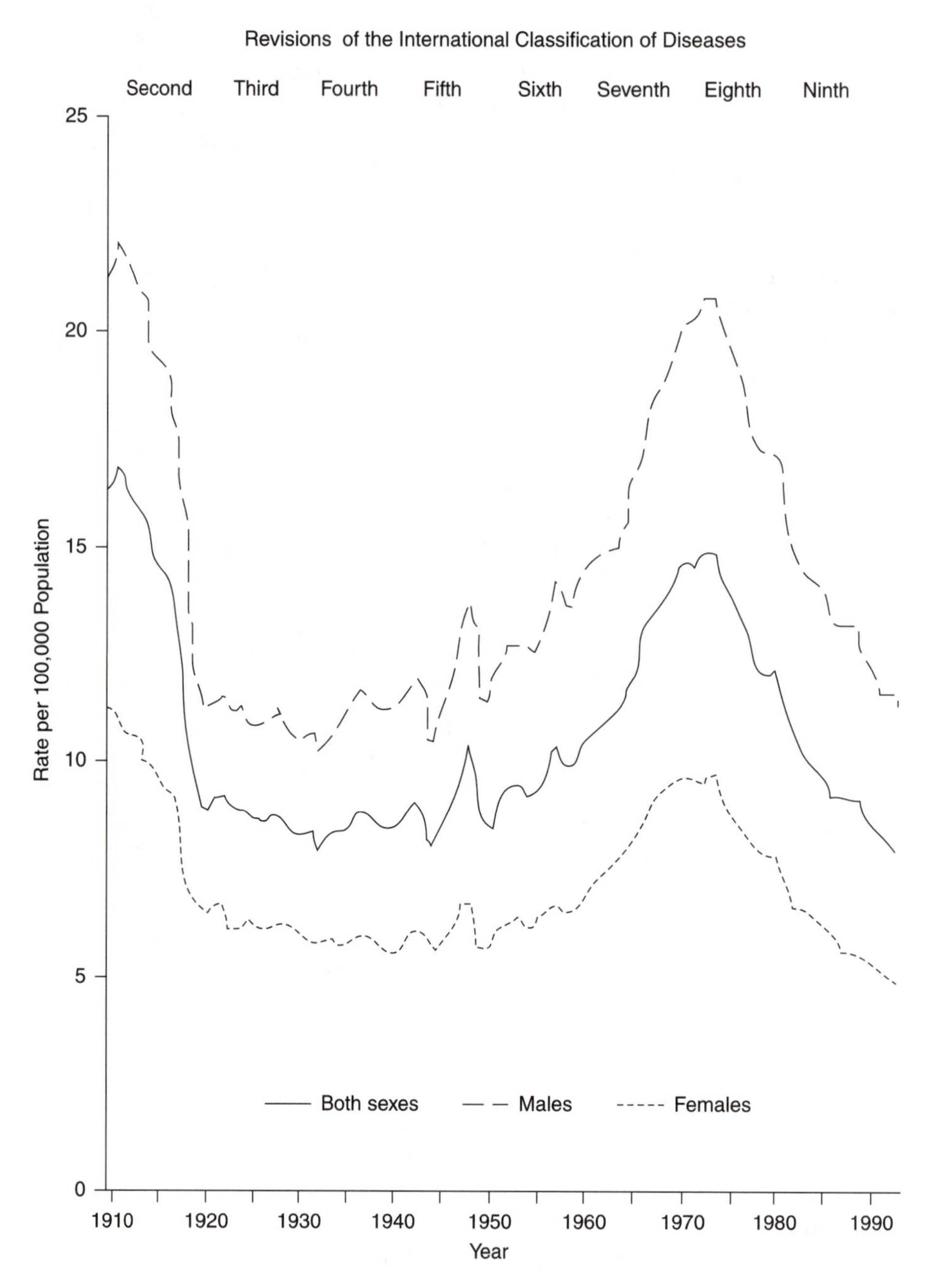

Figure 10–2 Age-adjusted death rates of liver cirrhosis by sex (death-registration states, 1910–1932, and United States, 1933–1993). *Source:* Reprinted from S.F. DeBakey, et al., *Liver Cirrhosis Mortality in the United States, 1970–1993*, NIAAA Surveillance Report No. 41, pp. 1–25, 1996, National Institute on Alcohol Abuse and Alcoholism.

---

transplacental or neonatal administration of alcohol. The studies have, for the most part, not produced an excess incidence of cancer. Studies have also been conducted to investigate the possibility that alcohol might enhance the carcinogenic activity of certain compounds. Experiments with various *N*-nitroso compounds generally failed to show that

Table 10–1 Alcohol Consumption Patterns by Gender

	Estimated Prevalence	
Alcohol Measure	*Males (%)*	*Females (%)*
Current drinking[1]	61.9	43.7
Binge drinking[2]	22.3	6.7
Chronic drinking[3]	5.4	0.8
Drinking and driving[4]	3.0	0.9

[1]Had alcoholic beverages during the past month.
[2]Five or more drinks on at least one occasion during the past month.
[3]Sixty or more drinks during the past month.
[4]Driving after having too much to drink one or more times.
Source: Reprinted from Behavioral Risk Factor Surveillance Data, 1997, the Centers for Disease Control and Prevention.

Exhibit 10–1 Experimental Studies of Alcohol and Cancer

Direct Feeding Experiments with Ethanol and Alcohol

- Most experiments involved oral administration of alcohol or alcoholic beverages to various strains of mice, rats, and hamsters; a few skin application experiments also have been conducted.
- Most studies show no statistically significant elevation in tumor incidence among exposed animals.

Alcohol in Combination with Known Carcinogens

- Some experiments showed an enhanced incidence of nasal cavity, forestomach, esophageal, and lung tumors in rodents exposed orally to alcohol, after injection with N-nitroso compounds; most studies showed no increased incidence associated with combined exposure to alcohol and N-nitroso compounds.
- Oral administration of vinyl chloride and ethanol increased the incidence of hepatocellular tumors and angiosarcomas of the liver.
- No enhanced carcinogenic effect was observed for combined exposure to alcohol and urethane.

Experimental Studies of Ethanol Metabolites

- Sufficient evidence exists for the carcinogenicity of acetaldehyde, a major metabolite of ethanol; an increased risk of adenocarcinomas of the respiratory tract was observed following inhalation of the chemical by experimental animals; particularly associated with squamous cell carcinomas of the nasal mucosa in rats and laryngeal carcinomas in hamsters.

The IARC working group has criticized many studies for

- failure to adequately report on study methods
- failure to conduct adequate histopathologic examinations of tumors
- small sample sizes and low statistical power
- small doses over short time periods
- inadequate follow-up periods
- absence of an untreated control group
- failure to control for important confounding factors

Source: Reprinted with permission from *Alcohol Drinking*, IARC Monographs on the Evaluation of Carcinogenic Risk to Humans, No. 44, pp. 71–321, © 1988, International Agency for Research on Cancer.

injecting rodents with these compounds in conjunction with feeding them alcohol had a carcinogenic effect. In several studies, the animals treated with a known carcinogen and alcohol actually experienced a lower incidence of various cancers than the animals treated only with the carcinogen. Rats exposed to vinyl chloride and ethanol experienced an increased incidence of hepatocellular carcinomas and angiosarcomas of the liver. Other experiments have failed to show an enhanced carcinogenic effect of urethane in the presence of alcohol. One study did show an increased number of pulmonary tumors among animals treated with urethane and alcohol in comparison with animals treated only with urethane. The carcinogenic potential of acetaldehyde, a major metabolite of ethanol, has been studied by exposing rats and hamsters via inhalation and intratracheal instillation. Inhalation of acetaldehyde produced an increased incidence of tumors of the respiratory tract in rats and hamsters and appeared to enhance the carcinogenic activity of benzo[*a*]pyrene, a potent carcinogen, but intratracheal instillation of the metabolite failed to produce an increased tumor incidence in hamsters.[8] IARC has determined that sufficient evidence exists to classify acetaldehyde as an animal carcinogen.[9,10]

These studies suffer from a number of methodological limitations, including the failure to report on study methods adequately, the failure to use an untreated control group, and the absence of careful histopathologic examinations of suspected tumors. This last limitation is important because of the difficulty of separating benign from malignant tumors in many animal species. Many of these studies also included small numbers of animals and may have lacked sufficient statistical power to detect a relationship between alcohol exposure and cancer. In addition, bias toward a negative finding may have resulted from the small dosages or the short testing or follow-up period. Some studies also failed to control for confounding variables such as nutrient intake.[8]

Descriptive Epidemiological Studies

Alcohol abuse has been causally linked to cancers of the oral cavity, esophagus, larynx, bladder, and liver. Secular incidence and mortality trends for esophageal cancers in the United States are presented separately for males and females in Figure 10–3. These data show a slow but steady increase in esophageal cancer incidence and mortality among males for the years 1973–1994. During this same time period, incidence and mortality rates for females remained fairly constant. The similarity of the incidence and mortality rates, particularly for males, is a clear indication of the poor chance of survival associated with these cancers. Data from the SEER program of population-based cancer registries show five-year survival rates for cancers of the oral cavity and pharynx, esophagus, and larynx to be 51.3%, 11.7%, and 64.6%, respectively.[11] These data also clearly demonstrate that males experience a significantly higher esophageal cancer disease burden than females.

Similar male excesses are observed for cancers of the oral cavity and pharynx, esophagus, and larynx (Figure 10–4). As previously noted, males are also more likely than females to report moderate to heavy alcohol use and to die from alcohol-related diseases such as cirrhosis of the liver. The data in Figure 10–4 also show that African Americans experience higher incidence rates for cancers of the aerodigestive tract than Caucasians, with the highest rate observed among African American males.

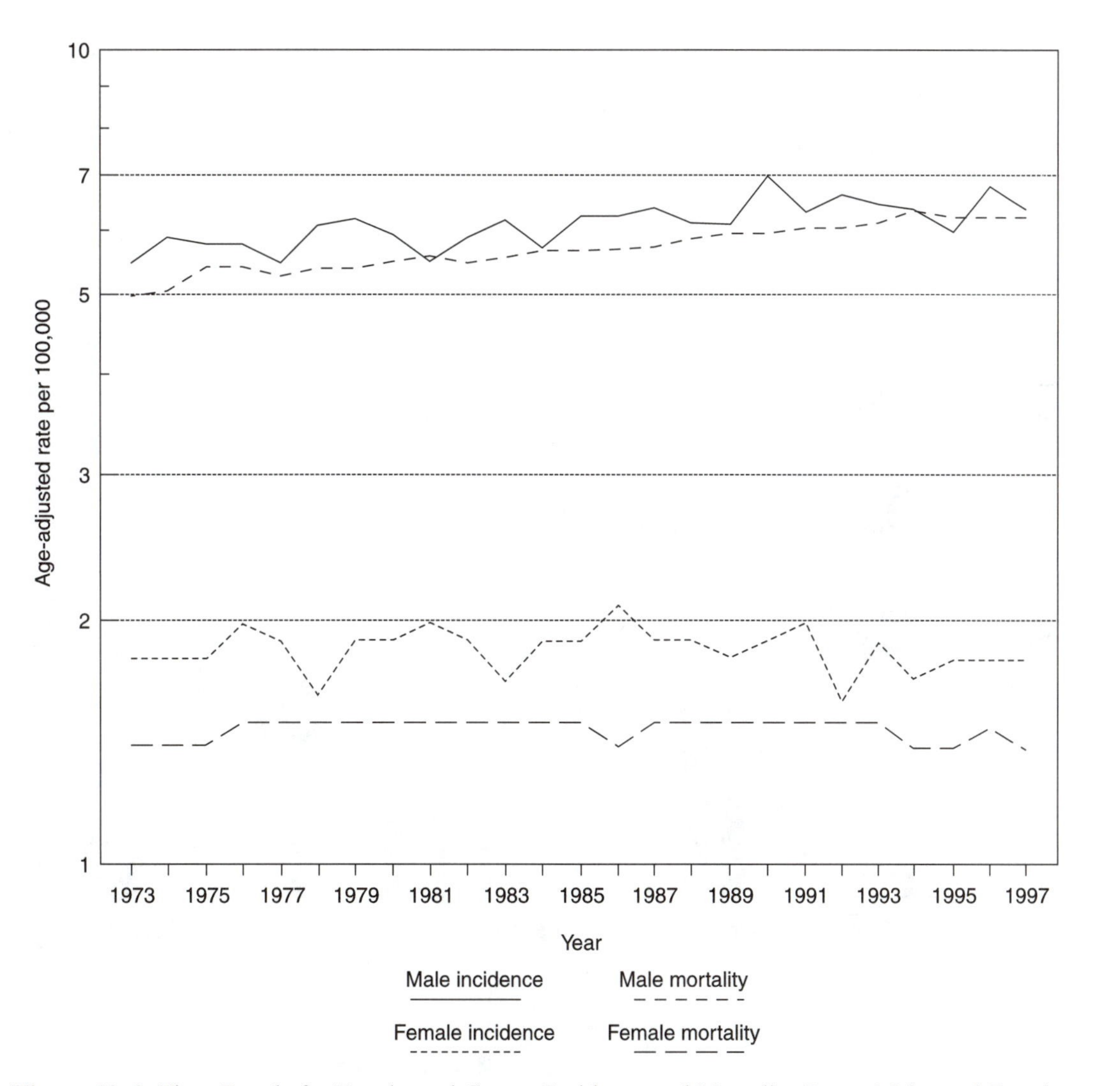

Figure 10–3 Time Trends for Esophageal Cancer Incidence and Mortality Rates, Males and Females, United States, 1973–1997. *Source:* Data from Surveillance, Epidemiology and End Results Program, National Cancer Institute.

Ecological studies have been conducted in which cancer incidence or mortality rates for selected cancers were compared to various measures of alcohol exposure in the same geographical subunits; these studies are summarized in Exhibit 10–2. Measures of alcohol exposure in each population were based on production or sales data or rates of other diseases already known to be associated with alcohol abuse.[8] Geographical correlation studies that compare disease rates and alcohol consumption measures for various countries[12] and for regions within a country[13–19] have also been conducted. Esophageal cancers were most strongly linked to alcohol consumption patterns, while weaker associations have been reported for cancers of the buccal cavity, pharynx, and larynx. Two studies showed a strong positive correlation between per capita beer consumption and

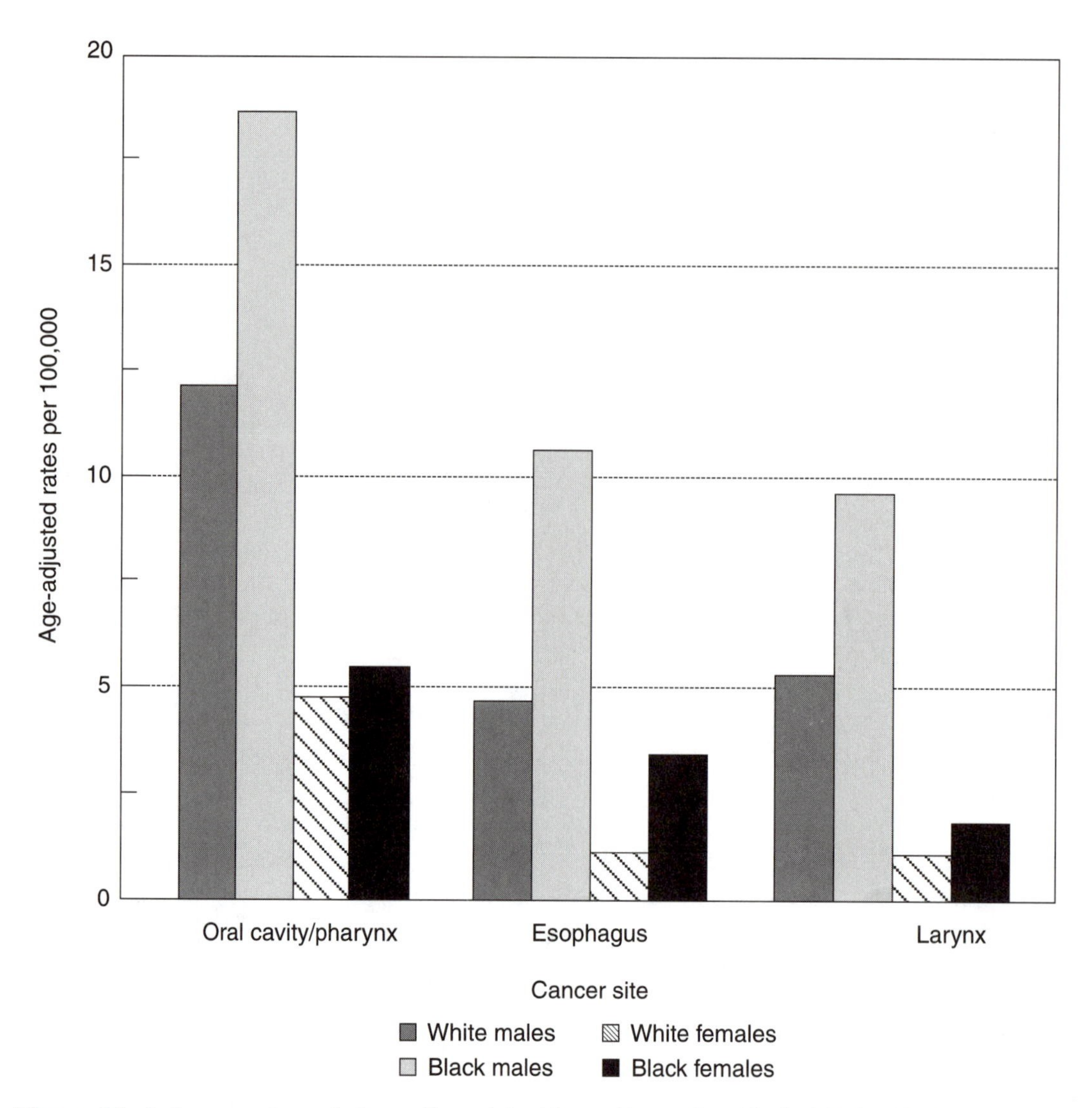

Figure 10–4 Average Annual Age-adjusted Incidence Rates for Alcohol-Related Cancers of the Aerodigestive Tract, United States, 1993–1997. *Source:* Data from Surveillance, Epidemiology and End Results Program, National Cancer Institute.

---

mortality from cancer of the rectum,[18,19] and another study suggested a possible association between alcohol use and stomach cancer.[16] In several studies, male:female ratios for selected cancers, such as cancers of the upper digestive tract and larynx, were similar to male:female ratios for alcohol-related diseases or for consumption of alcohol.[20–23]

A number of time trend analyses have also suggested concomitant variation over time in alcohol consumption patterns and mortality rates for cancers of the upper digestive tract, larynx, and colon.[24–31] Several investigators[32–34] have examined cancer mortality for birth cohorts in countries with high or increasing levels of alcohol consumption. After taking appropriate account of the latent period between first exposure and the onset of disease, these

Exhibit 10–2 Summary of Ecologic Studies Suggesting an Association between Alcohol Consumption and Various Forms of Cancer

International Comparisons

Positive correlations between per capita consumption of alcoholic beverages and cancers of the esophagus; associations weaker for cancers of the mouth, pharynx, and stomach; several studies show strong relation between per capita consumption of beer and cancer of the rectum.

Time Trend Studies

Results of time trend studies show results similar to those reported from international comparison studies; the male to female ratio of cancer mortality rates was similar to the male to female ratio for alcohol consumption patterns and for mortality from alcoholic liver cirrhosis.

Cancer Incidence and Mortality Rates in Religious Groups

Mormons, Seventh-Day Adventists, and other religious groups who abstain from alcohol and tobacco consumption show low incidence and mortality rates for cancers of the lung, oral cavity, pharynx, larynx, esophagus, and urinary bladder.

Source: Reprinted with permission from *Alcohol Drinking*, IARC Monographs on the Evaluation of Carcinogenic Risk to Humans, No. 44, pp. 71–321, © 1988, International Agency for Research on Cancer.

analyses showed increases in the mortality rates for cancers of the tongue,[32] esophagus,[33,34] oral cavity,[34] and larynx[34] in successive birth cohorts that were consistent with the existence of a causal relation between these cancers and alcohol consumption.

Descriptive studies of occupational groups have also suggested a causal relation between alcohol consumption and various cancers. McMichael et al[35] studied patterns of male mortality in Australia during the years 1968–1978. Death rates for liver cirrhosis, alcoholism, and alcoholic psychosis were elevated in various rural, service, and blue-collar groups. Mortality rates for cancers of the upper alimentary tract, larynx, and stomach were also elevated in these occupational groups. Lindsay et al[36] studied the mortality experience of 415,309 men enrolled in the Canadian Labor Force Ten Percent Sample Study. This record linkage study included 9,739 deaths attributed to cancer between 1965 and 1979 among men employed in 274 occupations and 294 industries. Thirty-three cancer sites were studied, and the investigators found that waiters, bartenders, and men working in breweries had elevated risks for cancers of the buccal cavity and pharynx.

The association between alcohol consumption and various cancers is further supported by studies of religious groups who abstain from consuming alcoholic beverages. These groups invariably show lower incidence and mortality rates for cancers of the aerodigestive tract than the general population. Reduced rates have been observed among Mormons[37–44] and Seventh-Day Adventists,[45–49] two religious groups who abstain from using either alcohol or tobacco. Several studies have also examined cancer incidence[41,42] and mortality[43] among Mormons based on the level of church activity. Gardner[41] examined cancer incidence rates for various cancer sites in three groups of male church members classified according to priesthood office. Men in the first group had never been ordained into any priesthood level or only into the Aaronic level, and such individuals are generally considered to be inactive as church members. Members of the second group were ordained as Elders and were probably active church members. The final group included those ordained as Seventies or High Priests, who are very likely to be active in the church. Decreased risks were observed among the Seventies and High Priests for cancers of the lip, oral cavity, pharynx, esophagus, and larynx. Comparisons of cancer incidence rates across the three priesthood levels showed a significant trend: Seventies and High Priests had the lowest risks, Elders had intermediate risks, and nonordained or Aaronic-ordained men had the highest risks for these cancers. A companion study of cancer incidence in Utah Mormon women[42] did not contain sufficient numbers of head and neck tumors for separate analysis, but the study did find lower rates of lung cancer among women with the highest estimated degree of adherence to church teaching.

Studies have also shown that Seventh-Day Adventists have lower risks for head and neck cancers than the general population. Mills et al[48] reported standardized mortality ratios (SMRs) for oral cavity cancers for 24 male and 41 female church members when compared to the general population. The SMRs for esophageal cancer were 0 and 42 for males and females, respectively. Reduced SMRs were also reported for cancers of the colon, rectum, stomach, and biliary passages and liver. Since more than 50% of Seventh-Day Adventists also adhere to a vegetarian diet, it is possible that abstinence from alcohol may be only one factor responsible for the reduced rate of gastrointestinal cancers in this group. Also of interest is a report by Hirayama[50] of a study of Japanese who follow a lifestyle similar to that of Seventh-Day Adventists, in that they abstain from alcohol, tobacco, and meat. This population showed significantly decreased risks for cancers of the oral cavity and esophagus.

Studies designed to detect correlations between disease and exposure measurements for countries or geographical regions within a country can be subject to ecological bias.[51] Disease and exposure measurements are not made on individuals, and it is altogether possible that individuals at high risk for the disease under study may not be the same individuals consuming large amounts of alcoholic beverages. In addition, these ecological studies usually rely on data from secondary sources and tend not to include data on other risk factors, which may act as important confounding variables. Because of their inability to control for confounding adequately, caution is warranted in interpreting data from these studies. Similarly, studies of occupational or religious groups also usually fail to take into account confounding by other factors. Ecological studies do provide reasonable opportunities for posing and initially testing a new hypothesis. Historically, the strong ecological relation between various cancers and alcohol consumption patterns and the significant decreases or increases in risk in subgroups with probable decreased or increased exposure to alcohol strongly suggested the need to conduct analytic epidemiological studies.

MEASURING ALCOHOL EXPOSURE IN EPIDEMIOLOGICAL STUDIES

Many of the early cohort studies of alcohol and cancer involved long-term follow-up of known alcoholics. The strengths and weaknesses of epidemiological studies conducted using a defined cohort of alcoholics are summarized in Exhibit 10–3. Little attention was paid to obtaining actual data on alcohol consumption patterns. Other cohort

Exhibit 10–3 Summary of Epidemiological Studies of Alcoholics

- Cohort studies of alcoholics have generally been noted for complete follow-up of cohort members to determine vital status and cancer occurrence.
- Few studies have information on the amount and type of beverages consumed by cohort members.
- Few studies included information on important confounding variables such as cigarette smoking, occupational exposures, and other risk factors.
- Excess risk was observed for cancers of the larynx and esophagus.
- Results for cancers of the stomach, colon, and rectum have been variable.
- Results for cancers of the pancreas and liver are based on small numbers of events and are difficult to evaluate.

Source: Reprinted with permission from *Alcohol Drinking*, IARC Monographs on the Evaluation of Carcinogenic Risk to Humans, No. 44, pp. 71–321, © 1988, International Agency for Research on Cancer.

studies utilized both diary and questionnaire methods to quantify the amount of alcohol subjects consumed, whereas the case-control studies relied primarily on the questionnaire approach. In the diary approach, the study subjects record detailed information on daily alcohol intake over a number of days, and they then repeat the process a number of times within a specified period. Food frequency questionnaires that contain detailed questions on the frequency and intensity of exposure to various types of alcoholic beverages have also been used in epidemiological research studies. In both the food frequency questionnaire and diet diary approaches, study subjects are usually asked to recall the number of drinks of different types of beverages they consumed each day. In order to calculate the overall amount of alcohol consumed each day, the cans or bottles of beer, glasses of wine, or shots of spirits are converted into the average amounts of alcohol contained in the types of beverage serving. US Department of Agriculture estimates of the alcohol content for each type of beverage are as follows: 12 fl oz of beer = 13 g of alcohol; 4 fl oz of wine = 10.8 g of alcohol; 1 fl oz of liquor = 10.1 g of alcohol.

The reliability and validity of alcohol intake data derived from these survey instruments have been extensively studied.[52–62] The reproducibility studies have involved administration of the same study instrument to the same group of subjects at different points in time. In a study of Finnish men,[53] a self-administered questionnaire was given three times to 121 men at 3-month intervals. In a separate substudy of 190 men, twelve 2-day diet diaries were completed in addition to the self-administered food frequency questionnaires. The investigators reported high levels of agreement between the alcohol consumption data provided by subjects through the three self-administered food frequency questionnaires. The data derived from the questionnaires also correlated strongly with the data obtained from the diet diaries. In a separate report,[54] the investigators reported that, despite the generally high correlation observed between the two data collection instruments, the questionnaire provided estimates of mean daily alcohol consumption that were only 60% of those reported in the diet diaries. The investigators also tested the use of two different questionnaires, one structured to target "light" drinking and the other structured to target " heavy" drinking.[55] The questionnaire developed to assess heavy drinking correlated more closely with the number of drinks associated with a hangover than the questionnaire oriented to light drinking. In addition, questionnaire and diet diary data were compared to various biological marker data measured in sera.[56] Statistically significant associations were found between highest daily intake reported from one of the diet diary periods and a number of serum markers, including mean cell volume (MCV), high-density lipoprotein cholesterol (HDL), and alkaline phosphatase (AFOS). No significant associations were detected between the diet diary data and several other serum markers used to monitor alcohol consumption as part of the clinical management of alcohol-related diseases, including serum gamma-glutamyl transferase (GGT), the HDL:total cholesterol ratio, and ferritin.

Giovannucci et al[57] selected samples of 173 women and 136 men from two large prospective cohort studies. The researchers compared alcohol intake figures obtained from a self-administered food frequency questionnaire given to women in 1980 and 1981 and to men in 1986 and 1987. The Spearman correlation coefficients ranged from 0.78 for liquor consumption in women to 0.92 for total alcohol consumption in men. The study also included the completion, over the one-year investigative period, of four dietary diaries by the women and two by the men. High correlation coefficients, in the range 0.69–0.90, were observed when alcohol consumption data from the food frequency questionnaire were compared to data obtained from the dietary diaries. Data were also available from the food frequency questionnaires administered in 1980, 1984, and 1986 to all 60,655 women free of cancer and heart disease. Data from the 1984 and 1986 questionnaires were highly correlated, and a value of 0.83 was obtained for all women in the cohort. Over the longer time period (from 1980 to 1986), the correlation coefficient remained high, at 0.75, for all cohort members. This study also showed a significant correlation between mean daily alcohol intake and high-density lipoprotein (HDL) cholesterol as measured from a single serum sample. HDL is an established biological marker known to increase in relation to the daily amount of alcohol consumed. The findings of the study suggest that the food frequency questionnaires provide data that are both reliable and valid. The investigators also examined the extent to which the questionnaires agreed with the dietary records with respect to patterns of drinking. In filling out the questionnaires, respondents tended to underestimate the mean number of days they drank in a typical week (assuming the diet diaries were accurate) and overestimate the largest number of drinks consumed on a single day over a one-month period.

Lee et al[58] reported similar results based on data derived from personal interviews conducted 12 years apart. In 1972, subjects were asked to report on their current use of alcohol and tobacco and their current amount of physical activity. During the 1983 interviews, subjects were asked to recall their 1972 levels of exposure and physical activity. High degrees of agreement were reported for alcohol consumption and tobacco use, whereas the physical activity data were found to be less reliable.

Longnecker et al[59] examined the reliability of self-reported alcohol use in 211 control subjects who participated in a case-control study of breast cancer in 1988–1991 in Massachusetts and Wisconsin. A questionnaire designed to assess mean daily alcohol consumption at various times in the women's lives was administered at the initial interview and a second time after an interval of 6 to 12 months. The data showed a high level of agreement for daily alcohol consumption as reported in the two interviews. The correlation coefficients for the various age periods covered in the questionnaire ranged from 0.75 to 0.84.

Giovannucci et al[60] also investigated the extent to which errors in reporting past alcohol consumption might bias the relation between alcohol and breast cancer in a large cohort study. The researchers used a nested case-control approach to assess the relation between breast cancer and alcohol. The study population consisted of 616 women diagnosed with breast cancer in the original cohort and a random sample of 1,277 cohort members who had not been diagnosed with breast cancer. The relation of breast cancer risk to alcohol consumption was calculated based on data from a questionnaire completed by all cohort members prior to the diagnosis of breast cancer and on data from a similar questionnaire completed by cases and controls after the breast cancer cases were diagnosed. The prospective data showed an elevated breast cancer risk among women who consumed 30 or more grams of alcohol per day (OR = 1.55; 95% CI = 1.01–2.39). The same analysis using the retrospective data produced a similar but slightly lower elevated risk (OR = 1.42; 95% CI = 0.85–2.40). These data show that recall bias had only a small effect on the observed association between high levels of alcohol consumption and breast cancer risk and that the bias tended to be in the direction of underestimating the risk.

More recently, Liu et al[61] reported on the reliability of alcohol intake data gathered through recall 10 years after initial data collection. The original and the recall data were obtained from 2,907 US adults who participated in the First National Health and Nutrition Examination Survey interviews during 1971–1975. Again, a high level of agreement was observed for all subjects when the alcohol consumption data collected 10 years later were compared to the original data.

Another approach involves examining the correlation between alcohol data and data collected through use of a standardized psychological scale of social desirability. Such scales are designed to measure the extent to which subjects are simply providing socially acceptable responses to questions about alcohol. Welte and Russell[62] administered the Marlowe-Crowne Social Desirability Scale (SDS) to 1,933 participants in a general population survey of alcohol consumption patterns. The investigators reported that the SDS did not correlate with gender or race but increased with age and decreased with socioeconomic status. Associations between alcohol consumption patterns and established risk factors were not significantly altered by controlling for the SDS score. The researchers concluded that social desirability response bias leads to an underestimation of heavy drinking but does not interfere with the study of predictors of heavy drinking.

Given that studies of alcohol and cancer often focus on anatomic sites for which the survival rates are low, investigators are often required to collect information on alcohol consumption through proxy interviews with next of kin. The ability of surrogates to accurately recall the drinking habits of family members is a concern in these studies. In an effort to provide some insight into this issue, Graham and Jackson[63] compared alcohol histories provided by proxy interviews with data obtained from the primary subjects. The investigators collected data on drinking frequency from 58 living case subjects diagnosed with a myocardial infarction and from the closest relative identified by each study subject. A similar approach was used with 456 control subjects and their nearest relatives. The alcohol consumption data were used to place study subjects into five categories (never drinker, ex-drinker, and three levels of drinking frequency) based on both primary and proxy data. Case subjects and their nearest relatives placed the subjects into the same exact drinking category 63.7% of the time, and control subjects and their relatives did it 62% of the time. Case subjects and relatives placed the case subjects within the same or a proximal drinking category 89% of the time (this percentage was the same for both case and control subjects). For 332 control subjects, the mean difference in the daily amount of alcohol consumption reported by the two sources was only 0.77 g. A larger difference was reported for case subjects (2.25 g), but it must be remembered that data were only available for 58 diseased subjects. These data and similar findings from two previous studies[64,65] suggest that proxy interviews provide alcohol consumption estimates that are similar to those provided by the primary subjects.

Overall, these studies suggest that diet diaries may be the best approach to collecting data on alcohol consumption levels and patterns. The food frequency questionnaires may tend to misrepresent certain drinking patterns and underestimate rates of heavy drinking. However, the food frequency questionnaire is the only practical instrument to use in case-control studies. Recall studies show that data from food frequency questionnaires are reliable over periods of up to 10 years. Given the long latency period between first exposure to alcohol and cancer diagnosis, additional research is needed to see if these questionnaires provide reliable data over longer time intervals. Questionnaire data also show high levels of agreement with data derived from diet diaries. Although questionnaire data may tend to underestimate the actual level of heavy drinking, the relative classification of study subjects may not be seriously compromised. In one study, the diet diary and questionnaire provided mean daily intake measurements that were highly correlated with HDL cholesterol. Although a number of serum biomarkers have been proposed to help monitor alcohol consumption among patients being treated for alcohol-related diseases, the utility of these markers in epidemiological research is yet to be demonstrated. One study showed only a weak correlation between alcohol consumption levels obtained from diet diaries and questionnaires and several serum markers commonly used in the clinical management of alcohol-related diseases. The lack of correlation between these serum markers and a range of alcohol exposure levels suggests that they may be of limited use in epidemiological research. The development of an exposure marker that is strongly correlated with epidemiological data on alcohol consumption would significantly add to our ability to sort out the nature of the relations between alcohol exposure and cancers at various sites.

ALCOHOL AND CANCERS OF THE ORAL CAVITY AND PHARYNX, ESOPHAGUS, AND LARYNX

Several major reviews[8,66–68] have presented detailed reports on the available data linking excess alcohol consumption to cancers of the upper aerodigestive tract. This section discusses the extent to which available data satisfy commonly accepted criteria for establishing causality. Supporting evidence is derived from the descriptive and ecological studies already discussed in this chapter and the large number of cohort and case-control studies reported in the literature. The cohort studies have included SMR studies in which observed numbers of site-specific cancer deaths occurring in alcoholics have been compared to the numbers expected to occur based on the mortality experience of the general population. These studies possess a number of strengths, including a focus on individuals with established excess exposure to the suspected etiologic agent and generally complete follow-up of cohort members over reasonable periods of time. Their weaknesses include the low numbers of the cancers of interest that occur in cohort members, the absence of data on potentially important confounding factors, and the absence of detailed alcohol consumption histories. The absence of detailed histories precludes the possibility of detecting any dose-response relation that may exist between the exposure and the disease. A second type of cohort study involves actually collecting data on past and current alcohol use patterns through the use of self-administered food frequency questionnaires and diet diaries. These and other study instruments are also completed by cohort members at specified intervals throughout the follow-up period to provide data on changes in alcohol consumption patterns or changes in the frequency or intensity of potentially important confounding factors.

The relation between alcohol and head and neck cancers has also been examined using case-control studies. These studies allow the investigator to collect detailed information on past alcohol consumption patterns and other potential confounding variables. They have usually had sufficient statistical power to provide reasonably precise estimates of the risk associated with any prior use of alcohol, varying levels of alcohol consumption, and interactions between alcohol consumption and other risk factors. The retrospective nature of the alcohol consumption histories creates a concern that bias may be present, particularly if the recall error occurs differentially between case subjects and control subjects. However, the reliability and validity studies cited above suggest that alcohol can be measured retrospectively and that the potential for bias needs to be weighed against the magnitude of the observed risk and other criteria.[66]

A number of cohort studies have demonstrated a strong association between alcohol use and cancers of the oral cavity and pharynx. A graphic summary of several of the cohort studies reviewed in the 1998 IARC report[8] is presented in Figure 10–5. Most studies show a large increased risk of oral and pharyngeal cancers in alcoholics or heavy drinkers and in brewery workers. Four- to sevenfold relative risks have been observed in alcoholics and heavy drinkers, and excess risks in brewery workers ranged from 0.8 to 1.9. Similar results have been observed in cohort studies for cancers of the esophagus and larynx.

Case-control studies have provided most of the data relating to level of drinking and risk of cancer. Most case-control studies have clearly demonstrated a gradient between mean daily amount of alcohol consumed and the level of excess risk for cancers of the oral cavity, pharynx, esophagus, and larynx. In Figure 10–6, the risk of pharyngeal cancer, as determined in various studies, is plotted against levels of alcohol use. Moderate to strong dose-response relations were observed in all studies, and several studies showed relative risks that exceeded 100 among subjects with the highest levels of alcohol consumption. All forms of alcohol consumption appear to confer an increased risk for these cancers. One study[69] showed that individuals who drink hard liquor only or hard liquor in combination with other alcoholic beverages appear to experience a higher risk than those who drink wine or beer. The beverage type–related differences remained even after the data were stratified according to daily dosage levels. However, overall assessment of results from all studies reported in the literature indicates that the excess risks for cancers of the oral cavity, pharynx, esophagus, and larynx are due to excess alcohol consumption per se irrespective of beverage type.[67]

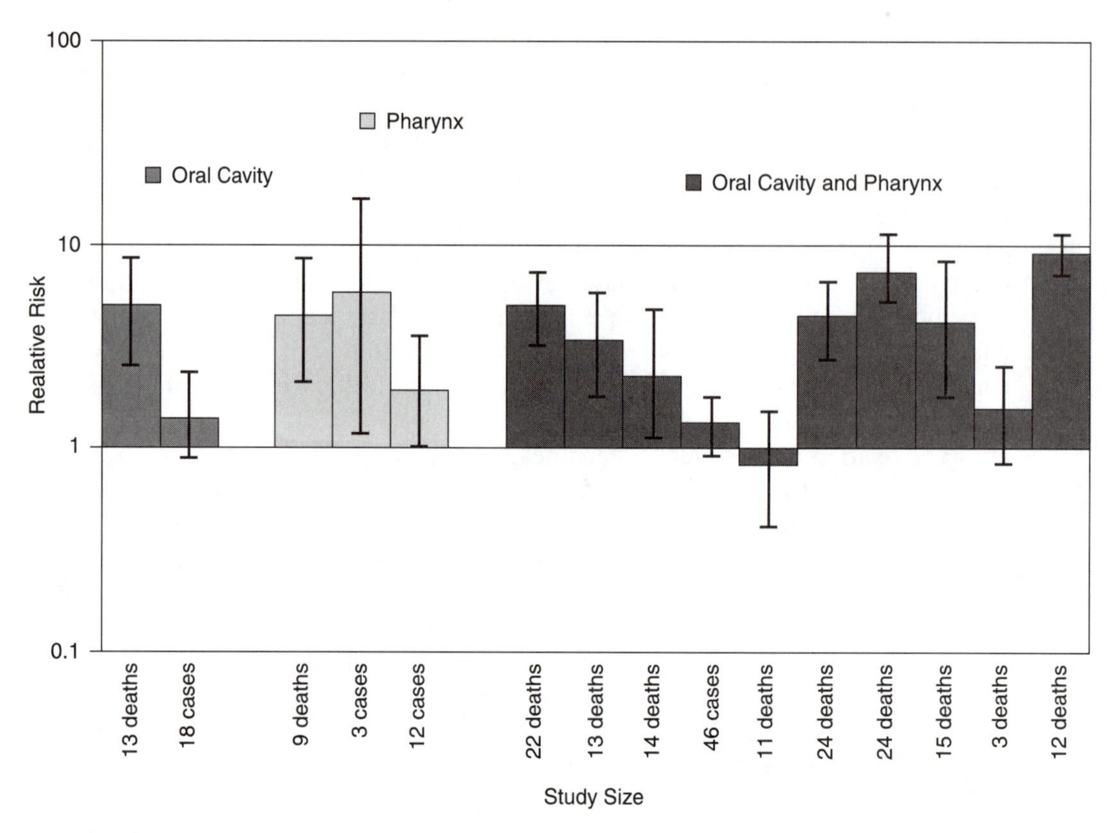

Figure 10–5 Relative risk (plotted on a log scale) of cancer of the oral cavity and pharynx from alcohol consumption. The results of various cohort studies are shown. Error bars represent 95% confidence intervals. *Source:* Adapted with permission from *Alcohol Drinking*, IARC Monographs on the Evaluation of Carcinogenic Risk to Humans, No. 44, pp. 71–321, © 1988, International Agency for Research on Cancer.

These studies have also controlled for confounding by cigarette smoking, poor dentition, and poor nutrition, the other strong risk factors for these cancers. Alcohol consumption appears not to be confounded by these other strong risk factors but rather to act synergistically with these factors to significantly increase risk. The interaction effects between alcohol consumption and cigarette smoking[70–73] and also with poor nutrition[74,75] appear to exceed additivity and are consistent with a multiplicative model (see Chapter 9). Graham et al[76] examined interactions between alcohol consumption, cigarette smoking, and poor dentition (Figure 10–7), and their findings suggest there are strong interactions between cigarette smoking and poor dentition and between alcohol consumption and poor oral health.

Several recent studies[77–79] have investigated interactions between genes and alcohol consumption and their effect on the risk of developing esophageal cancer. These studies were designed to assess changes in risk associated with alcohol exposure among subjects with different genotypes of the enzyme aldehyde dehydrogenase 2 (ALDH2). This ALDH2 enzyme system is polymorphic and is responsible for eliminating acetaldehyde from the body.[80] The mutant form of the gene is prevalent in Asian populations and leads

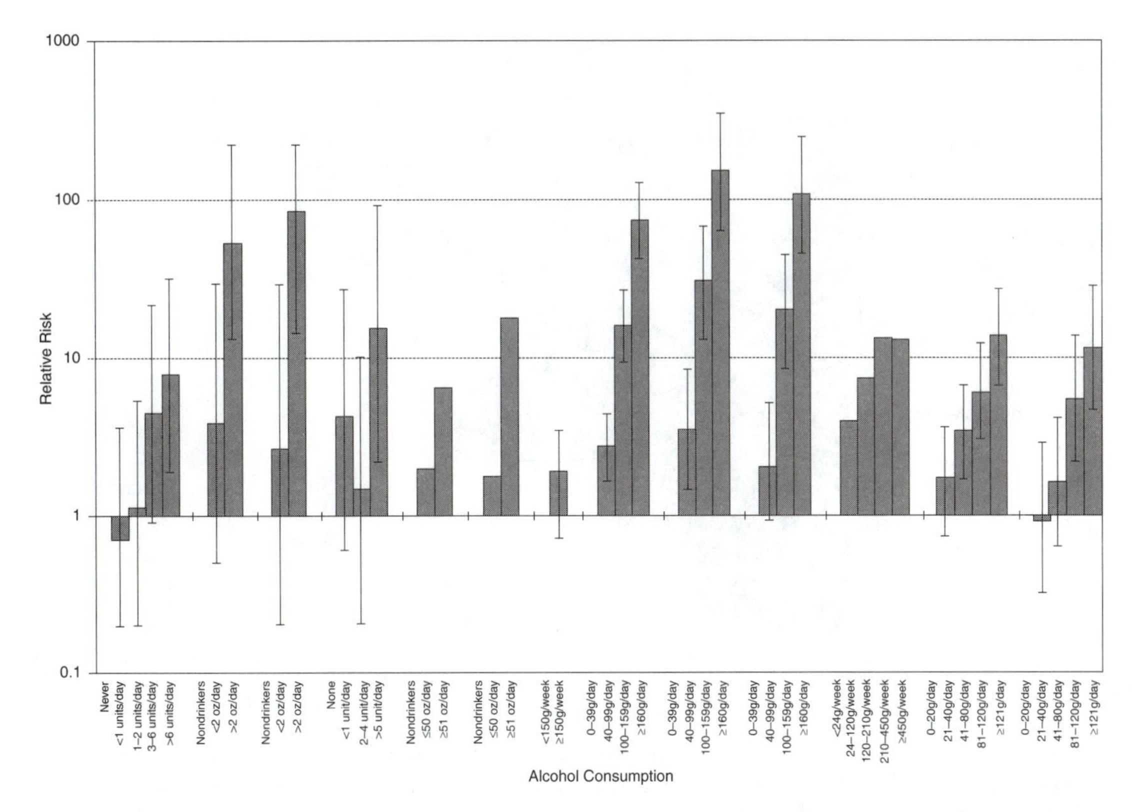

Figure 10–6 Relative risk (plotted on a log scale) of pharyngeal cancer by level of alcohol consumption. The results of various case-control studies are shown. Where available 95% confidence intervals are shown as error bars. *Source:* Adapted with permission from *Alcohol Drinking*, IARC Monographs on the Evaluation of Carcinogenic Risk to Humans, No. 44, pp. 71–321, © 1988, International Agency for Research on Cancer.

to enzyme inactivity. Acetaldehyde is a metabolite of alcohol that has been shown to be carcinogenic in several types of rodents. The studies mentioned above found esophageal cancer risk to be higher among subjects determined by genotyping to have the mutant form of the gene. In a screening program for esophageal cancer in alcoholic patients, the mutant form of the gene has been associated with an increased risk of multiple esophageal lesions. The studies used only small numbers of subjects, but they suggest that interactions between the *ALDH2* genotypes and alcohol consumption constitute a fruitful area for future research. In order to examine such interactions in larger populations, a method for reliably detecting the phenotype for the mutant form of the gene is needed. Yokoyama et al[81] recently reported on the reliability of a flushing questionnaire and the ethanol patch test in screening for the inactive form of the gene. The questionnaire was designed to identify individuals who experience facial flushing even after consuming one alcoholic beverage. The patch test is a cutaneous method for detecting the flushing response. Subjects were also genotyped for the *ALDH2* gene by technicians who were blinded to the questionnaire and patch test results. For subjects who always reported flushing after drinking, 94.4% were found to have the inactive (mutant) form of the

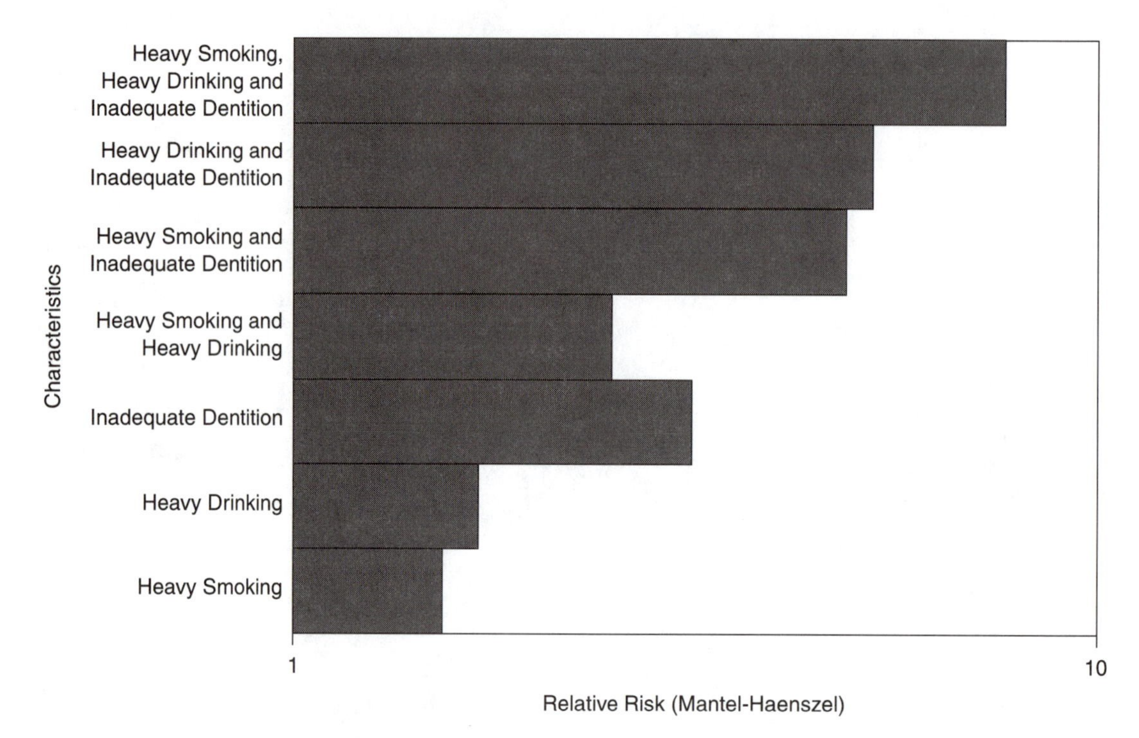

Figure 10–7 Relative risk (plotted on a log scale) of oral cancer for white males of various characteristics as compared with their complements, with adjustments for other study variables. Risks are calculated relative to light smoking (including nonsmoking), inadequate dentition, and light drinking (fewer than 7 drinks per week). *Source:* Adapted with permission from *Alcohol Drinking*, IARC Monographs on the Evaluation of Carcinogenic Risk to Humans, No. 44, pp. 71–321, © 1988, International Agency for Research on Cancer.

ALDH2 gene, while among those who sometimes experienced flushing, 47.7% had a mutant form. Among subjects who never reported flushing, 95.6% were found to have the active form of the gene. The sensitivity and specificity of the questionnaire was determined to be 96.1% and 79.0%, respectively, while comparable figures for the patch test were 72.4% and 71.4%. These data support the potential utility of the questionnaire in large-scale epidemiological studies, but the results need to be replicated in other Asian and non-Asian populations.

The exact mechanisms through which alcohol causes cancer in humans is not fully understood.[8,66–68,82] One possibility is that the cancer is caused by the various contaminants that have been detected in alcoholic beverages, many of which are known animal carcinogens. Acetaldehyde, a metabolite, has also been shown to be carcinogenic in several animal models. Another possibility is that alcohol enhances the absorption and action of other carcinogens. Alcohol may act topically to enhance the absorption of carcinogens in tobacco smoke, for example. Damage to the liver, a main site for detoxifying carcinogens, may also contribute to the development of cancer. Another possible factor is alcohol's ability to activate cytochrome P-450 enzyme activity in the liver, lung, esophageal, and intestinal tissues.[83] P-450 enzymes can, in some circumstances, increase the toxicity of some carcinogens.[84] In addition, given that alcoholics usually have poor diets, alcoholics may not be getting important nutrients that protect against the action of other carcinogens.[66]

The causal nature of the association between high levels of alcohol consumption and head and neck cancers is supported by the magnitude of the risks observed among excessive drinkers, the existence of a clear dose-response gradient, and strong interactions with other known human carcinogens. The consistency of the findings in a large number of cohort and case-control studies and the consistency between the analytical findings and descriptive epidemiological findings also suggest the relationship is causal. Although the mechanisms through which alcohol increases cancer risk in human populations have yet to be fully established, a number of reasonable biological hypotheses are compatible with the human and animal data collected thus far.

ALCOHOL AND CANCERS OF THE LOWER GASTROINTESTINAL TRACT

The association of alcohol consumption with cancers of the stomach, colon, rectum, liver, and pancreas is less well established. The findings from cohort studies of alcoholics, alcohol misusers, and brewery workers are summarized in Exhibit 10–4. Most of the cohort studies show relative risks for cancers of the stomach, colon, liver, and rectum that are close to unity. The numbers of observed and expected cancers in all studies combined also indicate there is only a small increase in risk for these cancers. A large excess of observed primary liver cancer is seen, along with a moderate but somewhat inconsistent increased risk for pancreatic cancer.

Case-control studies of stomach cancer[8,66–68,85,86] have generally not demonstrated an association between stomach cancer and alcohol consumption, although these studies did not consider subsites within the stomach. Four studies[87–90] showed an increased risk

---

Exhibit 10–4 Summary of Findings from Epidemiological Case-Control Studies of Alcohol Consumption and Cancers of the Larynx and Upper and Lower Digestive Tract

- Case-control studies have shown a strong relation between alcohol consumption and cancers of the oral cavity and pharynx, larynx, and esophagus.
- A strong dose-response relation has been shown between the reported daily amount of alcohol consumed and the risk of developing cancers of the oral cavity and pharynx, larynx, and esophagus.
- A strong interaction has been observed in some studies between alcohol consumption and tobacco smoking.
- No strong association has been observed between alcohol consumption and cancer of the stomach.
- Mixed results have been reported for cancers of the colon and rectum.
- A moderately increased risk has been noted for cancer of the liver.

Source: Reproduced with permission from *Environmental Health Perspectives*, Vol. 103, Supplement 8, D.B. Thomas, Alcohol as a Cause of Cancer, pp. 153–160, 1995.

for cancers of the gastric cardia but not for cancers in other subsites. However, two recent studies[91,92] failed to confirm these findings. A recent cohort study[93] also failed to find any association between alcohol and stomach cancer.

The case-control studies of alcohol and colorectal cancer[8,66–68,94,95] have been inconsistent. However, a number of recent case-control[96,97] and cohort studies[98–103] have reported a positive association between alcohol and colorectal cancer and between alcohol and hyperplastic polyps, a precursor of colon cancer. Several of these studies[96,97,101–103] found an increased risk among cohort members who consumed high levels of alcohol or had low levels of dietary folate. Kearny et al[100] reported an increased risk of hyperplastic polyps in both men and women who consumed 30 g or more of alcohol per day when compared with nondrinkers. High dietary folate was inversely related to polyp risk in both sexes. Giovannucci et al[101] found, in the same cohort, a twofold increase in the risk of colon cancer in men who were past drinkers or who reported drinking more than two drinks per day. Although folate and methionine intakes were only weakly associated with colon cancer risk, cohort members who did not report using aspirin on a regular basis and who had high alcohol consumption levels and low levels of these nutrients showed a significantly increased risk of colon cancer. The risk of cancer of the distal colon was particularly high for cohort members with this combination of factors (OR = 7.44; 95% CI = 1.58–6.88). Glynn et al[96] reported no statistically significant associations between serum folate and cancers of the colon or rectum in men but did observe an increased risk of colon cancer in relation to dietary folate. In addition, men who consumed high levels of alcohol and low levels of folate and protein showed a highly significant greater risk of developing colon cancer than men with low levels of alcohol consumption and high levels of folate and protein in their diet. Slattery et al[97] found only weak associations between colon cancer and alcohol or folate but did observe a moderately upward trend in colon cancer risk among subjects who had high levels of alcohol consumption and low levels of methionine, folate, and vitamins B_{12} and B_6 intake. Two recent cohort studies[98,99] showed a positive association between beer consumption and rectal cancer risk. One of these cohort studies[98] also showed a significant dose-response relation between the amount of beer consumed and rectal cancer risk. An association between beer consumption and rectal cancer risk has been observed in the majority of case-control studies conducted thus far.[8]

Alcoholics have been shown to be at increased risk for developing liver cancer. The extent of alcohol's effect on the risk of liver cancer is difficult to assess from these studies, since data on hepatitis B virus (HBV) infection were not collected.[66] Two case-control studies of liver cancer[104,105] showed an increased risk of liver cancer associated with alcohol after controlling for HBV infection, while two studies conducted in Japan[106,107] showed strong synergistic effects of alcohol and HBV infection on liver cancer risk. Significant interactions have also been shown for alcohol use and cigarette smoking.[67] Given the rarity of primary liver cancer in the United States, the public health impact of this cancer in this country is small relative to the other health effects of alcohol abuse. Additional studies of potential interactions between alcohol and other causes of liver cancer, including HBV, aflatoxin, and cigarette smoking, are warranted in countries where liver cancer is a major public health problem and the prevalence of these factors is high.[66, 67]

The epidemiological evidence linking alcohol consumption with cancer of the pancreas is generally weak.[66,67,108,109] Studies of pancreatic cancer in alcoholics show relative risks that are close to unity or only slightly elevated. Only one of the five cohort studies with internal controls that were reviewed in the 1988 IARC report[8] showed any evidence of an increased risk. Four more recent cohort studies[110–113] have also produced mixed results. Zheng et al,[110] in a cohort study of 17,663 white males in the United States, found a threefold increased risk for pancreatic cancer in subjects who reported consuming 10 or more drinks per month, but the dose-response trend was erratic. Shibata et al[111] found no consistent association between alcohol drinking and pancreatic cancer in a cohort of 13, 979 residents of a retirement community. A study conducted in a cohort of Swedish patients with chronic pancreatitis showed an approximately fourfold increased risk in the subcohort of patients who abused alcohol. Most recently, a cohort study of 33,976 postmenopausal Iowa women[112] showed a strong dose-response relation between the amount of alcohol consumed and pancreatic cancer risk. The risk increased approximately twofold in cohort members who drank more than two drinks per week and who were nonsmokers. Of the 23 case-control studies conducted thus far, only 4 provide even weak evidence of an association.[8,66,113–116]

The high case-fatality rate for cancer of the pancreas usually requires the collection of alcohol histories from family members. As previously discussed in this chapter, validation studies suggest that surrogates of deceased case subjects can provide alcohol consumption histories reasonably in agreement with the histories that the subjects would have provided. However, if alcohol has only a weak effect on pancreatic cancer risk, then even small errors in exposure assessment might obscure the association. The overall sense of the epidemiological data is that alcohol consumption is at best only a weak contributor to the development of cancer of the pancreas.

ALCOHOL AND BREAST CANCER

Several qualitative reviews,[66,67,109,117–119] three meta-analyses,[120–122] and a pooled data analysis of six cohort studies[123] of the possible causal nature of the association between alcohol consumption and female breast cancer have been published. A number of additional cohort[123,124] and case-control[125–134] studies have appeared in the literature since these reviews were published. Although negative cohort and case-control studies have been reported, the majority of studies have shown a moderately increased breast cancer risk among women consuming moderate to high levels of alcohol. Longnecker,[122] in his meta-analysis of 38 studies published prior to 1993, calculated a pooled dose-response trend that showed a modest association between daily alcohol consumption and breast cancer risk. The pooled relative risk was estimated to be 1.24 (95% CI = 1.15–1.34) among women consuming 26 g or more of alcohol per day. The association does not appear to be limited to any single type of alcoholic beverage. Smith-Warner et al,[123] in their analysis of pooled data from six cohort studies, found that the pooled relative risk increased linearly with increases in alcohol consumption. A pooled relative risk of 1.09 was observed for increments of 10 g of alcohol per day. The relative risk for women consuming between 30 g and 59 g of alcohol per day (2–5 drinks) was 1.41 (95% CI = 1.18–1.69).

Only two studies have examined the relation between breast cancer risk and duration of exposure, and both have failed to detect an effect. A large number of studies have reported conflicting results concerning possible interactions between alcohol and a number of variables, including age, menopausal status, body size, exogenous estrogen use, family history, and estrogen receptor status.[119] Reported studies have failed to demonstrate a consistent relationship exists between breast cancer risk and specific types of alcoholic beverages. The data suggest that ethanol per se or the metabolite acetaldehyde are responsible for the increased breast cancer risk, and they are consistent with beverage-specific data on alcohol and cancers of the aerodigestive tract.[67] However, the mechanism by which ethanol increases breast cancer risk (if it in fact does) is likely to be different from the mechanisms involved in aerodigestive tract cancers.

A review of the causal criteria usually employed in epidemiological research suggests caution is necessary in interpreting the existing data on alcohol and breast cancer. The low magnitude of the relative risks observed in most studies, coupled with some expected error in collecting alcohol consumption data, keeps open the possibility that the association is due to information bias. This is in sharp contrast to the findings for aerodigestive cancers, where the magnitude of the relative risk was large and unlikely to be an artefact of information bias. Although a dose-response relationship has been observed in a majority of the positive studies, the slopes of the response curves have generally been modest. Most studies have included extensive efforts to control for the possible confounding effects of established breast cancer risk factors. A number of studies were also able to control for dietary intake. Although a yet-to-be-identified confounder may be responsible for the association between alcohol and breast cancer, inclusion of known confounders in the analyses has failed to alter the association in positive studies. Ecological studies, both international and regional, have generally failed to show an association between alcohol consumption and breast cancer mortality. The fact that breast cancer mortality was used instead of incidence may have contributed to the failure to detect an association.[67] Ewertz and Duffy[135] recently used birth cohort analysis to show a strong positive temporal relation between breast cancer incidence and alcohol consumption in Denmark between 1943 and 1989.

A number of reasonable biological hypotheses have been presented to suggest that the association between alcohol and breast cancer may be causal. These include the effects of alcohol on the hepatic metabolism of carcinogens or procarcinogens, the effects on cell membranes and cell-to-cell communication, the production of cytotoxic protein products, immunological surveillance, and the effects on DNA repair and congener metabolism. The possible impact of alcohol on levels of estradiol and other steroid hormones is of prime importance given the wealth of epidemiological and experimental evidence linking these reproductive hormones to breast cancer etiology.[116] Several studies[136–142] have been conducted to determine the short-term effect of alcohol on the production of serum estradiol in women who imbibe four alcoholic drinks at one time. In three studies in which women received stimulation of the anterior pituitary,[136–138] estradiol levels increased significantly following ingestion of alcohol. Mixed results were observed in other studies not involving pituitary stimulation.[139–142] Another experimental study was conducted to determine the effect of alcohol on serum prolactin in menopausal women.[143] Women were given either alcohol or an isocaloric carbohydrate drink, and prolactin was measured in blood samples drawn 8 hours later. Two substudies were conducted, one in which a transdermal estradiol patch was administered a day before alcohol was consumed and was maintained until the blood samples were drawn and a second study in which the patches were removed after the alcohol or control drink was consumed. Both substudies showed significantly higher serum prolactin levels after the alcohol drink than after the isocaloric carbohydrate drink.

A number of recent studies[144–146] have also been conducted to determine the longer range effect of alcohol on estrogen production. A cross-sectional study[144] of 107 premenopausal women in Maryland compared alcohol consumption based on data from questionnaires and 7-day food records with hormones levels based on several fasting blood samples drawn at various times to reflect the follicular, midcycle, and luteal phase of the menstrual cycle. The investigators found no association between alcohol consumption and plasma estrogen levels. Hankinson et al[145] compared alcohol intake as measured during the previous year from semi-quantitative food frequency questionnaires with plasma hormones levels in stored sera from the Nurses' Health Study. After controlling for age, height, smoking, and body mass index, factors known to affect hormone levels, the researchers found a statistically significant association between alcohol and estrone sulfate but no association between alcohol and the other hormones measured.

Reichman et al[146] conducted a controlled diet experiment in which women were randomly assigned to two groups; one group consumed 30 g of alcohol per day for three menstrual cycles, and the other group received no alcohol. A crossover design was used, and after three menstrual cycles, the group of women who had been consuming alcohol abstained for the next three cycles and the initial control group began to consume alcohol. The women were all given a controlled caloric diet in order to maintain their baseline bodyweight. Hormonal assays were conducted on pooled sera and 24-hour urine specimens collected during the various phases of the menstrual cycle. Statistically significant increases in total estrogen level and amount of bioavailable estrogen were noted following alcohol intake.

The animal studies conducted thus far have been limited in number and have produced conflicting results. Three animal models have been utilized. The first involves mice of the C3H strain, which develop mammary tumors spontaneously as a result of an oncogenic RNA virus. The experiments using these mice were designed to determine if alcohol consumption significantly increased the incidence of spontaneous mammary tumors in these animals. No increased incidence of spontaneous mammary tumors was observed in any of the studies. One study showed a decreased latency period for spontaneous tumors, while a second study showed an increased latency period. The second model is designed to see if the administration of alcohol enhances tumor production in rats exposed to one of two potent carcinogenic agents, 7,12-dimethylbenz[*a*]anthracene (DMBA) or *N*-methyl-*N*-nitrosourea (MNU). Tumor incidence was higher in animals receiving both alcohol and either DMBA or MNU than in animals receiving only the carcinogen. However, no clear dose-response curves emerged from the data. In the third model, alcohol was shown to increase the number of lung metastases in rats with adenocarcinomas of the lung.[147] The observation is of interest given two recent epidemiological reports[128,134] showing an association between alcohol and breast cancer (limited to tumors with regional or distant spread).

Estrogen receptors (ER) provide a key mechanism through which estrogens stimulate the growth of breast cells,[148,149] and it is now an established practice to bioassay each newly diagnosed breast cancer in order to classify it as estrogen receptor positive (ER+) or estrogen receptor negative (ER-). The accumulating evidence that alcohol increases estrogen levels suggests that ethanol exposure might be more strongly linked to ER+ breast cancers than to ER- breast cancers. In vitro studies provide support for this hypothesis. Adding ethanol to cell cultures appears to selectively stimulate the proliferation of ER+ tumor cells.[150] Several epidemiological studies[151–155] have examined the association between alcohol and the risk of ER+ and ER- breast cancers. Nasca et al,[151] in a case-control study, showed that the association between alcohol consumption and breast cancer was limited to tumors classified as ER+. Enger et al[152] reported data on the relationship between alcohol consumption and the risk of breast cancers jointly classified by estrogen receptor and progesterone receptor (PR) status. These researchers observed that postmenopausal women who consumed more than 27 g of alcohol daily had an increased risk of breast cancer of the combined ER+ and PR+ subtype but not of breast cancer of other estrogen and progesterone receptor subtypes. Among premenopausal women, alcohol was not related to any of the estrogen and progesterone receptor subtypes. Three small studies that only included data on estrogen receptor assays have been conducted. These studies showed mixed result. One study[153] showed no association between alcohol and ER+ or ER- breast cancers, one study[154] showed positive associations between alcohol and both ER subtypes, and one study[155] showed an association between alcohol consumption and ER- breast cancers. The study by Potter et al[156] included both ER and PR assays and showed an association between alcohol and ER-/PR- tumors. There is clearly a need to conduct additional studies on the possible etiologic relationship between alcohol and specific estrogen and progesterone receptor breast cancer subtypes

SUMMARY

A large number of epidemiological and experimental studies, clearly show a causal relationship between high levels of alcohol consumption and cancers of the oral cavity, esophagus, and larynx. The relationship between alcohol and cancers of the lower digestive tract is less certain. The relationship between alcohol and breast cancer has drawn much attention, but its exact nature is still uncertain. The importance of understanding this relationship is underscored by the public health importance of breast cancer, the ubiquity of the exposure, and the potential for effective primary prevention.[118] The strong etiologic relationship between alcohol and certain cancers and the other established health consequences of alcohol misuse have led to public health warnings against the consumption high levels of alcohol. Knowing what public health recommendations to publicize regarding moderate alcohol consumption is more difficult given that recent data suggest that low levels of alcohol consumption may provide health benefits, particularly for cardiovascular disease. Fuchs et al[157] analyzed overall mortality in relation to dietary intake in a cohort of 85,709 women who were 34–59 years of age and did not have a history of cardiovascular disease upon entry into the study. The data showed a decreased risk of death from all causes combined among women who consumed 1.5–4.9 g of alcohol per day (one to three drinks per week) in comparison with nondrinkers (RR = 0.83; 95% CI = 0.74–0.93). Among those who consumed 5.0–29.9 g of alcohol per day, the relative risk was 0.88, but it climbed to 1.19 in women who consumed 30.0 g or more per day. The largest benefit associated with light to moderate drinking was with respect to deaths due to cardiovascular disease. Additional data of this type are needed to help formulate public health recommendations regarding alcohol consumption.

Discussion Questions

1. Discuss the strengths and weaknesses of the experimental studies intended to investigate the relationship between alcohol or its main metabolite and selected cancers.
2. Discuss the extent to which various methodological studies support the hypothesis that alcohol consumption can be measured in a reliable and valid manner in epidemiological studies.
3. Discuss how descriptive epidemiological studies helped to generate etiological hypotheses concerning alcohol and various cancer sites.
4. Discuss the strengths and weaknesses of ecological studies of alcohol consumption and cancer incidence and mortality.
5. Summarize the scientific evidence that supports the hypothesis that a causal relationship exists between excess alcohol consumption and cancers of the aerodigestive tract.
6. Summarize the extent to which the existence of a causal relationship between alcohol consumption and breast cancer is supported by current scientific evidence.

References

1. Williams GD, Stinson FS, Lane JD, et al. *Apparent Per Capita Alcohol Consumption: National, State, and Regional Trends, 1977–94.* Bethesda, MD: National Institute on Alcohol Abuse and Alcoholism; 1996. NIAAA Surveillance Report No. 39.
2. Bray RB, Kroutil LA, Wheeless SC, et al. Overview of trends in substance use and baseline measures for Healthy People 2000 Objectives. In: *Department of Defense Survey of Health Related Behaviors.* Department of Defense;1995.
3. Centers for Disease Control and Prevention. State- and sex-specific prevalence of selected characteristics: Behavioral Risk Factor Surveillance System, 1994 and 1995. *MMWR.* August 1, 1997;46:1–29.
4. Day N. Alcohol and mortality. Unpublished paper prepared for National Institute on Alcohol Abuse and Alcoholism under Contract No. NIA-76; 1977.
5. DeBakey SF, Stinson FS, Grant BF, DuFour MC. *Liver Cirrhosis Mortality in the United States, 1970–93.* Bethesda, MD: National Institute on Alcohol Abuse and Alcoholism; 1996. NIAAA Surveillance Report No. 41.
6. Harwood HJ, Napolitano DM, Kristiansen PL, Collins JJ. *Economic Costs to Society of Alcohol and Drug Abuse and Mental Illness, 1980.* Research Triangle Park, NC: Research Triangle Institute; 1984.
7. Rice DP, Kelman S, Miller LS, Dunmeyer S. *The Economic Costs of Alcohol and Drug Abuse and Mental Illness, 1985.* Rockville, MD: National Institute on Drug Abuse; 1990.
8. International Agency for Research on Cancer. *Alcohol Drinking.* Lyon, France: World Health Organization; 1988. IARC Monographs on the Evaluation of Carcinogenic Risks to Humans, No. 44.
9. International Agency for Research on Cancer. *Allyl Compounds, Aldehydes, Epoxides, and Peroxides.* Lyon, France: World Health Organization; 1985. IARC Monographs on the Evaluation of Carcinogenic Risks to Humans, No. 36.

10. International Agency for Research on Cancer. *Overall Evaluations of Carcinogenicity: An Updating of IARC Monographs Volumes 1 to 42.* Lyon, France: World Health Organization; 1987; Supplement 7. IARC Monographs on the Evaluation of Carcinogenic Risks to Humans.
11. Ries LAG, Kosary CL, Hankey BF, Miller BA, Harras BA, Edwards BK, eds. *SEER Cancer Statistics Review, 1973–1994.* Bethesda, MD: National Cancer Institute; 1997. NIH publication No. 97-2789.
12. La Vecchia C, Harris RE, Wynder EL. Comparative epidemiology of cancer between the United States and Italy. *Cancer Res.* 1988;48:7285–7293.
13. Lasserre O, Flamant R, Lellouch J, Schwartz D. Alcohol and cancer: study of geographical pathology in French departments [in French]. *Bulletin INSERM.* 1967;22:53–60.
14. Day NE, Munoz N, Ghadirian P. Epidemiology of esophageal cancer: a review. In: Correa P, Haenszel W, eds. *Epidemiology of Cancer of the Digestive Tract.* The Hague: Martinus Nijhoff; 1982:21–57.
15. Guo WD, Li JY, Blot WJ, et al. Correlations of dietary intake and blood nutrient levels with esophageal cancer mortality in China. *Nutr Cancer.* 1990;13:121–127.
16. Boing H, Martinez L, Frentzel-Beyme R, Oltersdorf U. Regional nutrition pattern and cancer mortality in the Federal Republic of Germany. *Nutr Cancer.* 1985;7:121–130
17. Blot WJ, Fraumeni JF Jr, Stone BJ, McKay FW. Geographic patterns of large bowel cancer in the United States. *J Natl Cancer Inst.* 1976;57:1225–1231.
18. Breslow NE, Enstrom JE. Geographic correlations between cancer mortality rates and alcohol-tobacco consumption in the United States. *J Natl Cancer Inst.* 1974;53:631–639.
19. Potter JD, McMichael AJ, Hartshorne JM. Alcohol and beer consumption in relation to cancers of bowel and lung: an extended correlation analysis. *J Chronic Dis.* 1982;35:833–842.
20. Flamant R, Lasserre O, Lazar P, et al. Differences in sex ratio according to cancer site and possible relationship with use of tobacco and alcohol: review of 65,000 cases. *J Natl Cancer Inst.* 1964;32:1309–1316.
21. Enstrom JE. Colorectal cancer and beer drinking. *Br J Cancer.* 1977;35:674–683.
22. Keller AZ. Alcohol, tobacco, and age factors in the relative frequency of cancer among males with and without liver cirrhosis. *Am J Epidemiol.* 1977;106:194–202.
23. Parrish KM, Higuchi S, Lucas LJ. Increased oesophageal cancer mortality rates in Japanese men. *Int J Epidemiol.* 1993;22:600–605.
24. Tuyns AJ, Pequignot G, Jensen OM. Oesophageal cancer in Ille-et-Vilaine in relation to alcohol and tobacco consumption [in French]. *Bull Cancer.* 1977;64:45–60.
25. McMichael AJ. Laryngeal cancer and alcohol consumption in Australia. *Med J Aus.* 1979;1:131–134.
26. McMichael AJ, Potter JD, Hetzel BS. Time trends in colorectal cancer mortality in relation to food and alcohol consumption: United States, United Kingdom, Australia and New Zealand. *Int J Epidemiol.* 1979;8:295–303.
27. Cheng KK, Day NE, Davies TW. Oesophageal cancer mortality in Europe: paradoxical time trend in relation to smoking and drinking. *Br J Cancer.* 1992;65:613–617.
28. Cayuela A, Vioque J, Bolumar F. Oesophageal cancer mortality: relationship with alcohol intake and cigarette smoking in Spain. *J Epidemiol Community Health.* 1991;45:273–276.
29. LaRosa F, Cresci A, Orpianesi C, et al. Esophageal cancer mortality: relationship with alcohol intake and cigarette smoking in Italy. *Eur J Epidemiol.* 1988;4:93–98.
30. MacFarlane GJ, MacFarlane TV, Lowenfels AB. The influence of alcohol consumption on worldwide trends in mortality from upper aerodigestive tract cancers in men. *J Epidemiol Community Health.* 1996;50:636–639.
31. Anglin L, Mann RE, Smart RG. Changes in cancer mortality rates and per capita alcohol consumption in Ontario, 1963–1983. *Int J Addict.* 1995;30:489–495.
32. Smith EM, An analysis of cohort mortality from tongue cancer in Japan, England and Wales and the United States. *Int J Epidemiol.* 1982;11:329–335.
33. Moller H, Boyle P, Maisonneuve P, et al. Changing mortality from oesophageal cancer in males in Denmark and other European countries, in relation to changing levels of alcohol consumption. *Cancer Causes Control.* 1990;1:181–188.
34. Devesa SS, Blot WJ, Fraumeni JF Jr. Cohort trends in mortality from oral, esophageal, and laryngeal cancers in the United States. *Epidemiology.* 1990;1:116–121.
35. McMichael AJ, Hartshorne JM. Mortality risks in Australian men by occupational groups, 1968–1978: variations associated with drinking and smoking habits. *Med J Aus.* 1982;1:253–256.

36. Lindsay JP, Stavraky KM, Howe GR. The Canadian Labour Force Ten Percent Sample Study: cancer mortality among men, 1965–1979. *J Occup Med.* 1993;35:408–414.
37. Lyon JL, Gardner JW, Klauber MR, Smart CR. Low cancer incidence and mortality in Utah. *Cancer.* 1977;39:2608–2618.
38. Lyon JL, Klauber MR, Gardner JW, Smart CR. Cancer incidence in Mormons and non-Mormons in Utah, 1966–1970. *N Engl J Med.* 1976;294:129–133.
39. Enstrom JE. Cancer and total mortality among active Mormons. *Cancer.* 1978;42:1943–1951.
40. Enstrom JE. Cancer mortality among Mormons in California during 1968–1975. *J Natl Cancer Inst.* 1980;65:1073–1082.
41. Gardner JW, Lyon JL. Cancer in Utah Mormon men by lay priesthood level. *Am J Epidemiol.* 1982;116:243–257.
42. Gardner JW, Lyon JL. Cancer in Utah Mormon women by church activity. *Am J Epidemiol.* 1982;116:258–265.
43. Enstrom JE. Health practices and cancer mortality among active California Mormons. *J Natl Cancer Inst.* 1989;81:1807–1814.
44. Lyon JL, Gardner K, Gress RE. Cancer incidence among Mormons and non-Mormons in Utah (United States), 1971–1985. *Cancer Causes Control.* 1994;5:149–156.
45. Wynder EL, Lemon FR, Bross IJ. Cancer and coronary artery disease among Seventh-Day Adventists. *Cancer.* 1959;12:1016–1028.
46. Lemon FR, Walden RT, Woods RW. Cancer of the lung and mouth in Seventh-Day Adventists: preliminary report on a population study. *Cancer.* 1964;17:486–497.
47. Phillips RL, Garfinkel L, Kuzma JW, et al. Mortality among Seventh-Day Adventists for selected cancer sites. *J Natl Cancer Inst.* 1980;65:1097–1107.
48. Mills PK, Beeson WL, Phillips RL, Fraser GE. Cancer incidence among California Seventh-Day Adventists, 1976–1982. *Am J Clin Nutr.* 1994;59(suppl):1136S–1142S.
49. Hirayama T. Mortality in Japanese with life-styles similar to Seventh-Day Adventists: strategy for risk reduction by life-style modification. *Natl Cancer Inst Monogr.* 1985;69:143–153.
50. Jensen OM. Cancer risk among Danish male Seventh-Day Adventists and other temperance society members. *J Natl Cancer Inst.* 1983;70:1011–1014.
51. Kelsey JL, Thompson WD, Evans AS. *Methods in Observational Epidemiology.* New York: Oxford University Press; 1986:204–208.
52. Williams GD, Aitken SS, Malin H. Reliability of self-reported alcohol consumption in a general population survey. *J Stud Alcohol.* 1985;46:223–227.
53. Pietinen P, Hartman AM, Haapa E, et al. Reproducibility and validity of dietary assessment instruments. I. A self-administered food use questionnaire with a portion size picture booklet. *Am J Epidemiol.* 1988;128:655–666.
54. Poikolainen K, Karkkainen P. Diary gives more accurate information about alcohol consumption than questionnaire. *Drug Alcohol Depend.* 1983;11:209–216.
55. Poikolainen K, Karkkainen P. Nature of questionnaire options affects estimates of alcohol intake. *J Stud Alcohol.* 1985;46:219–222.
56. Poikolainen K, Karkkainen P, Karkkainen J. Correlations between biological markers and alcohol intake as measured by diary and questionnaire in men. *J Stud Alcohol.* 1985;46:383–387.
57. Giovannucci E, Colditz G, Stampfer MJ, et al. The assessment of alcohol consumption by a simple self-administered questionnaire. *Am J Epidemiol.* 1991;133:810–817.
58. Lee MM, Whittemore AS, Jung DL. Reliability of recalled physical activity, cigarette smoking, and alcohol consumption. *Ann Epidemiol.* 1992;2:705–714.
59. Longnecker MP, Newcomb PA, Mittendorf R, et al. The reliability of self-reported alcohol consumption in the remote past. *Epidemiology.* 1992;3:535–539.
60. Giovannucci E, Stampfer MJ, Colditz GA, et al. Recall and selection bias in reporting past alcohol consumption among breast cancer cases. *Cancer Causes Control.* 1993;4:441–448.
61. Liu S, Serdula MK, Byers T, et al. Reliability of alcohol intake as recalled from 10 years in the past. *Am J Epidemiol.* 1996;143:177–186.
62. Welte JW, Russell M. Influence of socially desirable responding in a study of stress and substance abuse. *Alcohol Clin Exp Res.* 1993;17:758–761.
63. Graham P, Jackson R. Primary versus proxy respondents: comparability of questionnaire data on alcohol consumption. *Am J Epidemiol.* 1993;138:443–452.

64. Kolonel LN, Hirohata T, Nomura AMY. Adequacy of survey data collected from substitute respondents. *Am J Epidemiol.* 1977;106:476–484.
65. Marshall J, Priore R, Haughey B, et al. Spouse-subject interviews and the reliability of diet studies. *Am J Epidemiol.* 1980;112:675–683.
66. Thomas DB, Alcohol as a cause of cancer. *Environ Health Perspect.* 1995;103(suppl 8):153–160.
67. Jensen OM, Paine SL, McMichael AJ, Ewertz M. *Alcohol.* In: Schottenfeld D, Fraumeni JF Jr, eds. *Cancer Epidemiology and Prevention.* 2nd ed. New York: Oxford University Press; 1996:290–318.
68. Longnecker MP. Alcohol consumption and risk of cancer in humans: an overview. *Alcohol.* 1995;12:87–96.
69. Pottern LM, Morris LE, Blot WJ, et al. Esophageal cancer among black men in Washington, DC. I. Alcohol, tobacco, and other risk factors. *J Natl Cancer Inst.* 1981;67:777–783.
70. Wynder EL, Bross IG, Feldman RM. A study of etiological factors in cancer of the mouth. *Cancer.* 1957;10:1300–1322.
71. Keller AZ, Terris M. The association of alcohol and tobacco with cancer of the mouth and pharynx. *Am J Public Health.* 1965;55:1578–1585.
72. Rothman KJ, Keller AZ. The effect of joint exposure to alcohol and tobacco on risk of cancer of the mouth and pharynx. *J Chronic Dis.* 1972;25:711–716.
73. Tuyns AJ, Esteve J, Raymond L, et al. Cancer of the larynx/hypopharynx, tobacco and alcohol. *Int J Cancer.* 1988;41:483–491.
74. Ziegler RG. Alcohol-nutrient interactions in cancer etiology. *Cancer.* 1986;58:1942–1948.
75. Zheng W, Blot WJ, Shu X-O, et al. Diet and other risk factors for laryngeal cancer in Shanghai, China. *Am J Epidemiol.* 1992;136:178–191.
76. Graham S, Dayal H, Rohrer T, et al. Dentition, diet, tobacco, and alcohol in the epidemiology of oral cancer. *J Natl Cancer Inst.* 1977;59:1611–1618.
77. Yokoyama A, Muramatsu T, Ohmori T, et al. Esophageal cancer and aldehyde dehydrogenase-2 genotypes in Japanese males. *Cancer Epidemiol Biomarkers Prev.* 1996;5:99–102.
78. Yokoyama A, Muramatsu T, Ohmori T, et al. Multiple primary esophageal and concurrent upper aerodigestive tract cancer and the aldehyde dehydrogenase-2 genotype of Japanese alcoholics. *Cancer.* 1996;77:1986–1990.
79. Yokoyama A, Ohmori T, Muramatsu T, et al. Cancer screening of upper aerodigestive tract in Japanese alcoholics with reference to drinking and smoking habits and aldehyde dehydrogenase-2 genotype. *Int J Cancer.* 1996;68:313–316.
80. Crabb DW, Edenberg HJ, Bosron WF, Li T-K. Genotypes for aldehyde dehydrogenase deficiency and alcohol sensitivity. *J Clin Invest.* 1989;83:314–316.
81. Yokoyama A, Muramatsu T, Ohmori T, et al. Reliability of a flushing questionnaire and the ethanol patch test in screening for inactive aldehyde dehydrogenase-2 and alcohol-related cancer risk. *Cancer Epidemiol Biomarkers Prev.* 1997;6:1105–1107.
82. Blot WJ. Alcohol and cancer. *Cancer Res.* 1992;52:2119S–2123S.
83. Garro AJ, Lieber CS. Alcohol and cancer. *Annual Rev Pharm Toxocol.* 1990;30:219–249.
84. Garro AJ, Espina N, Lieber CS. Alcohol and cancer. *Alcohol Health and Research World.* 1992;16:81–86.
85. Murata M, Takayama K, Choi BC, Pak AW. A nested case-control study on alcohol drinking, tobacco smoking and cancer. *Cancer Detect Prev.* 1996;20:557–565.
86. Gajalakshmi CK, Shanta V. Lifestyle and risk of stomach cancer: a hospital-based case-control study. *Int J Epidemiol.* 1996;25:1146–1153.
87. Wu-Williams AH, Yu MC, Mack TM. Life-style, workplace, and stomach cancer by subsite in young men in Los Angeles County. *Cancer Res.* 1990;50:2569–2576.
88. Palli D, Bianchi S, Decarki A, et al. A case-control study of cancers of the gastric cardia in Italy. *Br J Cancer.* 1992;65:263–266.
89. Gonzales CA, Aguda A, Montes J, et al. Tobacco and alcohol intake in relation to adenocarcinoma of the gastric cardia in Spain. *Cancer Causes Control.* 1994;5:88–89.
90. Inoue M, Tjima K, Hirose K, et al. Lifestyle and subsite of gastric cancer: joint effects of smoking and drinking habits. *Int J Cancer.* 1994;56:494–499.
91. Zhang ZF, Kurtz RC, Sun M, et al. Adenocarcinomas of the esophagus and gastric cardia: medical conditions, tobacco, alcohol, and socioeconomic factors. *Cancer Epidemiol Biomarkers Prev.* 1996;5:761–768.

92. Ji BT, Chow WH, Yang G, et al. The influence of cigarette smoking, alcohol, and green tea consumption on the risk of carcinoma of the cardia and distal stomach in Shanghai, China. *Cancer.* 1997;77:2449–2457.
93. Nomura AM, Stemmermann GN, Chyou PH. Gastric cancer among the Japanese in Hawaii. *Jpn J Cancer Res.* 1995;86:916–923.
94. Potter JD, Slattery MI, Bostick RM, Gatspur SM. Colon cancer: a review of the epidemiology. *Epidemiol Rev.* 1993;15:499–545.
95. Gionannucci E, Willett WC. Dietary factors and risk of colon cancer. *Ann Med.* 1994;26:443–452.
96. Glynn SA, Albanes D, Pietinen P, et al. Colorectal cancer and folate status: a nested case-control study among male smokers. *Cancer Epidemiol Biomarkers Prev.* 1996;5:487–494.
97. Slattery ML, Schaffer D, Edwards SL, et al. Are dietary factors involved in DNA methylation associated with colon cancer. *Nutr Cancer.* 1997;28:52–62.
98. Goldbohm RA, van den Brandt PA, van't Veer P, et al. Prospective study on alcohol consumption and the risk of cancer of the colon and rectum in the Netherlands. *Cancer Causes Control.* 1994;5:95–104.
99. Gapstur SM, Potter JD, Folsom AR. Alcohol consumption and colon and rectal cancer in postmenopausal women. *Int J Epidemiol.*1994;23:50–57.
100. Kearny J, Giovannucci E, Rimm EB, et al. Diet, alcohol, and smoking and the occurrence of hyperplastic polyps of the colon and rectum. *Cancer Causes Control.* 1995;6:45–56.
101. Giovannucci E, Rimm EB, Ascherio A, et al. Alcohol, low-methionine, low-folate diets, and risk of colon cancer in men. *J Natl Can Inst.* 1995;87:265–273.
102. Glynn SA, Albanes D, Pietnen P, et al. Alcohol consumption and risk of colorectal cancer in a cohort of Finnish men. *Cancer Causes Control.* 1996;7:214–223.
103. Chyou PH, Nomura AM, Stemmermann GN. A prospective study of colon and rectal cancer among Hawaii Japanese men. *Ann Epidemiol.* 1996;6:276–282.
104. Austin H, Deizell E, Grufferman S, et al. A case-control study of hepatocellular carcinoma and the hepatitis B virus, cigarette smoking, and alcohol consumption. *Cancer Res.* 1986;46:962–966.
105. Mayans MV, Calvet X, Bruix J, et al. Risk factors for hepatocellular carcinoma in Catalonia, Spain. *Int J Cancer.* 1990;46:378–381.
106. Oshima A, Tsukuma H, Hiyama T, et al. Follow-up study of HB_bAg-positive blood donors with special reference to the effect of drinking and smoking on development of liver cancer. *Int J Cancer.* 1984;34:775–779.
107. Inaba Y, Maruchi N, Matsuda M, et al. A case-control study on liver cancer with special emphasis on the possible aetilogical role of schistosomiasis. *Int J Epidemiol.* 1984;13:408–412.
108. Gold EB. Epidemiology of and risk factors for pancreatic cancers. *Surg Clin North Am.* 1995;75:819–843.
109. Longnecker MP, Enger SM. Epidemiologic data on alcoholic beverage consumption and risk of cancer. *Clin Chim Acta.* 1996;246:121–141.
110. Zheng W, McLaughlin JK, Gridley G, et al. A cohort study of smoking, alcohol consumption, and dietary factors for pancreatic cancers. *Cancer Causes Control.* 1993;4:477–482.
111. Shibata A, Mack TM, Paganini-Hill A, et al. A prospective study of pancreatic cancer in the elderly. *Int J Cancer.* 1995;61:745–746.
112. Karlson BM, Ekbom A, Josefsson S, et al. The risk of pancreatic cancer following pancreatitis: an association due to confounding? *Gastroenterology.* 1997;113:587–592.
113. Friedman GD, van den Eeden SK. Risk factors for pancreatic cancer: an exploratory study. *Int J Epidemiol.* 1993;22:30–37.
114. Ji BT, Chow WH, McLaughlin JK, et al. Cigarette smoking and alcohol consumption and the risk of pancreatic cancer: a case-control study in Shanghai, China. *Cancer Causes Control.* 1995;6:369–376.
115. Lee CT, Chang FY, Lee SD. Risk factors for pancreatic cancer in Orientals. *J Gastroenterol Hepatol.* 1996;11:491–495.
116. Tavani A, Pregnolato A, Negri E, La Vecchia C. Alcohol consumption and risk of pancreatic cancer. *Nutr Cancer.* 1997;27:157–161.
117. Hiatt RA. Alcohol consumption and breast cancer. *Med Oncol Tumor Pharmacother.* 1990;7:143–151.
118. Rosenberg L, Metzger LS, Palmer JR. Alcohol consumption and risk of breast cancer: a review of the epidemiologic evidence. *Epidemiol Rev.* 1993;15:133–144.
119. Schatzkin A, Longnecker MP. Alcohol and breast cancer: where are we now and where do we go from here? *Cancer.* 1994;74(suppl):1101–1110.

120. Roth HD, Levy PS, Shi L, Post E. Alcoholic beverages and breast cancer: some observations on published case-control studies. *J Clin Epidemiol.* 1994;47:207–216.
121. Longnecker MP. Alcoholic beverage consumption in relation to risk of breast cancer: meta-analysis and review. *Cancer Causes Control.* 1994;5:73–82.
122. Tonnesen H, Moller H, Andersen JR, et al. Cancer morbidity in alcohol abusers. *Br J Cancer.* 1994;69:327–332.
123. Smith-Warner SA, Spiegelman D, Yaun SS, et al. Alcohol and breast cancer in women: a pooled analysis of cohort studies. *JAMA.* 1998;279:535–540.
124. van den Brandt PA, Goldbohm RA, van't Veer P. Alcohol and breast cancer: results from the Netherlands Cohort Study. *Am J Epidemiol.* 1995;141:907–915.
125. Freudenheim JL, Marshall JR, Graham S, et al. Lifetime alcohol consumption and risk of breast cancer. *Nutr Cancer.* 1995;23:1–11.
126. Longnecker MP, Newcomb PA, Mittendorf R, et al. Risk of breast cancer in relation to lifetime alcohol consumption. *J Natl Cancer Inst.* 1995;87:923–929.
127. Longnecker MP, Paganinni-Hill A, Ross RK. Lifetime alcohol consumption and breast cancer risk among postmenopausal women in Los Angeles. *Cancer Epidemiol Biomarkers Prev.* 1995;4:721–725.
128. Ranstam J, Olsson H. Alcohol, cigarette smoking, and the risk of breast cancer. *Cancer Detect Prev.* 1995;19:487–493.
129. Weiss HA, Brinton LA, Brogan D, et al. Epidemiology of in situ and invasive breast cancer in women aged under 45. *Br J Cancer.* 1996;73:1298–1305.
130. Haile RW, Witte JS, Ursin G, et al. A case-control study of reproductive variables, alcohol, and smoking in premenopausal bilateral breast cancer. *Breast Cancer Res Treat.* 1996;37:49–56.
131. Viladiu P, Izquierdo A, de Sanjose S, Bosch FX. A breast cancer case-control study in Girona, Spain: endocrine, familial, and lifestyle factors. *Eur J Cancer Prev.* 1996;5:329–335.
132. Levi F, Pasche C, Lucchini F, La Vecchia C. Alcohol and breast cancer in the Swiss Canton of Vaud. *Eur J Cancer.* 1996;32A:2108–2113.
133. Swanson CA, Coates RJ, Malone KE, et al. Alcohol consumption and breast cancer risk among women under age 45 years. *Epidemiology.* 1997;8:225–227.
134. Bowlin SJ, Leske MC, Varma A, et al. Breast cancer risk and alcohol consumption: results from a large case-control study. *Int J Epidemiol.* 1997;26:915–923.
135. Ewertz M, Duffy SW. Incidence of female breast cancer in relation to prevalence of risk factors in Denmark. *Int J Cancer.* 1994;56:783–787.
136. Mendelson JH, Mello NK, Teoh SK, Ellingboe J. Alcohol effects on luteinizing hormone-releasing, hormone-stimulated anterior pituitary and gonadal hormones in women. *J Pharmacol Exp Ther.* 1989;250:902–909.
137. Mendelson JH, Mello NK, Cristofaro P, et al. Alcohol effects on naloxone-induced stimulated luteinizing hormone, prolactin and estradiol in women. *J Stud Alcohol.* 1987;48:287–294
138. Mendelson JH, Mello NK, Cristofaro P, Skupny A. Alcohol effects on naltrexone-induced stimulation of pituitary, adrenal, and gonadal hormones during early follicular phase of the menstrual cycle. *J Clin Endocrinol Metab.* 1988;66:1181–1186.
139. Mendelson JH, Luka SE, Mello NK, et al. Acute alcohol effects on plasma estradiol levels in women. *Psychopharmacology.* 1988;94:464–467.
140. Mendelson JH, Mello NK, Ellingboe J. Acute alcohol intake and pituitary gonadal hormones in normal human females. *J Pharm Exp Ther.* 1981;218:23–26.
141. Valimaki M, Harkonen M, Ylikahri R. Acute effects of alcohol on female sex hormones. *Alcohol Clin Exp Res.* 1983;7:289–293.
142. Becker U, Gluud C, Bennett P, et al. Effect of alcohol and glucose infusion on pituitary-gonadal hormones in normal females. *Drug Alcohol Depend.* 1988;22:141–149.
143. Ginsburg ES, Walsh BW, Shea BF, et al. Effect of acute ethanol ingestion on prolactin in menopausal women using estradiol replacement. *Gynecol Obstet Invest.* 1995;39:47–49.
144. Dorgan JF, Reichman ME, Judd JT, et al. *Cancer Causes Control.* 1994;5:53–60.
145. Hankinson SE, Willett WC, Manson JE, et al. Alcohol, weight and adiposity in relation to estrogen and prolactin levels in postmenopausal women. *J Natl Cancer Inst.*1995;87:1297–1302.
146. Reichman ME, Judd JT, Longcope C, et al. Effects of alcohol consumption on plasma and urinary hormone concentrations in premenopausal women. *J Natl Cancer Inst.* 1993;85:722–727.

147. Singletary K. Ethanol and experimental breast cancer: a review. *Alcohol Clin Exp Res.* 1997;21:334–339.
148. Stanford JL, Szklo M, Boring CC, et al. A case-control study of breast cancer stratified by estrogen receptor status. *Am J Epidemiol.* 1987;125:184–194.
149. Habel LA, Stanford JL. Hormone receptors and breast cancer. *Epidemiol Rev.* 1993;15:209–219.
150. Singletary K, Yan W. Ethanol and proliferation of human breast cancer cells. *FASEB J.* 1996;10:712.
151. Nasca PC, Lie S, Baptiste MS, et al. Alcohol consumption and breast cancer: estrogen receptor status and histology. *Am J Epidemiol.* 1994;140:980–988.
152. Enger SM, Ross RK, Paganini-Hill A, Longnecker MP, Bernstein L. Alcohol consumption and breast cancer oestrogen and progesterone receptor status. *Br J Cancer.* 1999;79:1308–1314.
153. Cooper JA, Rohan TE, Cant EL, et al. Risk factors for breast cancer by oestrogen receptor status: a population-based case-control study. *Br J Cancer.* 1989;59:119–25.
154. McTiernan A, Thomas DB, Johnson LK, Roseman D. Risk factors for estrogen receptor–rich and estrogen receptor–poor breast cancers. *J Natl Cancer Inst.* 1986;77:849–854.
155. Holm LE, Callmer E, Hjalmar ML, et al. Dietary habits and prognostic factors in breast cancer. *J Natl Cancer Inst.* 1989;81:1218–1223.
156. Potter JD, Cerhan JR, Sellers TA, et al. Progesterone and estrogen receptors and mammary neoplasia in the Iowa Women's Health Study: how many kinds of breast cancer are there? *Cancer Epidemiol Biomarkers Prev.* 1995;4:319–26.
157. Fuchs CS, Stampfer MJ, Colditz GA, et al. Alcohol consumption and mortality among women. *N Engl J Med.* 1995;332:1245–1250.

Chapter 11

Ionizing, Nonionizing, and Solar Radiation and Cancer

Harris Pastides

Few causes of cancer are as verifiable as ionizing radiation. Evidence from studies of Japanese populations exposed to nuclear fallout during World War II, workers exposed to high levels of occupation-related radiation, and patients exposed to high levels of diagnostic or therapeutic radiation has confirmed that radiation can lead to cancers of multiple organs and various histologic origins. Radiation is prevalent in our environment, and "background levels" may also, potentially be a concern. It is difficult to determine the incidence of cancer attributable to ambient radiation, however. Radon is a major source of population exposure to ionizing radiation in certain geographic areas, and lung cancer is believed to be induced by sufficient radon levels. Nevertheless, the calculation of precise estimates of cancer risk due to radon is complicated by difficulties in determining cumulative individual exposure levels.

The potential carcinogenicity of nonionizing radiation, including electromagnetic radiation, is still in question. Epidemiological studies to date have provided conflicting data, but recent studies tend to cast doubt on the hypothesis that nonionizing radiation is carcinogenic. Excessive exposure to solar radiation, on the other hand, is believed to cause skin cancer, including squamous cell and basal cell carcinoma, and severe sunburning is associated with an increased risk of melanoma.

A central question of interest to epidemiologists that remains to be answered relates to the shape of the dose-response curve, that is, the risk associated with a variety of radiation doses, especially those at lower levels. Since it is impossible to shield ourselves from radiation completely, it is important to determine acceptable levels of population exposure to ionizing and nonionizing radiation.

Ionizing radiation is the most comprehensively understood cause of cancer. There is a vast body of experimental and epidemiological evidence documenting the carcinogenic potential of radiation exposure at high levels. Epidemiological information has been provided from studies of atomic bomb survivors in Japan following World War II, occupationally exposed workers, medically exposed individuals, and persons subjected to naturally occurring radiation such as radon. It is unfortunate that opportunities for primary prevention remain limited at the present time.

Cancers caused by radiation are called *radiogenic*. It is widely agreed that the great majority of types of human cancer are capable of being caused by ionizing radiation given a sufficient exposure dose. In fact, it would be far quicker to identify types for which there is no convincing evidence regarding ionizing radiation's effects (the list would include Hodgkin's disease and chronic lymphocytic leukemia).[1] Furthermore, epidemiological studies of radiation exposure in both general populations and specific occupational populations have led to quantitative estimates of the cancer risks associated with exposure.[2] Areas of radiation-induced carcinogenesis that are not clearly understood include the potentially risk modifying effects of genetic and environmental factors. Understanding these gene-environment interactions should, in the future, allow more precise quantification of risks at lower levels of exposure.

This chapter reviews the important sources of exposure to ionizing radiation and discusses the evidence implicating these sources as risk factors for cancer. It also describes the relationships, as currently understood, between nonionizing radiation and cancer and between solar radiation and cancer.

WHAT IS RADIATION?

Radiation is energy that is discharged from an object such as the sun, a radioactive element, a television studio's antenna, or a home electrical appliance. When the energy discharged has the property of being able to remove electrons from atoms, it is described as *ionizing*. Examples of ionizing radiation include X-rays and gamma rays. When atoms or cellular molecules absorb radiation energy, their electronic configuration and molecular structure is changed. It is plausible, therefore, that ionizing radiation can induce injury. The amount and type of injury to a cell is determined by the type of radiation, the rate at which it is deposited, how it is deposited throughout cells and tissue, and the duration of the exposure.[1] For many years, ionizing radiation was measured in rads. Currently, radiation dosage is given in grays (Gy). One gray equals 100 rads.

Nonionizing radiation refers to energy at the low-frequency end of the radiation spectrum (wavelengths > 200 nm). Nonionizing radiation does not alter the electronic configuration of atoms and cannot disrupt chemical bonds. It is therefore less potentially harmful to human cells and tissue than ionizing radiation on a dose-equivalent basis. Examples of nonionizing radiation include radio waves, microwaves, and extremely low frequency electromagnetic fields. Recently, questions about the health effects of extremely low frequency electromagnetic fields have created great public concern and inquiry because they are ubiquitous in our homes and workplaces. The potential cancer risk of electromagnetic fields will be discussed later in the chapter.

IONIZING RADIATION

Background Radiation

Most people are unaware that, for most populations, the greatest source of exposure to ionizing radiation is background radiation in the environment. (As shown in Table 11–1, for a resident of the United States, ionizing radiation from natural sources constitutes approximately 82% of the total from all sources.) Background radiation includes naturally occurring cosmic rays and radiation from decaying ground sources, such as uranium, radon, potassium, and other substances. Population exposure levels to background radiation vary widely and are related to the altitude of the location as well as the natural distribution of radioactive constituents in the earth. The average human exposure to

Table 11–1 Average Annual Effective Dose Equivalent of Ionizing Radiation to a Member of the US Population

	*Dose Equivalent**		*Effective Dose Equivalent*	
Source	*mSv*	*mrem*	*mSv*	*mrem*
Natural				
Radon†	24	2400	2.0	55
Cosmic	0.27	27	0.27	8.0
Terrestrial	0.28	28	0.28	8.0
Internal	0.39	39	0.39	11
Total natural	—	—	3.0	82
Artificial				
Medical				
X-ray diagnosis	0.39	39	0.39	11
Nuclear medicine	0.14	14	0.14	4.0
Consumer products	0.10	10	0.10	3.0
Other				
Occupational	0.009	0.9	<0.01	<0.3
Nuclear fuel cycle	<0.01	<1.0	<0.01	<0.03
Fallout	<0.01	<31.0	<0.01	<0.03
Miscellaneous‡	<0.01	<1.0	<0.01	<0.03
Total artificial	—	—	0.63	18
Total natural and artificial	—	—	3.6	100

*To soft tissues.

†Dose equivalent to bronchi from radon progeny. The assumed weighting factor for the effective dose equivalent relative to whole-body exposure is 0.08.

‡U.S. Department of Energy facilities, smelters, transportation, etc. Data from the National Council on Radiation Protection and Measurements.

Source: Reprinted from NCRP Report, 1997, with permission from the National Council on Radiation and Measurements.

naturally occurring background radiation is about 0.3 rem per year, according to the UN Scientific Committee on the Effects of Atomic Radiation,[3] an international body that periodically reviews the effects of ionizing radiation on the environment. The committee has predicted that the release of radioactive waste into the environment (ie, through depositing into landfills and surface waters) is likely to increase the levels of population exposure to radiation in the future.

It is extremely difficult to conduct epidemiological studies of the potential cancer risk from naturally occurring background radiation. One reason is that it is not possible to measure an individual's lifetime or cumulative exposure unless the individual has been monitored extensively for occupational exposures or for some other special reason. Most studies of the cancer risk from background radiation have been ecologic in nature. In particular, they have compared cancer rates between communities that have different background levels. Their strategy is to assign an average exposure level to everyone residing in one community. Obviously, migration patterns, occupational exposures, and the highly mobile nature of modern societies result in cumulative radiation exposure doses that vary widely within any community. Most of the ecologic studies to date have failed to demonstrate an elevated cancer risk as a result of residence in "high" rather than "low" background radiation areas. Notable is one large investigation comparing two sizable populations in China having substantially different average background exposures. While cancer incidence was not observed to differ meaningfully between the two populations, some increase in chromosomal anomalies in lymphocytes was noted in the population living in the area with the higher level of background radiation.[4]

Furthermore, ecologic studies usually do not take into account the possibility of confounding. In cases where population exposures vary, other cancer risk factors (eg, socioeconomic factors, diet, etc.) are likely to vary as well. Although prevention of or adjustment for confounding is fundamental in epidemiological studies, the ecologic nature of population data reflecting background levels poses special challenges to analysts.[5]

Nuclear Weapons

The tragic cancer experience of the victims of the atomic bombing of Nagasaki and Hiroshima by the United States toward the end of World War II serves as an unavoidable reminder of the carcinogenicity of ionizing radiation at high doses. Unlike experimental studies of animals or observational studies of highly select populations, such as workers or patients being treated with radiation, studies of the bombing victims had the advantage of study populations that were large and cross-sectional. In the years following the war, a registry of survivors was established for the purpose of monitoring the adverse health consequences of the high exposure to radioactivity, and follow-up has continued to the present time. Detailed analyses of the data have shown that persons exposed early in life suffered the greatest increase in cancer risk.[6] The first radiogenic cancer observed, leukemia, was noted to occur in excess of expected rates within the first decade of follow-up. Specifically, elevated risks were demonstrated for chronic myelocytic, myelogenous, and acute lymphocytic leukemias but not for chronic lymphocytic leukemia.[7] Victims exposed earlier in life were subject to sharper increases and more rapid declines in risk than those who experienced the bombing at later ages; males and females experienced similar relative risks.

Other sites of cancers clearly attributable to the atomic bombing of the two Japanese cities include the breast, lung, colon, ovary, stomach, and thyroid. In each case, age at exposure was a determinant of the magnitude of the excess risk. However, there was site-specific variability in terms of the shape of the dose-effect curve, indicating that genetic or other individual susceptibility factors could have enhanced or suppressed the influence of the ionizing radiation. For the solid tumors observed, most cell types were found to be elevated. In the case of radiogenic lung cancer, for example, cancers of the small cell and squamous cell types, as well as adenocarcinoma, were more common than normal.[8] The latency periods tended to be longer for solid tumors than for leukemias (the latency period for most solid tumors was at least 10 years).

Medical Treatment and Diagnosis

Examples of patients developing cancer following the employment of X-rays for diagnostic purposes or irradiation treatment for various illnesses have been known for a long time. For example, in the first volume of *The Lancet,* in 1955, Court Brown and

Abbatt demonstrated an increased incidence of leukemia following deep X-ray treatment for ankylosing spondylitis (a spinal deformity).[9] In the mid-1970s, Smith and Doll reported a threefold excess risk of dying from leukemia among women treated with radiation for excessive menstrual or intermenstrual bleeding.[10]

Therapeutic radiation dosages received by cancer patients are among the highest levels received by humans. There is incontrovertible evidence from clinical follow-up studies that a wide range of organs can develop cancers caused by radiation used in the treatment of a primary cancer. Investigating the risk of developing secondary cancers from radiation treatment is complicated by the potential for bias. For instance, secondary cancers may be causally linked to lifestyle and biological risk factors (eg, smoking, hormonal factors, etc.) or to chemotherapeutic agents being used to treat the primary site. Also, it is sometimes difficult to distinguish a second primary cancer from metastatic growth in an organ distant from the primary cancer.[11]

Children treated with external X-irradiation and by internal exposure to I^{131} (radioactive iodine) for enlarged thymus glands were observed to have developed papillary-follicular thyroid cancer after a latency of about 10 years.[12] The thyroid is particularly sensitive to the effects of ionizing radiation, especially when the exposure occurs during the early years, a truth demonstrated convincingly.[13] In fact, studies that examined highly divergent populations treated with radiation for a variety of illnesses and that employed different methodologies have consistently demonstrated the susceptibility of this target organ. Thyroid cancer risk has increased following treatment for skin disorders, enlarged tonsils, tinea capitis, and cervical lymphadenopathy. A hypothesis raised from time to time is that Jews are particularly susceptible to radiation-induced thyroid cancer.[14] The supporting evidence includes the observation that relatively high rates are seen in Israel and that thyroid cancer rates are higher among Jews than other religious groups in Los Angeles.[15] Other studies have not substantiated this hypothesis, however,[16,17] and the possibility of confounding should be carefully considered. Radiation-induced thyroid cancer is often bilateral.[18]

The treatment of selected medical conditions with radionuclides has created opportunities to conduct studies of the association of ionizing radiation and the development of cancer. Radionuclides are isotopes possessing the same number of protons as their parent elements but a different number of neutrons. Radionuclides that have been used effectively in medical management include phosphorous 32 (^{32}P), used for treating polycythemia vera; iodine 131 (^{131}I), used for nonmalignant thyroid disease as well as advanced-stage thyroid cancer; and radium 224 (^{224}R), used for tuberculosis involving the skeleton. Follow-up studies of patients treated with these substances have detected elevated rates of radiogenic cancers, especially leukemia.

The use of radiation for diagnostic reasons generally involves lower exposure levels. The lower levels may partly explain why studies of the cancer risks of individuals who have received large numbers of diagnostic X-rays have been inconsistent.[19,20] An additional problem is the difficulty of accurately estimating the radiation dosage through retrospective recall of the numbers of X-rays. Evidence regarding the cancer risk posed by dental X-rays remains similarly inconclusive.[21]

The public health community has engaged in vigorous promotion of periodic mammography for the secondary prevention of breast cancer. Secondary prevention is aimed at reducing the risk of mortality from breast cancer as well as the complications of late-stage cancer. To a large extent, health promotion activities targeted at breast cancer have been successful, although there is a nagging concern that mammograms expose patients to very low levels of ionizing radiation. In the early 1960s, an experimental study of 62,000 members of the Health Insurance Program of New York was carried out to evaluate the efficacy of periodic mammography at reducing the risk of dying from breast cancer.[22] Swedish researchers were also actively engaged in the evaluation of mammography as a screening tool.[23,24] Overall, randomized trials have included over half a million women.[25] Part of the reason for this focused attention is the particularly complex "risk versus benefit" issue that arises from subjecting healthy women to ionizing radiation, with known carcinogen potential, in order to diagnose a specific form of cancer at an early stage. Owing to a reduction in the amount of ionizing radiation that women are currently exposed to, coupled with tremendous improvement in the quality control aspects of screening mammography, there is little room for doubt that, in particular groups of women defined by age and personal risk profile, the benefits of mammography outweigh the risks. Debate about the exact age at which periodic mammography should begin and whether it should be undertaken by women aged 40–49 is still ongoing.

Overall, significant strides have been made in reducing patients' exposure to diagnostic and therapeutic ionizing radiation. Nevertheless, for most persons, diagnosis and therapy remain the most important source of exposure to ionizing radiation (apart from background radiation). Technological advances are likely to continue to reduce individuals' cumulative lifetime exposure levels. At the same time, effective communication strategies encouraging patients and clinicians to avoid exposing patients to unnecessary medical procedures involving ionizing radiation should be employed.

Occupational Exposures

Early in the 20th century, questions about radiation-associated cancer began to be asked, and radiologists became an obvious group to study. Through case reports, it became known that radiologists who were exposed to relatively high doses of X-ray without being shielded experienced serious skin cancers on their hands.[26] In international epidemiological studies of radiologists, other cancers observed to occur at increased frequencies included lung, pancreas, thyroid, bone, and breast cancers, although not all studies have been consistent.[27,28] As protective measures improved in radiology, cancer rates declined, but they remained slightly higher than in other medical specialties for many years.

Another unfortunate history of occupational exposure to radiation concerns the large number of young women, some of whom had recently emigrated from Europe, who found jobs in watch factories and were given the task of painting radium (^{226}RA and ^{228}RA) on watch dials in order to make them luminescent. Owing to the precision demanded by their work, they were in the habit of licking the tips of their radium-impregnated paintbrushes to make them sharper. Years later it was discovered that the observed incidence of osteosarcoma (cancer of the bone) among these workers was markedly elevated.[29]

More contemporary studies of occupational groups exposed to radiation have been conducted on nuclear shipyard and nuclear installation workers. The largest shipyard study did not attribute any elevated cancer risks to on-the-job radiation exposure.[30] Studies of employees at nuclear power installations have been more equivocal. Presently, it does not appear that a clear consensus can be reached based on the numerous studies done to date. It is difficult to determine whether the conflicting results are due to differences in exposure levels, ascertainment bias resulting from extremely rigorous follow-up of these groups, confounding factors, or other methodological characteristics of the research.

Radon

Radon-222 is a radionuclide that exists in the form of an inert gas created by decaying radioactive radium and uranium found in soil, rocks, and water. The fact that radon exposure increases the risk of lung cancer among underground miners has been known for many years, and additional evidence has been provided by the results of animal and epidemiological studies.[31] In 1987, IARC designated radon as an established human carcinogen.[32] However, extrapolating from the experience of miners to the risk for the general population, whose indoor exposure circumstances are very different from those in a mine, is fraught with difficulties. For one thing, miners sometimes have concomitant exposures to substances that are known causes of lung cancer, such as arsenic and silica.

The World Health Organization (WHO) has estimated that radon is the largest source of human exposure to ionizing radiation in most countries.[33] The US Environmental Protection Agency has asserted that indoor radon exposure is the second leading cause of lung cancer in the United States. This has led to a large number of epidemiological studies aimed at further quantifying the cancer risks as well as developing satisfactory measures for prevention. National Cancer Institute researchers have estimated that between 6,600 and 24,000 lung cancer deaths per year in the United States may be attributable to indoor radon.[34] Although most epidemiological studies done in Sweden, the United States, China, and elsewhere support a positive association, the level of the risk and the possibility that susceptible subpopulations exist are open to question. For example, a Swedish case-control study of 586 women and 774 men with lung cancer concluded that the risk of disease increased according to cumulative and time-weighted radon exposure. In this study, exposure levels were assessed by placing radon dosimeters in the living area and basement of all homes. At high residential exposure levels, the relative risk was 1.8, in the range of risk typical for workers exposed to radon in mines.[35] On the other hand, a case-control study performed in Winnipeg, Canada, came to a different conclusion: after adjusting for cigarette smoking and education, no radon-related increased lung cancer risk was identified.[36] The apparent contradiction led to cooperative pooling of data collected by different research teams. One analysis of the resulting large numbers of lung cancer cases among women failed to find a relationship between cancer and cumulative radon exposure dose.[37]

Inexpensive radon measurement devices and reasonably effective remediation techniques, including ventilation of high exposure areas and sealing of basement or foundation walls with impervious material, are readily available. Use of these devices and techniques should continue to be promoted with the goal of preventing new cases of lung cancer due to indoor radon exposure.

Nuclear Power Installations

Residents in communities where nuclear power plants are sited desire to know whether radioactive emissions from those plants, during normal operations as well as during upset conditions, could be increasing their likelihood of developing cancer. The question is certainly an important one, considering the number of new facilities that have been constructed in recent decades as well as the age and repair status of some of the older ones. However, arriving at an answer is a complex task. One reason is that the selection factors that determine where a nuclear power facility will be located are quite numerous; they undoubtedly include economic and political factors in addition to geographic, meteorologic, topographic, and demographic factors. This means that communities with these facilities are often different from communities without them, making the choice of comparison populations for estimating the expected cancer rates into a real challenge. An interesting methodological exercise was performed in England by Cook-Mozaffari et al,[38] who investigated cancer rates in communities where nuclear facilities were only recently built or were still being evaluated. They found elevated rates of leukemia and Hodgkin's disease in young persons and elevated rates of adult leukemia, a profile closely resembling that of communities where nuclear facilities had been operating for some time. Other challenges faced by studies of this type include the possibility of increased detection or reporting of cancer cases in communities where there is heightened concern due to some environmental factor. On the other hand, factors that might make it more difficult to establish a causal relationship between cancer and radiation from nuclear power facilities include the need to control for numerous other cancer risk factors, which can result in overmatching of subjects; difficulty in determining prevailing wind direction and other meteorologic phenomena, which can result in exposure misclassification; the size of the geographic area being evaluated, which may be too large to allow detection of cancer rate increases in small, more highly exposed areas; and the possibility that emissions may interact with personal or other environmental factors to provoke cancer only in particularly susceptible subgroups of the community.

In one of the largest epidemiological studies on this topic to date,[39] National Cancer Institute scientists compared cancer death rates in counties proximal to 62 nuclear facilities and cancer death rates in control counties with reasonably similar demographic factors. There was no evidence reported of an elevation in death rates for cancers at any site, including hematopoietic cancers in children and adults. Studies using similar ecologic approaches in Canada and Europe did not uncover elevations in cancer mortality rates, including for childhood cancers, which are often alleged to be related to environmental radiation.[40,41] However, one study by Bithell et al[42] did find elevated childhood leukemia around the Sellafield nuclear facilities in England.

One point frequently raised in attempting to explain the lack of evidence of an increase in cancer in communities containing nuclear power facilities is the relatively low level of the radiation exposure. The doses received during normal operating conditions are generally far below natural background levels.[43] Nevertheless, skepticism as to the safety of radiation from these facilities is prevalent, and pressure for continued epidemiological attention to this sensitive issue will continue to be levied.

The well-known nuclear reactor accidents at Three Mile Island and Chernobyl have vividly portrayed the potential for severe human health and environmental costs when accidental radiation releases occur. The Three Mile Island release was relatively small, and the population exposure levels have been characterized as less than background radiation levels. The magnitude of the exposure implies that any related cancer increases should be extremely small.[44] The aforementioned NCI study did not detect unusual cancer mortality patterns in the affected populations after accounting for latency. The radioactive release that occurred at Chernobyl, on the other hand, was unprecedented. To date, there has been a documented increase in thyroid cancer among children in the exposed populations[45] but no analogous or widespread increase of cancer incidence or mortality at other sites; neither has an increase in cancer at any site been demonstrated for adults. Clearly the case is not closed on this vital subject. Surveillance by the World Health Organization (WHO) and numerous other international scientific bodies is ongoing. Until longer latency periods have transpired and comprehensive evaluations are made of the range of residential populations and the hundreds of thousands of cleanup workers who were exposed, the full story will not be known.

Regardless of what the specific cancer risk is determined to be, safeguards against accidental releases from nuclear energy facilities should continue to be monitored and improved. If an accidental release does occur, the dose rates in the environment will depend on the quantities of specific radionuclides involved, the duration of the release, the initial dispersal and deposition patterns, and the subsequent redistribution of radionuclides by environmental processes over time.

The Importance of Dose

Figure 11–1 shows the relationship between mean bone marrow dose of ionizing radiation and the risk of dying from leukemia. As can be seen, the relationship is curvilinear and peaks around 300 rad (3 Gy). At higher doses, the risk may be reduced owing to a cell-sterilizing effect of the radiation.[46]

The shape of the dose-response curve at lower exposure levels is open to debate. In fact, the claim that low-dose exposures (< 0.2 Gy) can cause cancer remains unsupported.[1] Conclusions about the cancer-inducing potential of low-dose radiation are controversial and fertile ground for debate given the importance of this issue to society as a whole. A review of open questions regarding low-dose health effects, including the development of cancer, has been presented by Nussbaum and Kohnlein.[47] Their summarization of a number of major reports (by the Committee on the Biological Effects of Ionizing Radiation, the UN Scientific Committee on the Effects of Atomic Radiation, and the International Commission on Radiological Protection) identified several important unanswered questions, including the following:

- What is the shape of the dose-response curve for cancer induction?
- Does the linear, nonthreshold association between acute exposure and cancer mortality observed at levels above 0.2 Gy also occur below that level?

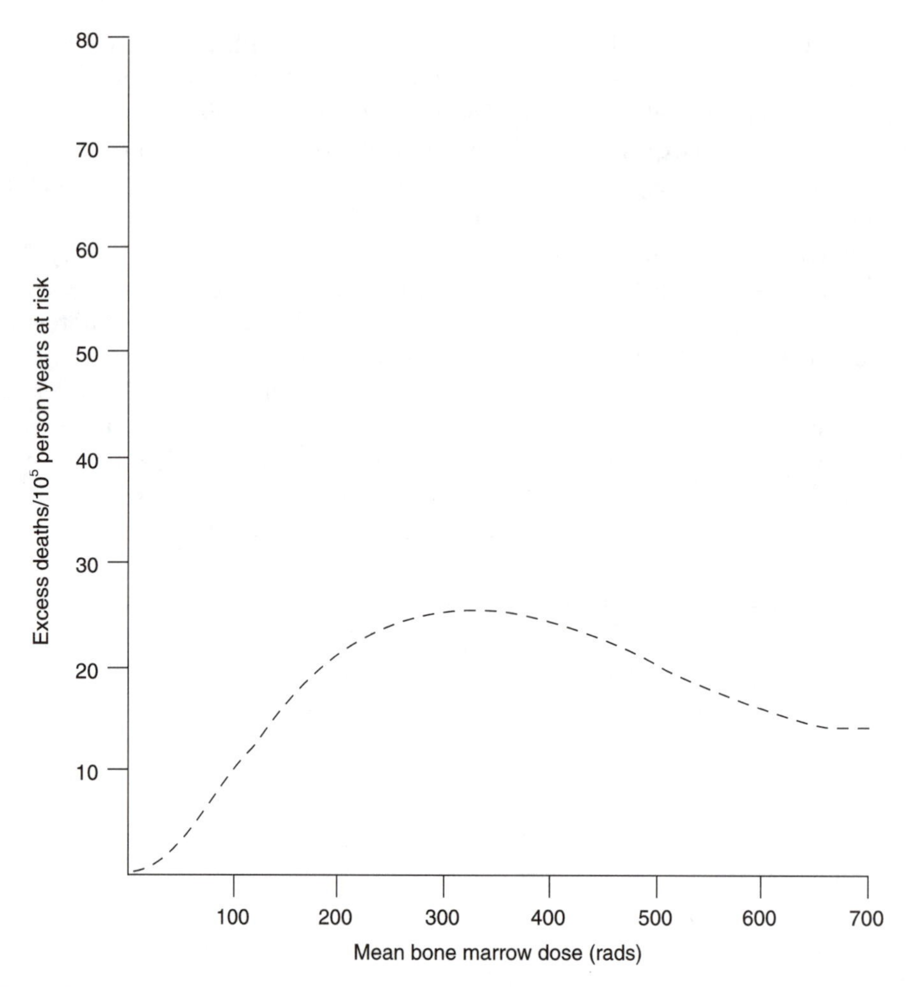

Figure 11–1 Excess death rate from leukemia among ankylosing spondylitics according to mean bone marrow radiation dose. *Source:* Adapted with permission from P.G. Smith and R. Doll, Mortality Among Patients with Ankylosing Spondylitis After a Single Treatment Course with X-ray, *British Medical Journal*, Vol. 284, pp. 449–460, © 1982, BMJ Publishing Group.

- What are the biological effects of X-rays as compared with gamma rays?
- What is entailed by the fact that the atomic bomb survivors were exposed to high-energy gamma rays while most human exposure to ionizing radiation involves X-rays?
- What is the role of free radicals in carcinogenesis?
- Can human exposure to repeated low doses of ionizing radiation result in tumor promotion through the mechanism of radiogenic free radical production?

Until answers to these questions are found, the issue of whether exposure to low-dose radiation presents a cancer risk will not be settled.

ELECTROMAGNETIC RADIATION

As mentioned previously, nonionizing radiation refers to energy at the low-frequency end of the radiation spectrum. It is composed of separate electrical fields and magnetic fields even though, colloquially, we refer to a single "electromagnetic field." It is a truism that wherever there is electrical wiring or equipment, such fields are prevalent. Strictly speaking, the fields generated are distinct from the radiant energy released from electrical sources. The distinction can be clarified by considering that radiation travels away from its source and continues to exist when the source is turned off. Electric and magnetic fields, in contrast, may exist near an electrical source and may disappear when the source is turned off.[48]

Few health topics engendered more public interest during the 1990s than the question of whether electromagnetic radiation is causally related to certain cancers. Since the early observation that residential exposure to weak electromagnetic fields surrounding power lines was associated with a small elevated risk of childhood cancers,[49] numerous epidemiological and laboratory studies have weighed in on the issue. The studies of the 1980s were generally supportive of a positive association between exposure to residential sources of electromagnetic radiation and leukemia and childhood cancers, although these studies tended to use a common exposure surrogate that resulted in some degree of exposure misclassification. These studies have been reviewed in detail,[50] and proposals have been offered for improvements in study design and conduct, including better exposure ascertainment, improved timing of the relevant exposure, examination of different populations, improved control selection, and better assessment of cancer endpoints.[51]

Biophysical mechanisms that might explain the positive findings of epidemiological studies have been suggested. Most of the hypotheses involve the adverse biological effects resulting from induced electrical currents, rearrangement of cellular materials caused by the presence of magnetic biological materials, changes in the rates of chemical reactions owing to free radical interference, or suppression of melatonin production. Critics of the hypotheses have noted that supporting evidence at the field levels found in residential and occupational settings is lacking.[48]

A recent, major epidemiological study may have helped stem the protracted debate.[52] In a case-control study of 629 children with leukemia and 619 control subjects, leukemia risk was not found to rise with electromagnetic field levels in the home. This study benefited from the assessment by technicians of the field levels in the homes where children had lived as well as, for part of the sample, in the homes of their mothers during pregnancy. Furthermore, the technicians were unaware of the case-control status of the resident. This "blinding" was not a universal feature of the early epidemiological studies.

Accompanying the report of this study was an editorial entitled "Power Lines, Cancer, and Fear,"[53] in which the author reviewed the public acceptance of the early findings that followed Wertheimer and Leeper's original paper. The author attributed a large degree of responsibility for the spreading of alarm to journalist Paul Brodeur, who in 1989 published three articles on the supposed risks of electromagnetic radiation in *The New Yorker*. Brodeur portrayed the scientific establishment as conservative, allied with industry, and unwilling to accept the scientific evidence at hand. Public suspicions became directed at many home appliances as well as video display terminals and cellular telephones. Studies were launched in an effort to uncover potential cancer risks to multiple organs, especially those for which the etiology of cancers remain largely unknown. As a consequence of the ensuing debate, some individuals living near power lines or other sources of low-frequency radiation sold their homes, and many moved their children from schools sited near such sources. In Sweden, the government nearly legislated the relocation of students from schools situated within 1,000 meters of large power lines.[53]

In 1997, the National Research Council of the US National Academy of Sciences concluded that the data relating high-voltage power lines to one or more health hazards were not convincing.[54] On the other hand, this body found no consistent bias or other methodological factor that explained the positive findings of earlier studies. Given the uncertainty that remains, it is unlikely that public and scientific attention will be moved away from this perceived environmental health problem in the immediate future. Fears will be largely allayed only if carefully performed epidemiological and laboratory investigations begin to offer consistently negative evidence and scientists put forth other credible theories of the etiology of leukemia, brain cancer, and other cancers for which little causal information currently exists.

SOLAR RADIATION

Studies of the health of migrant populations have long demonstrated the potential for harm from excessive exposure to the sun. Migrant groups with fairer skin who moved to regions nearer the equator, such as the northern Europeans who emigrated to Australia and the central Europeans who departed for Israel, have generally faced accelerated skin damage. Additionally, rates of skin cancer, including squamous cell and basal cell carcinoma, have been found to be dramatically increased in these groups.

Melanoma, the most insidious skin cancer, is also known to be increased in these groups, but, except for lentigo malignant melanoma, which usually occurs on the hands or face, the role of sunlight in the development of melanoma is not conclusive.[55] Severe sunburning is associated with an increased risk of melanoma, while long-term consistent sun exposure inhibits melanoma.[56] Melanoma incidence is increasing worldwide more rapidly than any other cancer; mortality rates are also increasing by about 2% per year.[57] In 1996, the lifetime risk of developing malignant melanoma for a person living in the United States was about 1 in 87.[58]

While the exact mechanism by which cancers are induced by solar radiation remains elusive, it is clear that sunlight can affect cell, tissue, and organ function. First, sunlight can inhibit melatonin production by the pineal gland. When melatonin production is decreased, skin color becomes lighter, the person may become sluggish, and reproductive functions may be inhibited.[59] Also, immune function has been shown to be affected by sunlight. Ultraviolet radiation (UVA) can suppress cellular immunity, and the suppression of immunity has been postulated as a factor in tumor growth.[60] DNA damage can also be caused by ultraviolet radiation exposure.[61]

It has also been suggested that sunlight may protect against cancer development. The descriptive epidemiology of cancers of the prostate, breast, and colon suggests an inverse relationship exists between sunlight exposure and the incidence and mortality rates of these diseases.[62,63] Also, it has been noted that there is a statistical correlation between race and cancer "aggressiveness" at certain sites. Studzinski and Moore[59] have suggested that the poorer prognosis of African American women following a diagnosis of breast cancer as well as the higher incidence of more aggressive prostate cancer in African American men may be partially explained by a protective role played by sunlight among people with lighter skin. Specifically, they hypothesize that sunlight-generated vitamin D metabolites can retard the progression of cancer and that African Americans experience less of this metabolic activity. Of course, differences in access to, and use of health services between diverse racial and ethnic groups would need to be taken into account in epidemiological studies designed to address the role of sunlight as an agent of cancer prevention—a substantial methodological challenge.

In addition to the descriptive epidemiological data, there is experimental evidence that sunlight or vitamin D intake retards the growth of colon and breast cancer cells.[64] Also, vitamin D metabolites have been shown to promote differentiation of leukemia and lymphoma cells. Abe et al[65] and Mangelsdorf et al[66] have shown that mouse and human cancer cells can return to normal morphology following administration of these metabolites. Sunlight's efficient role in vitamin D activation is well known, and research to try to unravel the potential relationship between sunlight, vitamin D, and the etiology of cancer is ongoing.

A better understanding the specific physiological consequences of exposure to excessive sunlight will come from further research. In the meantime, the public health community has much to do if it is to reduce substantially the harm that currently results from exposure to solar radiation. Many societal influences are present that encourage people, especially the young, to be deeply tanned and to get tanned quickly. Perhaps it will be necessary to borrow the approach used in antismoking campaigns and more effectively portray the "unattractive" consequences of tanning. It may also behoove officials to quantitate the recommended exposure to sunlight. Unlike in the case of tobacco products, where the message can be "zero tolerance," it would be inappropriate to tell people with no or little skin damage that they should not expose themselves to sunlight at all. In other words, the challenge of understanding the potential health and cancer consequences of low- versus high-dose exposure to solar radiation and communicating these to the public is similar to the challenge that exists with respect to ionizing radiation.

SUMMARY

The carcinogenicity of high levels of ionizing radiation is not open to question. Epidemiological and experimental studies have convincingly shown the health consequences of exposure to radiation from nuclear weapons, diagnostic and therapeutic X-rays, radionuclides, radiation from the nuclear reactor accidents (as at Chernobyl), occupation-related ionizing radiation, and sunlight (in the case of susceptible individuals). The evidence presented by these studies should not, however, leave the reader with the impression that there is little left to learn from continued monitoring of exposed populations and carefully designed analytic studies. Questions that remain to be answered include the shape of the dose-response curve, the risk associated with residential exposure to radon, and the potential interaction between radiation and chemical and other carcinogenic agents. While the opportunities for primary prevention are probably not as numerous for this risk factor as for others discussed in this book, there is still ample room for education, especially of occupationally exposed individuals.

Discussion Questions

1. Give several explanations for why such a wide variety of cancers can be induced by high levels of radiation. Can you think of other causes of cancer that are responsible for such a diversity of cancers?
2. Contrast the challenges presented by conducting cumulative, individual exposure assessments of radiation from the bombing of Hiroshima and Nagasaki, from occupational exposures in mining, and from household radon.
3. Suppose you are designing an epidemiological study to investigate the incidence of certain kinds of cancer in a particular community. How would you attempt to address the contribution of background radiation to the cancer rates in (1) an ecological study and (2) a study conducted at the level of the individual.

References

1. Boice JD, Land CE, Preston DL. Ionizing radiation. In: Schottenfeld D, Fraumeni JF Jr, eds. *Cancer Epidemiology and Prevention.* 2nd ed. New York: Oxford University Press; 1996
2. Samet JM. Epidemiologic studies of ionizing radiation and cancer: past successes and future challenges. *Environ Health Perspect.* 1997;105(suppl 4):883–889.
3. United Nations Scientific Committee on the Effects of Atomic Radiation (UNSCEAR). *Sources and Effects of Ionizing Radiation.* UNSCEAR 1996 Report to the General Assembly, with Scientific Annex.New York: United Nations; 1996. UN sales publication No. E.96.IX.3.
4. Wei L, Zha Y, Tao Z, et al. Epidemiological investigation of radiological effects in high background radiation areas of Yangjiang, China. *J Radiat Res.* 1990;31:119–136.
5. Corvalan C, Nurminen M, Pastides H. *Linkage Methods for Environment and Health Analysis: Technical Guidelines.* Geneva: World Health Organization; 1997.
6. Thompson DE, Mabuchi K, Ron E, et al. Cancer incidence in atomic bomb survivors. Part II. Solid tumors, 1958–1987. *Radiat Res.* 1994;137:S17–S67.
7. Preston D, Kusumi S, Tomonaga M, et al. Cancer incidence in atomic bomb survivors. Part III. Leukemia, lymphoma and multiple myeloma, 1958–1987. *Radiat Res.* 1994;137:S68–S97.
8. Yamamoto T, Kopecky KJ, Fujikura T, et al. Lung cancer incidence among Japanese A-bomb survivors, 1950–80. *J Radiat Res.* 1987;28:156–171.
9. Court Brown WM, Abbatt JD. The incidence of leukemia in ankylosing spondylitis treated with X-rays: a preliminary report. *Lancet.* 1955;1:1283–1285.
10. Smith PG, Doll R. Late effects of X-irradiation in patients treated for metropathia haemorrhagica. *Br J Radiol.* 1976;39:224–232.
11. Boice JD, Land CE, Preston DL. Ionizing radiation. In: Schottenfeld D, Fraumeni JF Jr, eds. *Cancer Epidemiology and Prevention.* 2nd ed. New York: Oxford University Press; 1996.
12. Greenwald ED, Greenwald ES. *Cancer Epidemiology.* New Hyde Park, NY: Medical Examination Publishing Co; 1983.
13. Wakabayashi T, Kato H, Ikeda T, Schull WJ. Studies of the mortality of A-bomb survivors. Report 7, Part III. Incidence of cancer in 1959–1978. *Radiat Res.* 1983;93:112–146.
14. Shore RE, Hildreth N, Dvoretsky P. Benign thyroid adenomas among persons irradiated in infancy for enlarged thymus gland. *Radiat Res.* 1993;134:217–223.
15. Preston-Martin S, Menck HR. The epidemiology of thyroid cancer in Los Angeles County. *West J Med.* 1979;131:369–372.
16. Pottern LM, Kaplan MM, Larsen PR, et al. Thyroid nodularity after irradiation for lymphoid hyperplasia: a comparison of questionnaire and clinical findings. *J Clin Epidemiol.* 1990;43:449–460.
17. Ron E, Kleinerman RA, Boice JD Jr, et al. A population-based case-control study of thyroid cancer. *J Natl Cancer Inst.* 1987;79:1–12.

18. Samaan NA, Schultz PN, Ordonez NG, et al. A comparison of thyroid carcinoma in those who have and have not had head and neck irradiation in childhood. *J Clin Endocrinol Metab.* 1987;64:219–223.

19. Linos A, Gray JE, Orvis AL, et al. Low-dose radiation and leukemia. *N Engl J Med.* 1980;302:1101–1105.

20. Gibson R, Graham S, Lilienfeld A, et al. Irradiation in the epidemiology of leukemia among adults. *J Natl Cancer Inst.* 1972;48:301–311.

21. Preston-Martin S, Thomas DC, White SC, et al. Prior exposure to medical and dental X-rays related to tumors of the parotid gland. *J Natl Cancer Inst.* 1988;80:943–949.

22. Shapiro S. *Periodic Screening for Breast Cancer: The Health Insurance Plan Project and Its Sequelae, 1963–86.* Baltimore: Johns Hopkins University Press; 1988.

23. Holmberg LH, Tabar L, Adami HO, et al. Survival in breast cancer diagnosed between mammographic screening examinations. *Lancet.* 1986;2:27–30.

24. Andersson I, Aspegren K, Janzon L, et al. Mammographic screening and mortality from breast cancer: the Malmo mammographic screening trial. *BMJ.* 1988;297:943–948.

25. Fletcher SW, Black W, Harris R, et al. Report of the international workshop on screening for breast cancer. *J Natl Cancer Inst.* 1993;85:1644–1656.

26. National Academy of Sciences. *Committee on the Biological Effects of Ionizing Radiation, 1980.* Washington, DC: National Academy Press; 1980.

27. Matanoski GM, Seltser R, Sartwell PE. The current mortality rates of radiologists and other physician specialists: specific causes of death. *Am J Epidemiol.* 1975;101:199–210.

28. Wang JX, Inskip PD, Boice JD Jr, et al. Cancer incidence among medical diagnostic X-ray workers in China. *J Natl Cancer Inst.* 1990;82:478–485.

29. Stebbings JH, Lucas HF, Stehney AF. Mortality from cancer of major sites in female radium dial workers. *Am J Ind Med.* 1984;5:435–459.

30. Matanoski G. Nuclear shipyard workers study. *Radiat Res.* 1993;133:126–127.

31. National Academy of Sciences. *Health Effects of Radon and Other Internally Deposited Alpha-Emitters.* Washington, DC: National Academy Press; 1988. BIER Report IV.

32. International Agency for Research on Cancer. *Man-Made Mineral Fibers and Radon.* Lyon, France: International Agency for Research on Cancer;1987. IARC Monographs on the Evaluation of Carcinogenic Risks to Humans, No. 43.

33. World Health Organization Regional Office for Europe. *Air Quality Guidelines for Europe.* Bilthoven, Netherlands: World Health Organization; 1987. Series No. 23.

34. Lubin JH, Boice JD Jr. Estimating Rn-induced lung cancer in the United States. *Health Phys.* 1989;57:417–427.

35. Pershagen G, Akerblom G, Axelson O, et al. Residential radon exposure and lung cancer in Sweden. *N Engl J Med.* 1994;330:159–164.

36. Letoumeau EG, Krewski D, Goddard MJ, et al. Case-control study of residential radon and lung cancer in Winnipeg, Manitoba, Canada. *Am J Epidemiol.* 1994;140:310–322.

37. Lubin JH, Liang Z, Hrubec Z. Radon exposure in residences and lung cancer among women: combined analysis of three studies. *Cancer Causes Control.* 1994;5:114–128.

38. Cook-Mozaffari P, Darby S, Doll R. Cancer near potential sites of nuclear installations. *Lancet.* 1989;2:1145–1147.

39. Jablon S, Hrubec Z, Boice JD Jr. Cancer in populations living near nuclear facilities: a survey of mortality nationwide and incidence in two states. *JAMA.* 1991;265:1403–1408.

40. McLaughlin JR, Clarke EA, Nishri D, et al. Childhood leukemia in the vicinity of Canadian nuclear facilities. *Cancer Causes Control.* 1993;4:51–58.

41. Hattchouel, J, Laplanche A, Hill C. Cancer mortality around French nuclear sites. *Ann Epidemiol.* 1996;6:126–129.

42. Bithell JF, Dutton SJ, Neary NM. Distribution of childhood leukemias and non-Hodgkin's lymphomas near nuclear installations in England and Wales. *BMJ.* 1994;309:501–505.

43. Darby SC, Doll R. Fallout, radiation doses near Dounreay, and childhood leukemia. *BMJ.* 1987;294:603–607.

44. Upton AC. Health impact of the Three Mile Island accident. *Ann NY Acad Sci.* 1981;365:63–75.

45. Stsjazhko VA, Tsyb AF, Tronko ND, et al. Childhood thyroid cancer since accident at Chernobyl. *BMJ.* 1995;310:801.

46. Major IR, Mole RH. Myeloid leukemia in X-ray irradiated VBA mice. *Nature.* 1978;272:455–456.

47. Nussbaum RH, Kohnlein W. Inconsistencies and open questions regarding low-dose health effects of ionizing radiation. *Environ Health Perspect.* 1994;102:656–667.
48. Moulder JE, Foster KR. Biological effects of power-frequency fields as they relate to carcinogenesis. *Society for Experimental Biological Medicine.* 1995;209:309–324.
49. Wertheimer N, Leeper E. Electrical wiring configurations and childhood cancer. *Am J Epidemiol.* 1979;109:273–284.
50. Savitz DA. Overview of epidemiologic research on electric and magnetic fields and cancer. *Am Ind Hyg Assoc J.* 1993;54:197–204.
51. Savitz DA. Epidemiologic studies of electric and magnetic fields and cancer: strategies for extending knowledge. *Environ Health Perspect.* 1993;101(suppl 4):83–91.
52. Linet MS, Hatch EE, Kleinerman RA, et al. Residential exposure to magnetic fields and acute lymphoblastic leukemia in children. *New Eng J Med.* 1997;337:1–7.
53. Campion EW. Power lines, fear, and cancer. *New Eng J Med.* 1997;337:1–7. Editorial.
54. National Research Council. Possible health effects of exposure to residential electric and magnetic fields. Washington, DC: National Academy Press; 1997.
55. Koh HK. Cutaneous melanoma. *New Eng J Med.* 1991;325:171–182.
56. Ainsleigh HG. Beneficial effects of sun exposure on cancer mortality. *Prev Med.* 1993;22:132–140.
57. Grin CS, Rigel DS, Friedman RJ. Worldwide incidence of malignant melanoma. In: Balch CM, Houghton AN, eds. *Cutaneous Melanoma.* Philadelphia: JB Lippincott Co; 1992.
58. Rigel DS, Friedman RJ, Kopf AW. The incidence of malignant melanoma in the United States: issues as we approach the 21st century. *J Am Acad Dermatol.* 1996;34:839–847.
59. Studzinski GP, Moore DC. Sunlight—can it prevent as well as cause cancer? *Cancer Res.* 1995;55:4014–4022.
60. Hersey P, Hasic E, Edwards A, et al. Immunological effects of solarium exposure. *Lancet.* 1983;1:545–548.
61. Kripke ML. Ultraviolet radiation and immunology: something new under the sun. *Cancer Res.* 1994;54:6102–6105.
62. Gorham FC, Garland CF, Garland, FC. Acid haze air pollution and breast and colon cancer mortality in 20 Canadian cities. *Can J Public Health.* 1989;80:96–100.
63. Schwartz GG, Hulka BS. Is vitamin D deficiency a risk factor for prostate cancer? (Hypothesis). *Anticancer Res.* 1990;10:1307–1312.
64. Ansleigh HG. Beneficial effects of sun exposure on cancer mortality. *Prev Med.* 1993;22:132–140.
65. Abe E, Miyaura C, Sakagami H, et al. Differentiation of mouse myeloid leukemia cells induced by 1a,25-hydroxyvitamin D_3. *Proc Natl Acad Sci USA.* 1981;78:4990–4994.
66. Mangelsdorf DJ, Koeffler HP. 1a,25-Hydroxyvitamin D_3 induced differentiation in a human promyelocytic leukemia cell line. *J Cell Biol.* 1984;98:391–398.

Chapter 12

Viruses and Cancer

Philip C. Nasca

This chapter provides an overview of the methodological issues involved in investigating the etiologic relationship between a virus and one or more human cancers. It illustrates these issues through a detailed description of the role of hepatitis B and C viruses in the etiology of liver cancer and of the dominant role that human papillomavirus has been discovered to play in the etiology of cancer of the uterine cervix. Additional sections focus on the relationship between Epstein-Barr virus and selected cancers and the role of human T-cell lymphotropic virus in the etiology of adult T-cell leukemias. The chapter as a whole provides an introduction to the descriptive and analytic epidemiological studies that have helped to establish a causal relationship between viral agents and types of cancer. The importance of new molecular biological techniques for ensuring reliable identification of viral subtypes and the importance of new methods for collecting biological specimens are also discussed. Finally, the chapter reviews the biological mechanisms identified for each of the virus-cancer relationships described.

A number of viruses are etiologically related to various types of cancer. Chapter 3 describes the molecular basis of viral carcinogenesis, and Chapter 13 covers the effects of human immunodeficiency virus (HIV) on the immune system and the associated increased risk of Kaposi's sarcoma, non-Hodgkin's lymphoma, and other cancers. The focus of this chapter is on several viruses that, according to a substantial body of evidence, are implicated in the development of various cancers. Virus-cancer associations include hepatitis B virus (HBV) and hepatitis C virus (HCV) and liver cancer, Epstein-Barr virus (EBV) and nasopharyngeal carcinoma, Burkitt's lymphoma and Hodgkin's disease, human papillomavirus (HPV) and cancer of the uterine cervix and anal canal, and adult T-cell leukemia virus and adult leukemias and lymphomas. The discussion covers linkages between epidemiological data, animal models, and cellular biology.

GENERAL PRINCIPLES

In 1990, Evans and Mueller[1] presented an overview of various problems that might be encountered when attempting to relate human cancers to viral infections (Exhibit 12–1). First, viruses, like chemical carcinogens, produce cancer in the host only after a substantial incubation or latency period. The latency period usually extends for years, thus making it difficult to conduct studies that allow the linking of a particular viral exposure with a particular cancer. The long latency period between infection with HBV and the development of liver cancer is a prime example. A second obstacle is that the viral infection may be extremely common whereas the related cancer may be uncommon. Epstein-Barr virus is a good example of an agent that often presents as a subclinical primary

Exhibit 12–1 Problems in Relating Viruses to the Causation of Human Cancers

- The long incubation or induction period between initial infection with the putative virus and the cancer(s) with which it is associated.
- The common and ubiquitous nature of most candidate viruses and the rarity of the cancer with which they are associated.
- The initial infection with the candidate virus is often sub-clinical, so that the time of infection can not be established by clinical features.
- The need for cofactors in most viral-related cancers.
- The causes of cancer may vary in different geographic areas or by age.
- Different viral strains may have different oncogenic potential.
- The human host plays a critical role in susceptibility to cancer, especially the age at the time of infection, the genetic characteristics, and the status of the immune system.
- Cancers result from a complex and multistage process, in which a virus may play a role at different points in pathogenesis in association with alterations in the host's immune system, oncogenes, chromosomal translocations, and a variety of events at the molecular level.
- The inability to reproduce many human cancers in experimental animals with the putative virus.
- The recognition that a virus, toxin, chemical, altered gene, or other causal factor may all be capable of initiating or promoting the processes that result in a cancer with the same histologic features.

Source: Reprinted from *Annals of Epidemiology*, Vol. 1, A.S. Evans and N.E. Mueller, Viruses and Cancer: Causal Associations, pp. 71–92, Copyright 1990, with permission from Elsevier Science.

infection and is much more common than nasopharyngeal carcinoma, the cancer it is etiologically associated with, which is quite rare. In addition, cancers related to a particular virus may also be related to other cofactors, and the relationships between these factors and the viral exposure need to be sorted out. Various host factors may be of great importance. For example, patients treated with immunosuppressive drugs experience activation of EBV and a subsequent increased risk of non-Hodgkin's lymphoma. Interactions between viral infections and other environmental exposures may also be important. As shown in the next section, liver cancer is clearly related to hepatitis B virus infection early in life. These cancers are also related to the consumption of foods contaminated with aflatoxins. Individuals with both HBV infection and exposure to aflatoxins are at extremely high risk for developing liver cancer. Attention must also be paid to various strains or serological subtypes of the virus. When technology to subtype the various HPV strains was developed and incorporated into epidemiological research studies, cancer of the uterine cervix was discovered to be related more strongly to some viral subtypes than to others. The complex, multistage nature of various cancers is now firmly established, and determining when and how, in the process of malignant transformation, the virus affects the target cell is essential. The mechanisms through which these agents contribute to cellular transformation are beginning to be understood in the case of some viruses but not others, even though the viral-cancer relationship has been clearly established.

Evans and Mueller[1] also presented epidemiological and virological guidelines for assessing whether a causal relationship between a putative virus and a human cancer exists (Exhibit 12–2). These guidelines encompass standard epidemiological criteria for assessing causality, including the coherence between the hypothesis and the known distribution of the agent and the disease in different populations, a large magnitude of effect, and the proper temporal relationship. Since infection with some of these agents can be prevented by vaccination, the effect of prevention measures on the incidence of a particular cancer can be observed in some instances. The virological guidelines indicate the importance of coherence between the epidemiological findings and experimental findings.

HEPATOCELLULAR CARCINOMA AND HEPATITIS VIRUSES B AND C

Several lines of epidemiological and experimental evidence have firmly established a causal role for HBV and HCV in the development of hepatocellular carcinoma (HCC).[2–7] HBV is a DNA virus of the hepadnaviruses, which, as the name suggests, have an affinity for hepatic cells. The viruses in this family all have the same gene structure and replicate in the same manner.[7] In Asia, where infection rates are extremely high, the primary route of transmission is from infected mothers to their offspring. This route of exposure usually occurs in the neonatal period but can also occur in utero.[8–12] The vertical transmission leads more often to persistent lifelong infection than does horizontal

---

Exhibit 12–2 Guidelines for Relating a Virus to a Human Cancer

Epidemiological

- The geographic distribution of infection with the virus should be similar to that of the tumor with which it is associated when adjusted for the age of infection and the presence of cofactors known to be important in tumor development.
- The presence of the viral marker (high antibody titers or antigenemia) should be higher in cases than in matched controls in the same geographic setting, as shown in case-control studies.
- The viral marker should *precede* the tumor, and a significantly higher incidence of the tumor should follow in persons with the marker than in those without it.
- Prevention of infection with the virus (vaccination) or control of the host's response to it (such as delaying the time of infection) should decrease the incidence of the tumor.

Virological

- The virus should be able to transform human cells in vitro into malignant ones.
- The viral genome or DNA should be demonstrated in tumor cells and not in normal cells.
- The virus should be able to induce the tumor in a susceptible experimental animal and neutralization of the virus prior to injection should prevent development of the tumor.

Source: Reprinted from *Annals of Epidemiology*, Vol. 1, A.S. Evans and N.E. Mueller, Viruses and Cancer: Causal Associations, pp. 71–92, Copyright 1990, with permission from Elsevier Science.

transmission to adults through contaminated blood products.[4] Although males and females are equally likely to be infected at birth, males are significantly more likely to suffer from chronic active hepatitis. Males are three times more likely than females to develop cirrhosis and six times more likely to develop HCC.[4,13,14] Clinical and experimental evidence suggests that these gender differences may be hormonal. A high incidence of HCC has been observed among patients treated with methyl testosterone for aplastic anemia. Strains of rats with high spontaneous HCC incidence also show a male predominance, which declines if the males are castrated. Female rats experience disease rates close to males if they are treated with male hormones.[3]

HCV is an RNA virus with a molecular structure similar to the family of flaviviruses that cause yellow fever or Dengue fever and the pestiviruses that cause various animal diseases.[7] Unlike HBV, HCV is not commonly transmitted vertically from mother to child. Horizontal transmission through transference of contaminated blood products is the most common route, and intravenous drug users, hemodialysis patients, and recipients of blood transfusions are at highest risk. Sexual transmission may also occur, and it is common for infected patients to fall outside all of these risk categories.[7,15,16] The prevalence of HCV is higher in developed countries and lower in developing countries, but the prevalence of HBV tends to be higher in these latter countries.

Descriptive Epidemiology

The first suggestion that HBV might be etiologically related to HCC came from data showing striking geographical similarities in the worldwide distribution of HBV and HCC. Data on HCC derived from population-based cancer registries maintained by various countries were compared to HBV infection data collected through serological prevalence studies. The distributions of HCC and HBV by country are shown in Figures 12–1 and 12–2.[4] The figures show the highest HBV prevalence rates occur in China and Southeast Asia and sub-Saharan Africa. Intermediate HBV prevalence rates are seen in the Indian subcontinent and South America. The HCC rates are highest in areas with the highest HBV prevalence rates, and a considerable degree of overlap exists for countries with intermediate HBV and HCC rates.

Qiao et al[17] compared primary HCC death rates and HBV prevalence rates in 30 countries. These authors reported a statistically significant correlation between HBV and HCC ($r = 0.53$) after controlling for each country's mean annual per capita consumption of alcohol. Regression analyses showed that the relation between HCC and HBV was independent of alcohol and that HBV infection was a more important determinant of the HCC death rate than drinking patterns. Variations between HCC and HBV have also been examined within regions of a country. Hsing et al[18] examined liver cancer mortality rates and HBV prevalence rates in 65 counties in China. Counties with the highest rates of HCC and the highest rates of HBV overlapped extensively, and the overlap was observed for both males and females. Lamont et al[19] reported concomitant secular trends for primary liver cancer rates and HBV prevalence rates in Scotland from 1972 to 1985. Significant geographical correlations between primary liver cancer incidence and HBV incidence were also observed in the various parts of the country, which has a low rate of HBV infection.

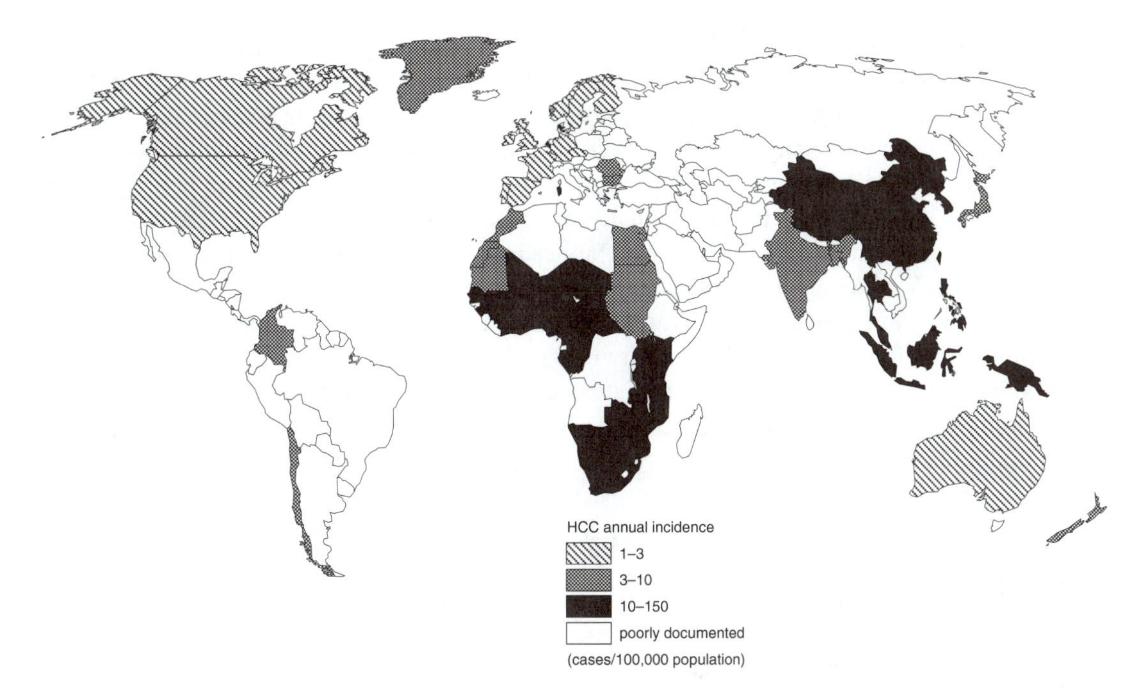

Figure 12–1 Annual incidence of HCC in the world. *Source:* Reprinted with permission from J.L. Melnick, Hepatocellular Carcinoma Caused by Hepatitis B Virus, in *Viral Infections in Humans: Epidemiology and Control, 3rd Edition*, A.S. Evans, ed., pp. 769–780, © 1989, Plenum Publishing Corporation.

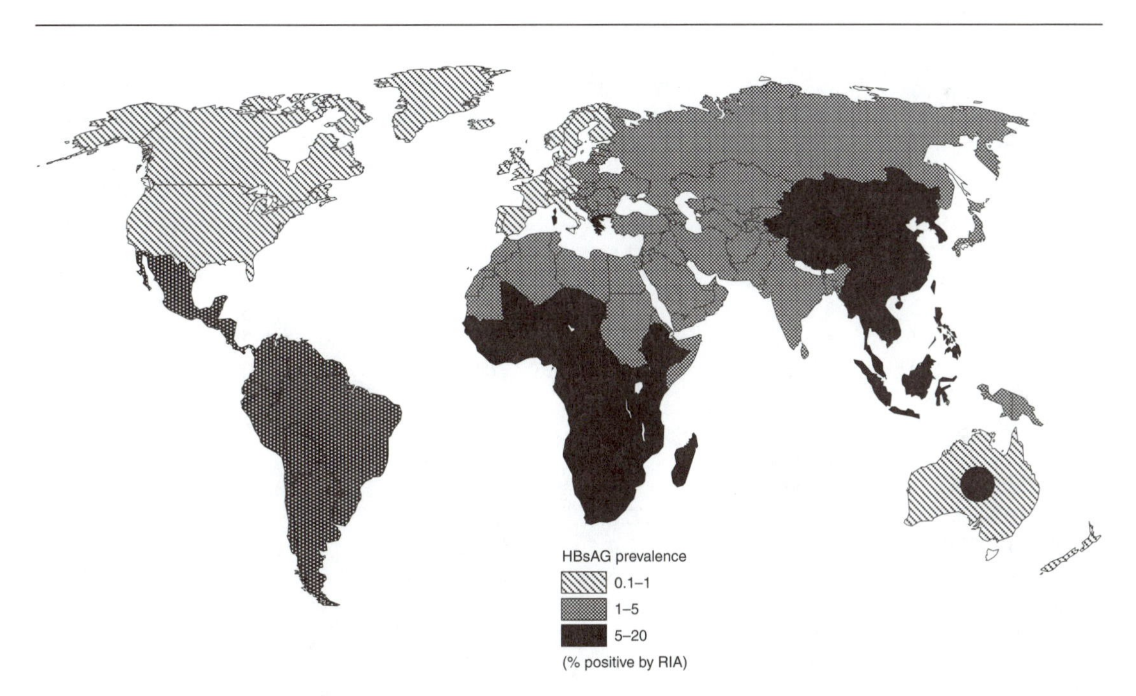

Figure 12–2 Prevalence of HbsAG in the world. *Source:* Reprinted with permission from J.L. Melnick, Hepatocellular Carcinoma Caused by Hepatitis B Virus, in *Viral Infections in Humans: Epidemiology and Control, 3rd Edition*, A.S. Evans, ed., pp. 769–780, © 1989, Plenum Publishing Corporation.

Given the worldwide distribution of HBV, it is not surprising to see significant racial differences in the incidence of HCC. Chinese males who immigrated to New York City show HCC mortality rates that are 10 to 40 times higher than the males in other ethnic groups in the city.[20] Since a large number of these men lived in the United States for 10 years or more prior to dying from HCC, the data support the idea that infection with HBV occurs early in life and that early infection confers a lifelong increased risk of HCC. Rosenblatt et al[21] also reported higher HCC incidence rates among males and females born in Asia. The annual incidence rates per 100,000 for males born in China, Japan, the Philippines, and the United States were 26.5, 16.5, 11.4, and 6.5, respectively. Smaller differences were observed when males of Asian descent born in the United States were compared to US–born Caucasian men. Similar high rates of HBV and HCC have been reported among immigrants from the Indian subcontinent to England and Wales,[22] among Alaskan natives,[23] and among the circumpolar Inuit.[24]

Analytic Studies of HCC and Hepatitis Viruses

Blumberg and London[25,26] reviewed results from case-control studies conducted prior to 1982. The large number of case-control studies of HBV and HCV conducted from 1982 through 1996 are summarized in Table 12–1. These studies uniformly show a

Table 12–1 Summary of Results from Serological Case-Control Studies of Hepatocellular Carcinoma and Hepatitis B Virus (HBV) and Hepatitis C Virus (HCV), 1982–1996

		HBV		*HCV*	
First Author (Year)	*Country*	*Odds Ratio*	*(95% CI)*	*Odds Ratio*	*(95% CI)*
Lam (1982)[27]	China	21.3	(10.1–45.9)		
Yeh (1985)[28]	China	17.0	NA		
Trichopoulos (1987)[29]	Greece	13.7	(8.0-23.5)		
Tanaka (1988)[30]	Japan	31.0	NA		
Tsukuma (1990)[31]	Japan	14.3	(5.7–36.3)		
Yu (1990)[32]	US	7.0	(3.1–16.1)	10.5	(3.5–31.3)
Kaklamani (1991)[33]	Greece			6.3	NA
Srivatanakul (1991)[34]	Thailand	12.0	(2.9–50.4)	1.3	(0.2–8.7)
Stroffolini (1992)[35]	Italy	13.3	(5.5–32.2)	21.3	(8.8–51.5)
Zavitsanos (1992)[36]	Greece			10.4	(4.2–26.0)
Tanaka (1992)[37]	Japan	13.8	(5.9–32.5)		
Chang (1994)[38]	Taiwan			88.2	NA
Pyong (1994)[39]	Japan*	58.2	NA	92.4	NA
Tanaka (1995)[40]	Japan†	42.4	(11.2–160.2)		
Hadziyannis (1995)[41]	Greece	18.8	(8.2–43.2)	7.7	(1.7–35.1)
Nomura (1996)[42]	US‡	43.0	(5.7–325.5)		
Silini (1996)[43]	Italy			1.7	NA
Sun (1996)[44]	Taiwan	24.6	(9.5–64.1)	4.0	(0.7–24.0)

*Koreans living in Japan.
†Women only.
‡Only one control and no cases had antibodies to HCV.

substantially elevated risk of HCC associated with HBV infection. The odds ratios observed in these studies range from 7.0 to 58.2. The range of findings for HCC and HCV are broader, with some studies showing only marginal associations and some reporting extremely low HCV prevalence. In the study by Nomura et al[42] of Japanese Americans, only one control subject and none of the case subjects showed antibodies to HCV. However, the majority of studies show strong associations between HCC and HCV.

Despite the magnitude of the risk observed in these case-control studies, they cannot establish the necessary temporal relationship between viral infection and development of HCC. Researchers, however, have conducted a number of cohort studies[45–51] in which viral infection was identified many years in advance of the diagnosis of HCC. The results of seven cohort studies are summarized in Table 12–2. The large prospective study by Beasley et al[45] was the first epidemiological investigation to establish that a temporal relationship between the infection and HCC clearly exists. Beasley and his associates studied 22,707 Taiwanese male civil servants who were 40–59 years of age at the time of initial recruitment. A total of 19,253 men tested HBV negative and 3,454 tested HBV positive at the beginning of the study. After 10 years of follow-up, the HBV-positive men showed an HCC incidence rate of 494.5 per 100,000, whereas the HBV-negative men showed a rate of only 5.3. The relative risk for the HBV-positive men was

Table 12–2 Cohort Studies of Hepatocellular Carcinoma among Subjects Serologically Positive for Hepatitis B Virus, 1984–1993

First Author (Year)	*Country*	*Subjects*	*Follow-up (Years)*	*Comparison Group*	*Relative Risk*
Beasley (1981)[45]	Taiwan	22,707 HBV male carriers	8.9	HBV NC*	98.4
Iijma (1984)[46]	Japan	495 HBV male carriers	10.0	Population†	10.4
Oshima (1984)[47]	Japan	8,646 HBV male carriers	6.2	Population	6.6
Tu (1985)[48]	China	12,222 HBV male carriers	3.0	HBV NC	6.7
Tokudome (1987)[49]	Japan	2,595 HBV male carriers	7.0	Population	7.3
Tokudome (1988)[50]	Japan	3,769 HBV female carriers	8.0	Population	5.6
Tsukuma (1993)[51]	Japan	917 patients chronic liver disease; HBV or HCV carriers	3.0	HBV NC HCV NC	6.9 4.1

*HBV or HCV noncarriers.

†Observed numbers of hepatocellular cancers compared with number expected based on disease rates in the general population.

98.4. Some of the subjects who were serologically negative at baseline probably converted to a positive serology as the study progressed. The extremely large relative risk is probably an underestimate of the true relative risk. In addition to demonstrating the study's internal validity, the authors also provided data to suggest that the study results might be extrapolated to other populations with high HBV rates. Although the civil servants tended to be better educated and in better health than the population as a whole, rates of HBV, HCC, and cirrhosis in the study population and the general population were similar.

Other cohort studies in populations with high HBV prevalence have also established a clear temporal relation between HBV infection and the risk of developing HCC. These studies have reported relative risks in the range of 4.1 to 10.4. The low relative risks observed in these studies, as compared with the study by Beasley and his coworkers, are probably due to nature of the comparison groups. These studies used HCC incidence or mortality rates in the general population to create numbers of HCC cases or deaths expected to occur among the HBV-positive cohort members. These disease rates are derived from populations with high HCC incidence and mortality rates, and the expected numbers are based on events that occur among a mixed population of HBV positives and negatives. It is therefore not unexpected that the relative risks observed in these studies would be lower than the relative risks observed by Beasley and others who compared HCC incidence in HBV-positive and -negative study members. Despite the attenuation, the relative risks associated with HBV are still of a moderate to large magnitude and provide support for the existence of a causal relationship between HCC and HBV.

A retrospective cohort study of US Army veterans provides additional support. Norman et al[52] conducted a study of veterans who were given yellow fever vaccine contaminated with HBV in 1942. A total of 69,988 veterans were divided into three subcohorts: men hospitalized with hepatitis in 1942, men subclinically infected in 1942, and control subjects who began their service after 1942. Men in the subclinical infection group showed higher rates of liver cancer mortality than the control subjects, but no differences were observed between those diagnosed with hepatitis and the control subjects. A nested case-control study conducted within this cohort showed a threefold increased risk of dying from liver cancer associated with the receipt of contaminated vaccine.

Vaccination for HBV and Reductions in HCC Incidence

The evidence in support of a causal relation between HBV and a particular cancer would be strengthened if protection from HBV infection was to result in a significant reduction in the occurrence of the cancer. A large nationwide hepatitis B vaccination program was implemented in Taiwan in 1984.[53] During the first two years of the program, vaccination was provided to neonates whose mothers were HBV carriers. The program was extended to all neonates in 1987, to primary school children in 1988, to middle school children in 1989, and to adults in 1990. Data on liver cancer in children aged 6–14 years were collected for the years 1981–1994 from the Taiwan National Cancer Registry and from a record review at Taiwan's 17 major medical centers. The prevalence of HBV positivity in six-year-olds declined from a high of 10.6% in 1982 to 0.8% in 1994. The liver cancer incidence rates for children who reached the age of 6–9 years after the vaccination program was initiated were dramatically lower than the rates for children who had reached that age prior to the start of the program. The data are summarized in Table 12–3. Liver cancer incidence rates in all children aged 6–9 declined from a preprogram rate of 0.52 per 100,000 children to a rate of 0.13 per 100,000 children in the after-program cohort. Declines in liver cancer incidence were observed in each single year of age.

Experimental Data

Experimental studies have also provided strong support for the existence of a causal relationship between HBV and HCC.[54–64] Hepadnaviruses that affect various animal species are similar in structure to the human HBV.[54] The prevalence of hepadnavirus infection has been shown to be high in ground squirrels,[55,57] ducks,[58–60] and woodchucks.[61–65] These species also experience high rates of spontaneous liver cancer and persistent infection with the virus. Subsequent high rates of liver cancer can be induced by experimentally challenging uninfected animals with HBV. Almost all experimentally challenged and persistently infected animals develop HCC, while HCC occurs in only a low percentage of animals with transient viral infections. These studies as well as experiments utilizing chimpanzees[65–67] have been extremely useful in helping to develop vaccines for HBV and for investigating therapies for virally induced liver hepatoma.[68]

The biological mechanism through which HBV causes hepatocellular cancer in humans has not been determined. Molecular studies have shown that the viral genome is integrated into the host DNA.[69–74] However, the integrations have been found in many locations throughout the host DNA, making it difficult to link these integrations with an adjacent cellular oncogene.[4,7] In 1987, Zhou et al[75] reported finding HBV DNA on chromosome 17p near the p53 gene, sparking interest in the possible effects of HBV on this human tumor suppresser gene.[76–78] Other areas of research include the possible capacity of HBV to foster genetic instability in the DNA repair process.[79]

Table 12–3 Incidence of Liver Cancer per 100,000 Children in Birth Cohorts Determined According to the Date of Implementation of the Hepatitis B Vaccination Program

	Before-Program Cohort (July 1974–June 1984)		*After-Program Cohort (July 1984–June 1986)*	
Age at Diagnosis (Years)	*Population*	*No. of Cancers (Incidence)*	*Population*	*No. of Cancers (Incidence)*
6	3,940,747	18 (0.46)	648,642	0 (0.00)
7	3,938,119	21 (0.53)	647,051	1 (0.15)
8	3,931,983	19 (0.48)	644,892	2 (0.31)
9	3,928,721	24 (0.61)	340,521*	0 (0.00)
Total	15,739,570	82 (0.52)	2,281,106	3 (0.13)†

*This value is based on data for the cohort born from July 1984 to June 1985.

†$p < 0.001$ for the comparisons between birth cohorts.

Source: Reprinted with permission from Chang, et al., Universal Hepatitis B Vaccination in Taiwan and the Incidence of Hepatocellular Carcinoma in Children, *The New England Journal of Medicine*, Vol. 336, pp. 1855–1859,

HUMAN PAPILLOMAVIRUSES

Epidemiological Studies

Human papillomaviruses (HPVs) are DNA viruses that have been causally linked to cancers of the uterine cervix[80–83] and are suspected to be causally related to anal cancers[84] and cancers of the aerodigestive tract.[85] The focus here is on the relation between HPVs and cancers of the uterine cervix and anus.

Epidemiological studies conducted from the 1950s through the 1970s strongly suggested that cancer of the uterine cervix was caused by an agent passed from men to women during sexual intercourse. The venereal nature of this cancer was suggested by the high disease risks observed among women who experienced first coitus at an early age, had multiple sexual partners, and had a history of other sexually transmitted diseases, and the high risk observed among prostitutes and the low risk observed among nuns were taken as further support for this view. Experimental studies during the 1970s and early 1980s demonstrated the presence of the HPV in dysplastic, in situ, and invasive cervical lesions.[86] HPV was shown to have the capability of transforming human epithelial cells in vitro.[87] Recent studies have shown that HPV encodes for two transforming genes that create proteins that interact with products formed by the p53 and pRB tumor suppresser genes and cause these products not to function.[88] The identification of various subtypes of HPV eventually led to the recognition that certain subtypes, namely, 16 and 18, were more strongly linked to cervical cancer than other types.

The discovery that HPV might well be a carcinogenic agent for cervical cancer led to the development of a large number of case-control studies of invasive cervical cancers and the spectrum of preinvasive lesions thought to be part of the natural history of these cancers. (The preinvasive lesions are referred to as *cervical intraepithelial neoplasia [CIN]*, and are now graded according to severity as CIN I through CIN III.)[89] Results from the early epidemiological studies were inconsistent and failed to uncover a coherent relation between sexual activity, HPV infection, and cervical cancer risk. The lack of coherence was probably due to the inability of the serological tests used in these studies to correctly categorize case and control subjects with regard to infection status.[90–92] Analysis of the possible effects of HPV measurement error on the observed odds ratios suggested that even low levels of misclassification might lead to underestimation of the relation between HPV and sexual activity. Misclassification would make it difficult to examine the relation between sexual activity and disease status while attempting to exercise statistical control over HPV infection status.[91] The problem was eventually solved with the development of new molecular probes, which possessed greater sensitivity and specificity than previous methods. The development of the polymerase chain reaction (PCR) technique made it possible to detect multiple copies of the virus in samples obtained from cervical swabs. The PCR approach has been shown to be superior to other methods, such as the Southern hybridization method.[93]

The effect of measurement error was clearly demonstrated by Schiffman and Schatzkin,[92] who compared results from two case-control studies of HPV and cancer of the uterine cervix that used similar designs. The major difference between these two studies was that the earlier employed a laboratory technique, the Southern blot hybridization technique, that was inferior to the one used in the later study. The Southern blot hybridization technique showed modest repeatability and poor interlaboratory agreement when applied to specimens from the same aliquots. The data suggest that study subjects had a high likelihood of being misclassified with respect to HPV infection status. The second study used the PCR technique, which was found to be significantly superior in terms of repeatability and interlaboratory agreement. In addition, whereas an odds ratio of 3.7 (95% CI = 2.6–5.3) was observed in the first study, the study using the PCR technique showed an odds ratio of 20.1 (95% CI = 14.1–28.0). Further, the first study showed a weak association between HPV infection and lifetime number of sexual partners, but the second study showed a clear dose-response relationship between the percentage of HPV-positive subjects and lifetime number of sexual partners. Finally, it had long been suspected that a risk factor such as lifetime number of sexual partners increases the risk of cancer of the uterine cervix by increasing a woman's probability of being exposed to HPV. If this hypothesis is correct, controlling for HPV infection at the data analysis phase of the study would eliminate the association between cervical cancer and measures of sexual activity. Controlling for HPV infection in the study that employed the Southern blot technique failed to attenuate this association; in the study using the PCR technique, however, controlling for HPV infection completely eliminated the association.

Concerns about the classification of CIN lesions have also been raised. Kato et al[94] reported high levels of agreement among a panel of three cytopathologists for invasive carcinomas and normal or inflammatory tissues but somewhat lower levels of agreement for CIN III. The final consensus diagnosis by the panel showed near perfect agreement with the diagnosis originally made by the local cytopathologists. In addition, the odds ratios for various risk factors were not seriously affected by the error rate for CIN III.

The advent of infection classification methods led to the development of a number of case-control studies clearly demonstrating HPV to be a likely cause of most cervical neoplasia.[95–108] In 1993, Schiffman et al[95] conducted a carefully designed case-control study that overcame many of the methodological problems encountered in previous studies and showed an unequivocal etiologic relation between HPV and CIN. These investigators conducted a case-control study of 500 women with CIN and 500 control subjects who had been receiving cytological screening as members of a large prepaid health plan. HPV infection status and subtyping were determined by testing cervicovaginal lavage specimens for gene amplification using the PCR approach. A number of approaches were used to ensure that study subjects were correctly classified as cases and controls. A sample of 250 cervical smears were selected for cytological review, including 200 smears from borderline lesions, where the potential for misclassification was greatest. None of the cases originally reported as CIN were found to be misclassified. The distribution of 363 cases by severity of disease was determined through colposcopically directed biopsies, and the distribution was found to be similar to the distribution that might be expected in an unselected series of US cases. By reducing the probability of misclassifying the HPV infection and disease status of study subjects, the stage was set for examining the relations between HPV infection and established risk factors, such as sexual activity, cigarette smoking, oral contraceptive use, parity, and measures of socioeconomic status. The investigators reported the expected bivariate relation between HPV and the risk of CIN, with HPV types 16 and 18 showing a relative risk of 51.0 when compared with those with negative tests. Types thought to confer intermediate and lower levels of risk showed relative risks of 33.0 and 8.7, respectively. Elevated relative risks were also observed for the established CIN risk factors. The associations either disappeared or were greatly attenuated when the investigators controlled for HPV status. The data clearly demonstrated that HPV significantly increased the risk of CIN independently of any other known risk factors. Similar findings have been reported from studies conducted in the United States, South America, and Europe.

Several studies also focused on determining the male role in transmitting HPV to their sexual partners.[104–108] Bosch et al[104] studied the husbands of women participating in two case-control studies in Spain. In addition to interviewing the husbands about their sexual practices, the investigators collected cytological specimens from the distal urethra and the surface of the glans penis of 183 husbands of case subjects and 171 husbands of control subjects. Using the PCR technique, the investigators found that the presence of HPV DNA in a husband's cytological sample conferred a nearly fivefold increased risk for cervical cancer on his wife. A ninefold increased risk of cervical cancer was observed in women whose husbands were infected with type 16 HPV. A woman's risk was also strongly related to the number of extramarital sexual partners (OR = 11.0; 95% CI = 3.0–40.0) reported by the husband and the number of times the husband reported having sexual relations with a prostitute (OR = 8.0; 95% CI = 2.9–22.2). A similar study of the husbands of control subjects enrolled in four case-control studies in Colombia and Spain showed a close correspondence between the countrywide risk of cervical neoplasia and the probability that the husband was infected with HPV.[106] Husbands of controls living in Colombia, a high-risk country, were five time more likely to have a positive PCR test for HPV than husbands in Spain, a low-risk country. Among Spanish husbands, a strong dose-response relation was observed between HPV prevalence and various measures of sexual activity. No association was observed between HPV prevalence and sexual practices in Colombia. According to the data from these case-control studies, poorly educated men were two to five times more likely than highly educated men to have penile samples that tested positive for HPV.[104]

Prevalence surveys conducted in various countries suggest that HPV is likely to be a major cause of cervical neoplasia in all parts of the world. Bosch et al[108] collected over 1,000 specimens from patients diagnosed with invasive cervical cancer in 32 hospitals in 22 countries. PCR techniques revealed HPV DNA in 93% of all invasive cancers, with 50% showing infection with type 16. This high-risk type was the predominant form of the virus in all countries with the exception of Indonesia, where type 18, another high-risk variant, was most common. These results strongly suggest that HPV plays a key role in the development of invasive cervical cancer in a large number of diverse populations.

Cofactors

The relationship between HPV and other infectious agents has also been investigated. Jha et al[109] tested serum samples from 219 women with cervical cancer and 387 female control subjects for antibodies to HPV 16 and 18, herpes virus (HSV) types 1 and 2, *Chlamydia trachomatis*, cytomegalovirus (CMV), and Epstein-Barr virus (EBV). In addition to the expected increased risk among HPV-positive women, the assays also showed increased risks for women who tested positive for HSV and *Chlamydia trachomatis*. However, the associations between cervical cancer and these other infectious agents disappeared when the analysis was limited to HPV-positive cases and controls.

Virus-induced immunosuppression appears to have an effect on the relation between HPV and cervical and anal neoplasia, and a number of studies have shown higher HPV prevalence in patients who tested positive for the human immunodeficiency virus (HIV).[110–113] Sun et al[113] collected two or more semiannual cervicovaginal lavage specimens from 220 women infected with HIV and 231 women who tested negative for HIV. At each examination, women with HIV were more likely to test positive for HPV. Persistent HPV infection was observed in 24% of women who were seropositive for HIV and in only 3% who were seronegative. These findings suggest an interaction between immune suppression and infection with HPV exists and is probably responsible for the higher rates of CIN observed in HIV-positive women.

Other cofactors that have been studied include smoking, oral contraceptive use, and pregnancy. A number of early studies showed a two- to threefold increased risk among cigarette smokers compared with nonsmokers. This association persisted after controlling for measures of sexual activity. However, in subsequent studies, the association between smoking and cervical cancer was found to be inconsistent after controlling for HPV infection. A number of laboratory studies have shown that smokers are more likely than nonsmokers to have mutagenic cervical fluids. It has also been suggested (1) that smoking may have an immunologic effect that allows HPV to persist in cervical cells and (2) that smoking may contribute to chromosomal instability.[114,115] A more detailed account of the possible relationship between smoking and cancer of the uterine cervix is presented in Chapter 9.

The relation between oral contraceptive use and cervical cancer is controversial.[114,115] In a large case-control study in Latin America, the HPV-adjusted risk for adenocarcinoma of the uterine cervix was 2.4, but the adjusted relative risk for squamous cell carcinomas was only 1.1.[116] Similar results have been reported from several cohort studies in which adjustment for HPV infection significantly attenuated or eliminated the association between oral contraceptive use and cervical cancer.[95,117,118] Parity has long been recognized as a risk factor for cancer of the uterine cervix. The association between parity and uterine cancer exists among HPV-positive and -negative subjects, and parity has been shown to be an independent risk factor even after adjustment for HPV.[119]

More recently, investigators have explored the extent to which the relation between HPV and cervical cancer might be modulated by dietary factors. Potischman and Brinton[120] have written an extensive review of the literature on the relation between nutrition and cervical neoplasia. The authors view the current literature as providing reasonably consistent support for the hypothesis that women consuming low levels of vitamin C and carotenoids are at increased risk for cervical neoplasia. The evidence for an association between the risk of cervical neoplasia and vitamin E and folate is weaker, but further research on these nutrients is clearly justified. A number of small trials of the effect of β-carotene supplementation on CIN progression or regression have already been conducted. Because of the small numbers of subjects and short follow-up periods, the results have been inconsistent. The true effect of nutrition supplementation should emerge from a number of larger trials currently being conducted. A key issue that needs to be addressed is the extent to which various nutrients interact with HPV to increase the risk of CIN lesions. To date, most studies have either used surrogate measures of HPV infection, such as sexual activity, or imprecise laboratory methods for determining HPV infection. Consequent high levels of measurement error may be partially responsible for the inconsistent results reported thus far. Butterworth[121] reported an interaction between low folate and infection with HPV-16 among women with cervical neoplasia, but Potischman[122] found no interaction between folate and HPV among women with invasive carcinomas. The prospect that nutrient supplements could be used to stem the progression of CIN toward invasive disease is an exciting one and offers a fertile area for additional research.

The natural history of CIN is not entirely understood at this time. One model suggests that most CIN I lesions regress and that affected tissues return to normal. The remaining CIN I lesions are thought to progress from low grade to high grade in the face of persistent HPV infection. These high-grade lesions can, if left untreated, progress to frankly invasive carcinoma. A second model proposes that most CIN I lesions regress but that new higher-grade lesions can appear on other areas of the cervix as a result of persistent HPV infection.[82,123] In the second model, a continuum from CIN I to CIN III is not always present. Two cohort studies[118,124] provided some insight into the natural history of these lesions. Koutsky et al[118] followed a cohort of 241 women with negative cervical cytology. Every four months, the women received cytological and colposcopic examinations of the uterine cervix and HPV DNA testing. The cumulative incidence of CIN over two years was found to be 28% in women infected with HPV but only 3% in women who tested negative for HPV. The relative risk for CIN was 11 (95% CI = 4.2–26) in women with HPV subtypes 16 or 18, and the estimated attributable risk was 52%. The authors concluded that CIN is an early and frequent consequence of infection with these HPV subtypes. Ho et al[124] applied a statistical model to data derived from a 15-month study of 70 women diagnosed with cervical dysplasia. The women were examined every three months using cervical cytology and colposcopy and were tested for HPV DNA. The authors found that chronic cervical lesions did not correlate with age, ethnicity, education, sexual behavior, smoking, or the use of oral contraceptives. However, the data do show that persistent infection with a high viral load produces chronic cervical lesions. Coker et al[125] conducted a case-control study encompassing a cohort of 5,995 women who had received cervical cytological examinations during a family planning visit. Random samples of women with cytological diagnoses of CIN II/III, CIN I, atypia, infection or inflammation, and normal cervical cytology were selected for HPV DNA testing. The percentage of women found to be HPV positive was directly correlated with the degree of cytological abnormality. The odds ratios for CINII/III, CIN I, atypia, infection or inflammation were 21.9, 11.7, 3.0, and 2.6, respectively.

Although HPV has been firmly established as the major cause of cervical neoplasia, additional studies are needed to further clarify the natural history of the disease process and develop and test new screening strategies and technologies. A large population-based study is currently being conducted in Costa Rica with these goals in mind.[126] A random sample of 10,738 resident women 18 years of age and older has been selected. After completing an epidemiological questionnaire, sexual active women are offered pelvic and cytological examinations, colposcopy, and HPV DNA testing. A serum sample is also being taken for immunologic and micronutrient measurements. The cohort will be followed at one-year intervals and will also serve as the source for subjects for a prevalence case-control study.

HPV has also been identified as a possible cause of anal cancer. In 1987, Daling et al[127] conducted a case-control study of 148 subjects with anal cancer and 166 colon cancer control subjects. Receptive anal intercourse was a high risk factor for anal cancer in men but was only weakly related to anal cancer in women. Anal cancer was also found to be strongly related to a history of genital warts, seropositivity for herpes simplex type 2, *Chlamydia trachomatis,* and current cigarette smoking. Two other case-control studies[128,129] also found strong associations between these factors and anal cancer risk. More recently, Frisch et al[130] conducted a case-control study of 324 women and 93 men diagnosed with invasive or in situ carcinoma of the anal canal, 534 rectal cancer control subjects, and 554 population control subjects. Epidemiological data were collected through telephone interviews. The investigators were also able to obtain paraffin-embedded biopsy specimens for anal cancer subjects and rectal cancer control subjects. The findings in this study were similar to those reported from previous case-control studies: anal cancer was shown to be associated with various measures of sexual promiscuity in both men and women. HPV DNA was detected in the tumor specimens of 93% of the women and 69% of males diagnosed with anal cancer. None of the rectal cancer specimens were positive for HPV. Eighty-four percent of all anal cancer specimens were positive for high-risk types of HPV, particularly type 16. The epidemiological and laboratory data are complementary and strongly suggest that HPV infection is etiologically related to anal cancer.

Serious consideration is now being given to the development of a prophylactic vaccine against HPV. Initial immunization programs will probably focus on creating a vaccine targeted at subtypes 16, 18, 31, and 45, which are known to be causative agents for human cancers.[131] Sherman et al[131] have also speculated that immunization programs will be aimed toward adolescents who have not yet first engaged in sexual activity. The extent to which a vaccine might provide some protection from cancer for women already infected with the virus is not known.

EPSTEIN-BARR VIRUS

Epstein-Barr virus (EBV) has been linked to Burkitt's lymphoma and other B-cell lymphomas and nasopharyngeal cancer. EBV is also a suspected agent in the development of Hodgkin's disease.[132] EBV is a double-stranded DNA virus that multiplies in B lymphocytes. Once infected, B lymphocytes become immortalized and can grow continually in a cell culture where they lose contact inhibition and develop new surface antigens. The virus has been shown to have the capability to cause malignant lymphoma in several primate species. EBV can cause a number of host responses, including subclinical infections and infectious mononucleosis, after which the virus can remain in a latent state within the epithelial cells.[7]

Given the widespread distribution of the virus and the rarity of the cancers associated with it, cofactors apparently are involved in the carcinogenic process. Immunosuppression can lead to reactivation of latent EBV, leading to excess numbers of non-Hodgkin's lymphomas in renal transplant patients, patients with in-born immunodeficiency disorders, and patients with immunodeficiency due to AIDS.[133–137] Cofactor interactions with EBV have also been identified for nasopharyngeal carcinomas and Burkitt's lymphomas.

Nasopharyngeal cancer is rare among North American and European whites but is more common among Chinese, Malaysians, Greenland Eskimos, and native Hawaiians.[138] Among Chinese males, the age-adjusted incidence rate is as high as 28 per 100,000 population, while the rate for women ranges from 3 to 11 per 100,000.[7] Several lines of evidence support a causal relation between EBV and nasopharyngeal carcinoma. Both case-control and cohort studies have shown an association between these cancers and the virus. In 1970, Henle et al[139] conducted a series of serological case-control studies in East Africa, Hong Kong, India, and France. Sera of nasopharyngeal carcinoma cases, a series of oncologic controls, and a series of nonneoplastic controls were tested for the presence of anti-EBV titers. The findings from this study are summarized in Figure 12–3. The data show that most nasopharyngeal carcinoma patients have titer readings of 160 or above whereas most patients with the other tumors have titer readings less than 160. The anti-EBV titers in the two control groups are shifted toward the lower values, while the curve for the nasopharyngeal carcinoma patients is shifted to the right. These differences were observed not only in the combined data but in each of the country-specific data sets.

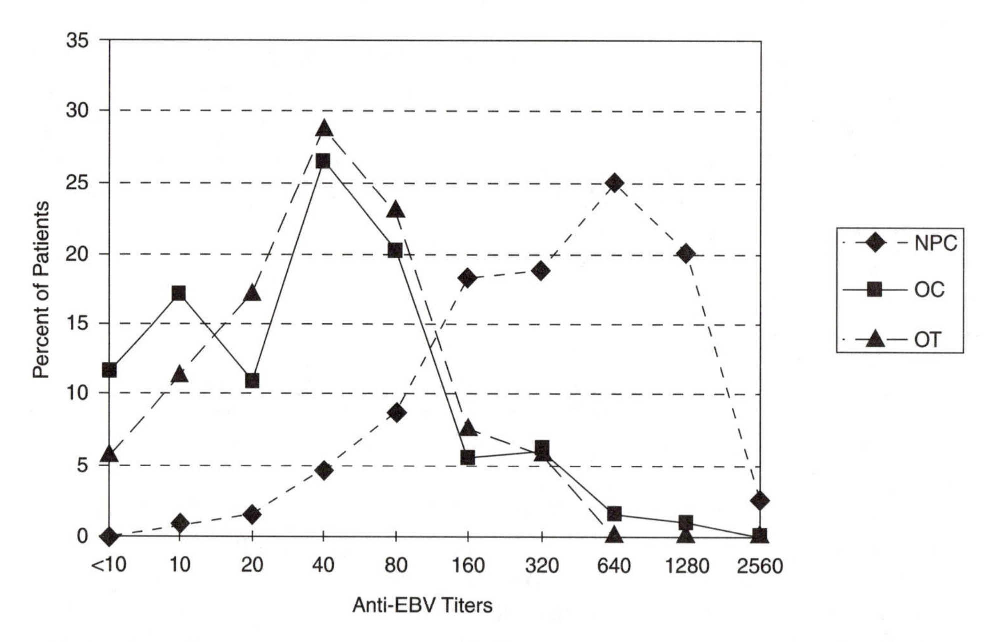

Figure 12–3 Anti-EBV titers among patients with carcinoma of the nasopharynx (NPC), patients with carcinomas arising from all other sites of head and neck (OC), and patients with tumors other than carcinomas (OT). *Source:* Adapted from Henle, et al., Antibodies to Epstein-Barr Virus in Nasopharyngeal Carcinoma, Other Head and Neck Neoplasms, and Control Groups, *Journal of the National Cancer Institute*, Vol. 44, pp. 225–231, 1970, National Cancer Institute.

In 1985, Zeng et al[140] reported the results of a prospective study of 1,136 persons found positive for EBV IgA/VCA antibody among 20,726 people screened. After four years of follow-up, the nasopharyngeal carcinoma incidence rate in the EBV-positive group was 18 times higher than in the entire screened population. Experimental studies have shown that nasopharyngeal carcinomas carry EBV in all tumor cells,[141,142] which indicates that the cancers arise from clonal expansion of a single infected cell. Pathmanathan et al[143] screened 5,326 biopsy specimens and identified 11 specimens with dysplasia or carcinomas in situ without adjacent invasive carcinoma. All 11 specimens contained evidence of EBV infection, and all samples tested contained the EBV-transforming gene *LMP-1*. Further, the investigators found that the lesions contained many abnormal cells that emerged from a single infected cell. The identification of clones of EBV-infected cells in premalignant lesions and the observation that five of eight cases with premalignant lesions developed nasopharyngeal carcinoma within a year provide further support for the hypothesis that a causal relation between EBV and nasopharyngeal carcinoma exists.[144] The carcinogenic potential of EBV may be influenced by a number of factors already shown to be risk factors for these malignancies. Given the geographic focus of high nasopharyngeal carcinoma incidence in southern China, both genetic susceptibility[145] and dietary exposures[146] have been implicated.

Evans and de-The[147] published a detailed history of the early epidemiological and experimental studies that led to our current knowledge of Burkitt's lymphoma, EBV, and various cofactors. A summary of that history is presented below. In 1958, Denis Burkitt published the first paper to clinically describe a jaw tumor that African children suffered from.[148] Two years later, O'Conor and Davies[149] described the distinctive histological pattern of the tumor when viewed under low magnification as a "starry sky" pattern resulting from macrophage infiltration. Burkitt then attempted to determine the geographic distribution of the tumor, first by mailing notices to physicians throughout Africa and then by visiting 60 hospitals in 10 countries of east Africa.[150] Burkitt's tumor safaris were later extended to western and central Africa. His efforts produced a clear picture of the geographic distribution of Burkitt's lymphoma across the African continent (Figure 12–4). As the figure shows, Burkitt's lymphoma was restricted to the sub-Saharan regions of Africa, and the cases tended to occur in areas of low altitude, high annual rainfall, and high temperatures and humidity.[151] Although the data observations initially suggested that an insect vector might play a role in Burkitt's lymphoma, it was eventually recognized that the geographic distribution of Burkitt's lymphoma cases matched that of endemic malaria.[152]

Eventually, Epstein and Barr[153] and Pulvertaft[154] were able to grow human lymphoblasts in culture and to detect virus particles in lymphoblasts from Burkitt's lymphoma.[155] The development of an immunofluorescent antibody test made it practical to conduct population-based epidemiological studies of EBV and Burkitt's lymphoma.[156] One early case-control study showed that Burkitt's lymphoma patients were significantly more likely than controls to have antibodies to EBV.[157] The evidence that EBV might be related to human cancers was strengthened when EBV DNA was discovered in biopsies from Burkitt's lymphomas and nasopharyngeal cancers[158] and when inoculation with EBV was shown to produce reticuloproliferative disease and malignant lymphomas in primate species.[159,160] A large prospective study was launched in Uganda in 1972 by

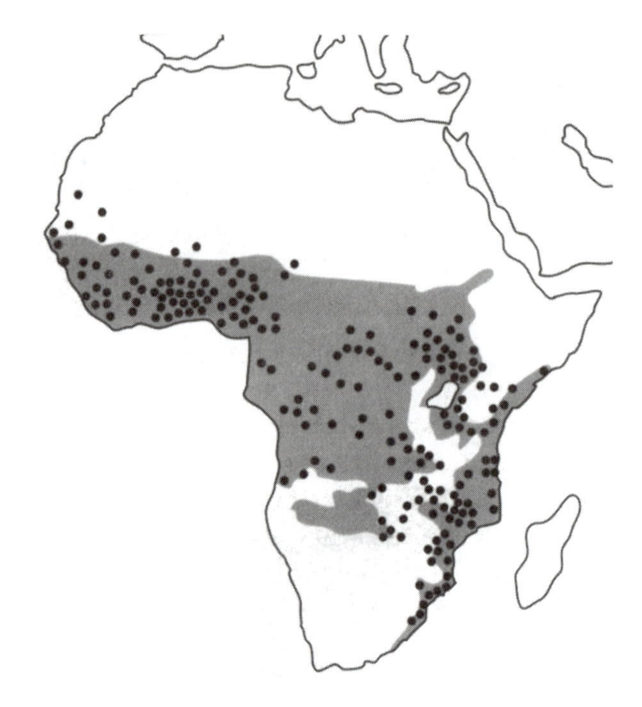

Figure 12–4 The distribution of malaria in Africa (shaded area) and distribution of the cases of Burkitt's lymphoma documented by Denis Burkitt in 1962 (dots). *Source:* From GENES AND THE BIOLOGY OF CANCER by Varmus and Weinberg © 1993 by Scientific American Library. Used with permission of W.H. Freeman and Company.

de-The et al.[161] Between 1972 and 1974, these investigators took blood from 42,000 children aged 0–8, and they then followed these children until 1979. A total of 14 subjects developed Burkitt's lymphoma during the follow-up period, for an incidence rate of 7 per 100,000 per year. In each case, antibodies to EBV were present in the original blood sample. The titers for these 14 subjects were also significantly higher than those for a control group of children who had not developed Burkitt's lymphoma during the follow-up period (RR = 30). In addition, 9 of 10 Burkitt's lymphoma cases showed viral DNA sequences in the host genome, and in many tumors there were large numbers of multiple copies. Other studies demonstrated that Burkitt's lymphoma cells frequently contain chromosomal translocations, supporting the assumption that the etiological factors leading to Burkitt's lymphoma clearly involved the host DNA.[162–164] Approximately 75% of Burkitt's lymphoma cases show chromosomal translocations between the long arms of chromosomes 8 and 14, with less frequent translocations between the long arm of chromosome 8 and either the short arm of chromosome 2 or the long arm of chromosome 22. These translocations occur at a point on the chromosome where genes for the human immunoglobulins and the c-*myc* oncogene are located.

Although Burkitt's lymphoma is endemic in tropical Africa, it does occur sporadically in western Europe and North America and with intermediate frequency in Egypt,[165] China,[166,167] Brazil,[168–170] Turkey,[171] Mexico,[172] and other parts of the world. In areas where it is endemic, most people with the disease exhibit positive serological evidence of EBV infection. In areas where it is sporadic, approximately 20% of those with the disease are EBV positive, and the incidence rates for EBV infection are even higher in areas in which Burkitt's lymphoma occurs at an intermediate level. Araujo et al[168] found PCR evidence of EBV in 47 of 54 Brazilian children with Burkitt's lymphoma (80%) but such evidence in only 2 of 10 German children diagnosed with the disease.

EBV is not a complete carcinogen but appears to be part of a multistep carcinogenic process.[173–175] In endemic areas, EBV infection at an early age immortalizes lymphocytes and leads to polyclonal expansion of EBV-infected cells. EBV expresses 11 viral genes, only some of which are actually involved in transformation (*EBNA-2, EBNA-3A, EBNA-3C, LMP-1,* and *LMP-2*). These genes produce proteins that cause cells to grow by modifying cell signal pathways.[176] Malarial infection acts as a cofactor by depressing cytotoxic T-cell clones, which would normally control the proliferation of EBV-infected B cells. Activation of the c-*myc* oncogene results from somatic mutations involving the chromosomal translocations previously mentioned, thus completing the transformation process.[175] Jox et al[177] noted that integration of EBV into the host genome causes a gap (or "vulnerable site"), which after long-term in vitro cultivation leads to the deletion of the integrated genome, including the *LMP* and *EBER* encoding genes. This raises the possibility that the failure to identify EBV in all tumors may result from a hit-and-run mechanism in some cases.

Both epidemiological and experimental data suggest that an infectious agent might contribute to the development of Hodgkin's disease. Mueller reviewed findings from molecular studies that indicate that the Reed-Sternberg cells, the type of lymphoid cells used by pathologists to help establish a diagnosis of Hodgkin's disease, are "frozen in a state of activation."[132(p23)] In addition, nonrandom chromosomal translocations, seen in other hematological disorders, are regularly observed in Hodgkin's disease. Mueller noted that these observations are consistent with the hypothesis that Hodgkin's disease involves chronic antigenic stimulation (see Chapter 13 for further discussion of chronic antigenic stimulation) and pointed out that the epidemiological literature provides support for this hypothesis. In upper socioeconomic populations, the age-incidence curve for Hodgkin's disease is bimodal. The incidence rate is low during childhood, it increases rapidly during the teen years and peaks at around age 25, it plateaus until around age 50, and then begins rising again until it reaches a second peak at age 80. McMahon[178] suggested that the curve indicated the existence of two separate disease processes, with Hodgkin's disease in young adults being related to an infectious agent. In lower socioeconomic groups, the age-incidence curve lacks the peak during young adulthood.

Hodgkin's disease might be a rare outcome of a common infection more likely to occur in individuals who are not exposed until they are past early childhood. Support for this hypothesis comes from a number of epidemiological observations and from the analogy with paralytic polio. Studies have shown that the risk of Hodgkin's disease decreases as sibship size and housing density increase. The risk of Hodgkin's disease increases as parental income increases.[179,180] These relations have been observed in young adult and middle-aged patients but not in older patients, again suggesting a separate etiologic mechanism. The findings for sibship size, housing density, and parental socioeconomic status are consistent with delayed exposure to infectious agents, possibly including the agent responsible for Hodgkin's disease. Mueller[132] pointed out that infection by common viruses at a later age often results in more severe symptoms, alteration of immune control, and chronic antigenic stimulation.

The potential role of EBV as the putative viral agent is less certain. A number of observations support an etiologic role for EBV in Hodgkin's disease. Patients diagnosed with infectious mononucleosis, a disease caused by EBV, experience a threefold increased risk of developing Hodgkin's disease.[7] In addition, serologic studies have consistently reported higher EBV titers in Hodgkin's disease study subjects than in control subjects.[132] A nested case-control study[181] based on blood samples drawn from a cohort of 240,000 persons showed a significantly elevated risk of Hodgkin's disease among subjects with serological evidence of EBV infection. The association was strongest for cases occurring at least three years after the sera were originally collected. Studies conducted in the late 1980s and early 1990s used PCR testing to detect EBV DNA sequences in 13% to 29% of Hodgkin's disease biopsy specimens, specifically in the Reed-Sternberg cells.[132] Newer studies show that approximately 40% of Hodgkin's disease cases occurring in developed countries are associated with EBV.[182] However, more recent analysis of EBV infection in relation to various sociodemographic factors and histologic subtypes suggests that EBV is unlikely to be the viral agent involved in the development of Hodgkin's disease among young adults. The nodular sclerosis subtype of Hodgkin's disease occurs most frequently in young adults, whereas the mixed cellularity form of the disease is more likely to occur in older patients. An analysis of data from the SEER program for the years 1973–1977, 1978–1982, and 1983–1987 showed significant secular increases in the incidence of the nodular sclerosis subtype but stable incidence rates for the mixed cellularity subtype.[183] Glaser et al[184,185] studied EBV tumor status in relation to various socioeconomic characteristics and histologic subtypes. The risk of EBV-associated Hodgkin's disease was found to be greater among Hispanics than whites, greater among children from poor countries than children from more economically developed nations, and greater among young males than young females. EBV-associated Hodgkin's disease was also more likely to be associated with the mixed cellularity subtype than the nodular sclerosis type. The data fail to support a role for EBV in young adult–onset Hodgkin's disease and suggest that, although EBV may be related to Hodgkin's disease, the relationship is complex.

HUMAN T-CELL LYMPHOTROPIC VIRUS AND ADULT T-CELL LEUKEMIAS

Adult T-cell leukemia (ATL) in Japan was first described by Takatsuki et al[186] in 1977. Clinically, the disease is characterized by hypercalcemia with or without the presence of skin lesions, lymphadenopathy, and immune suppression.[187,188] Levine et al[189] developed a working four-point disease classification scale that was designed to help facilitate the comparison of data from epidemiological studies conducted in different countries. In 1980, Poiesz et al[190] isolated the human T-cell lymphotropic virus (HTLV-I) that contributed to the development of human T-cell leukemias. Subsequent studies showed that the virus was primarily spread horizontally from husband to wife through transmission in semen and vertically from mother to children, with breast milk being a likely vector.[191,192] The low rate of seroconversion after age 40 suggests that infection at an early age is likely to be etiologically important.[193] One study showed that patients who test negative for HTLV-I when standard serological techniques are applied also tend to test negative when PCR techniques are applied, indicating that seronegative carriers are rare in areas where the virus is endemic.[194]

The most striking feature of ATL is the geographic clustering of cases in Japan (Figure 12–5).[195,196] The highest incidence rate occurs on the southern Japanese island of Kyushu, but high rates also occur on the islands of Okinawa, Shikoku, and the far northern island of Hokkaido. The annual incidence rate for ATL is estimated at 0.6 per 1,000 adult HTLV-I carriers. Although the data may underestimate the true incidence of ATL in Japan,[197] ATL is obviously a rare outcome of a fairly common viral infection. In Kyushu, the incidence rate increases dramatically between the ages of 40 and 65 years and then declines steadily thereafter. Men have a higher ATL incidence rate throughout the age range for the disease than women.[187] The total number of HTLV-I carriers in Japan was estimated to be 1.2 million persons in 1987, with 50% of the carriers living in

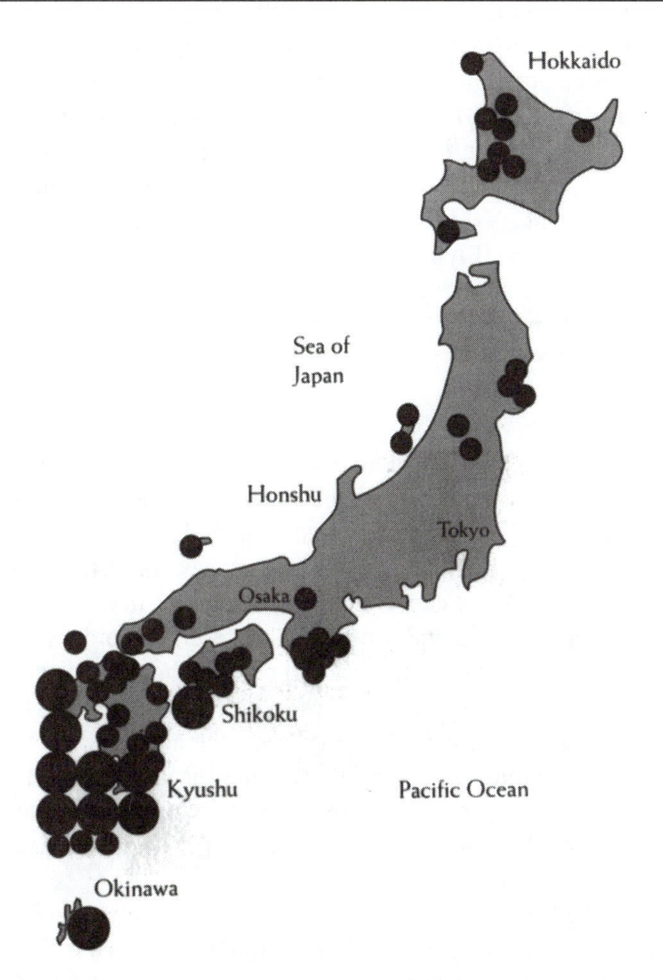

Figure 12–5 Map of Japan showing distribution of adult T-cell leukemia (larger dots indicate more cases). *Source:* From VIRUSES by Levine © 1992 by Scientific American Library. Used with permission of W.H. Freeman and Company.

Kyushu and 30% in the large metropolitan areas of Tokyo, Nagoya, and Osaka. Persons in these urban areas who are HTLV-I positive tend to have migrated from areas where HTLV-I viral infection is endemic.[198]

ATL is also found in other parts of the world, most notably among Japanese living in other parts of Asia and among central Africa blacks, blacks from the Caribbean, Melanesians in Papua New Guinea, and natives of the Andean regions of South America.[199,200] The overall lifetime risk of ATL is between 2% and 6% in persons who are persistent carriers of HTLV-I. The incidence of ATL in the United States is sporadic, and most cases occur among immigrants from the Caribbean or other countries where the virus is endemic. A large cluster of ATL cases in Brooklyn has been reported, and most of those with the disease migrated to the area from the Caribbean.[201,202] In the Kinmen Islands of China, risk of HTLV-I infection is significantly associated with living along the eastern coastal areas, where contact with infected Japanese sailors and fisherman may be more likely.[203]

Given that a large percentage of patients with ATL have relatives with ATL, other lymphomas, or other hematopoietic neoplasms, the possibility of a genetic susceptibility to HTLV-I has been entertained.[196] Attempts to associate ATL with the HLA phenotype have produced inconsistent findings.[7] In addition, no consistent pattern of cytogenetic abnormalities has been seen in ATL.[204] The biological role of HTLV-I in ATL is still poorly understood, but given the rarity of the disease in the presence of a common exposure, it is likely that HTLV-I is only part of a multistep carcinogenic process. Like EBV, HTLV-I can immortalize B lymphocytes in culture. The HTLV-I tax gene is thought to be directly involved in this process and may have indirect effects through interactions with other cellular transcription proteins.[205,206]

SUMMARY

Evans and Mueller[1] presented an overview of various problems that might be encountered when attempting to establish a relationship between a viral infection and a human cancer (Exhibit 12–1). These problems include the often long latency period between the initial infection and the development of the cancer, the possible ubiquity of the infection and the rarity of the cancer, and the possibility that cofactors play a role in the etiology of the cancer. Evans and Mueller also presented epidemiological and virological guidelines for assessing whether a causal relationship between a putative virus and a human cancer exists (Exhibit 12–2). These guidelines encompass standard epidemiological criteria for assessing causality, including the coherence between the hypothesis and the known distribution of the agent and the disease in different populations, the observation of a large magnitude of effect, and the temporal precedence of the agent. Consistency between the epidemiological and experimental findings is also essential for substantiating a possible relationship.

Persistent infection with hepatitis viruses is a primary cause of hepatocellular carcinoma in areas of the world where this form of malignancy is a major public health problem, including China, Southeast Asia, Africa, and the Indian sub-continent. Public health control of the effects of these viruses may be achieved over a number of years by widespread immunization at an early age. The biological mechanisms through which

HBV and HCV operate are not fully understood at this time. It is not clear whether these viruses simply interact with cofactors through their ongoing damage to hepatic tissues or whether other cellular interactions also play a role in carcinogenesis. HPV has been firmly linked with cancer of the uterine cervix and other cervical neoplasms, and the virus probably plays a causal role in cancers of the anal canal. HPV appears to have a deleterious effect on at least two suppressor genes. Now that the etiologic importance of HPV is well established, new strategies can be developed for screening, treating, and preventing these neoplasms.

Experimental and epidemiological data have clearly demonstrated that EBV is part of a multistage carcinogenic process leading to Burkitt's lymphomas and nasopharyngeal cancer. The link between EBV and Hodgkin's disease is less well established. HTLV-I is clearly related to the risk of ATL but also appears to act as an incomplete carcinogen. Overall, viruses have been shown to be important contributors to the development of several cancers that are major public health problems in underdeveloped and economically emerging countries. The complex, multistage nature of various cancers has been confirmed, and determining when and how, in the process of malignant transformation, the virus affects the target cell is an important research goal. The mechanisms through which some viruses contribute to cellular transformation are beginning to be understood, but the etiological mechanisms for other viruses are still a mystery.

Discussion Questions

1. Discuss the basic issues and problems involved in attempting to find a link between a virus and a cancer using HTLV and adult T-cell leukemias as an example (see Exhibit 12–1).
2. Discuss the epidemiological and virological criteria that might be used to establish a causal relationship between a virus and a cancer using HBV and hepatocellular carcinoma as an example (see Exhibit12–2).
3. Discuss the epidemiological and virological criteria that might be used to establish a causal relationship between a virus and a cancer using EBV and nasopharyngeal cancer as an example (see Exhibit12–2).
4. Discuss how the use of new methods for collecting biological specimens and for subtyping viruses has led to a clearer sense of the relationship between HPV and cancer of the uterine cervix.
5. Discuss the role of cofactors in the relationship between HPV and various cancers.

References

1. Evans AS, Mueller NE. Viruses and cancer: causal associations. *Ann Epidemiol.* 1990;1:71–92.
2. Blumberg BS, London WT. Hepatitis B virus and the prevention of primary cancer of the liver. *J Natl Cancer Inst.* 1985;71:267–273.
3. Beasley RP. Hepatitis B virus: the major etiology of hepatocellular carcinoma. *Cancer.* 1988;61:1942–1956.
4. Melnick JL. Hepatocellular carcinoma caused by hepatitis B virus. In: Evans AS, ed. *Viral Infections of Humans: Epidemiology and Control.* 3rd ed. New York: Plenum Medical Book Co; 1989:769–780.
5. Zur Hausen H. Viruses in human cancers. *Science.* 1991;254:1167–1173.

6. Bosch FX. HCV and liver cancer: the epidemiological evidence. *Princess Takamatsu Symposia.* 1995;25:15–25.
7. Mueller NE, Evans AS, London WT. Viruses. In: Schottenfeld D, Fraumeni JF Jr, eds. *Cancer Epidemiology and Prevention.* 2nd ed. New York: Oxford University Press; 1996:502–531.
8. Stevens CE, Beasley RP, Tsui J, Lee WC. Vertical transmission of hepatitis B antigen in Taiwan. *N Engl J Med.* 1975;292:771–774.
9. Schweitzer IL. Infection of neonates and infants with the hepatitis B virus. *Prog Med Virol.* 1975;20:27–48.
10. Larouze B, London WT, Saimot G, et al. Host responses to hepatitis-B infection in patients with primary hepatic carcinoma and their families: a case-control study in Senegal, West Africa. *Lancet.* 1976;2:534–538.
11. Okada K, Kamiyama I, Inomata M, et al. E antigen and anti-e in the serum of asymptomatic carrier mothers as indicators of positive and negative transmission of hepatitis B virus to their infants. *N Engl J Med.* 1976;294:746–749.
12. Beasley RP, Trepo C, Stevens CE, Szmuness W. The e antigen and the vertical transmission of hepatitis B surface antigen. *Am J Epidemiol.* 1977;105:94–98.
13. Blumberg BS, London WT. Hepatitis B virus and hepatocellular carcinoma: relationship of "icrons" to cancer. In: Essex M, Todara G, Zur Hausen H, eds. *Viruses in Naturally Occurring Cancers.* Cold Spring Harbor, NY: Cold Spring Harbor Laboratory; 1980:401–421.
14. Tong MJ, Thursby MW, Lin J-H, et al. Studies on the maternal-infant transmission of the hepatitis B virus and HBV infection within families. *Prog Med Virol.* 1981;27:137–147.
15. Alter MJ, Margolis HS, Krawczynski K, et al. The natural history of community-acquired hepatitis C in the United States: The Sentinel Counties Chronic Non-A, Non-B Hepatitis Study Team. *N Engl J Med.* 1992;327:1899–1905.
16. Stevens CE, Taylor PE. Perinatal and sexual transmission of HCV, a preliminary report. In: Hollinger FB, Lemon SM, Margolis HS, eds. *Viral Hepatitis and Liver Disease.* Baltimore: Williams & Wilkins; 1991:407–409.
17. Qiao ZK, Halliday ML, Rankin JG, Coates RA. Relationship between hepatitis B surface antigen prevalence, per capita alcohol consumption and primary liver cancer death rate in 30 countries. *J Clin Epidemiol.* 1988;41:787–792.
18. Hsing AW, Guo W, Chen J, et al. Correlates of liver cancer mortality in China. *Int J Epidemiol.* 1991;20:54–59.
19. Lamont DW, Buchan KA, Gillis CR, Reid D. Primary hepatocellular carcinoma in an area of low incidence: evidence for a viral aetiology from routinely collected data. *Int J Epidemiol.* 1991;20:60–67.
20. Szmuness W, Stevens CE, Ikram H, et al. Prevalence of hepatitis B virus infection and hepatocellular carcinoma in Chinese-Americans. *J Infect Dis.* 1978;137:822–829.
21. Rosenblatt KA, Weiss NS, Schwartz SM. Liver cancer in Asian migrants to the United States and their descendants. *Cancer Causes Control.* 1996;7:345–750.
22. Swerdlow AJ, Marmot MG, Grulich AE, Head J. Cancer mortality in Indian and British ethnic immigrants from the Indian subcontinent to England and Wales. *Br J Cancer.* 1995;72:1312–1319.
23. Lanier AP, McMahon BJ, Alberts SR, et al. Primary liver cancer in Alaskan natives, 1980–1985. *Cancer.* 1987;60:1915–1920.
24. Storm HH, Nielsen NH. Cancer of the digestive system in circumpolar Inuit. *Acta Oncol.* 1996;35:553–570.
25. London WT, Blumberg BS. Comments on the role of epidemiology in the investigation of hepatitis B virus. *Epidemiol Rev.* 1985;7:59–79.
26. Blumberg BS, London WT. Primary hepatocellular carcinoma and hepatitis B virus. *Curr Probl Cancer.* 1982;6:3–23.
27. Lam KC, Yu MC, Leung JW, Henderson BE. Hepatitis B virus and cigarette smoking: risk factors for hepatocellular carcinoma in Hong Kong. *Cancer Res.* 1982;42:5246–5248.
28. Yeh FS, Mo CC, Luo S, et al. A serological case-control study of primary hepatocellular carcinoma in Guangxi, China. *Cancer Res.* 1985;45:872–873.
29. Trichopoulos D, Day NE, Kaklamani E, et al. Hepatitis B virus, tobacco smoking and ethanol consumption in the etiology of hepatocellular carcinoma. *Int J Cancer.* 1987;39:45–49.
30. Tanaka K, Hirohata T, Takeshita S. Blood transfusion, alcohol consumption, and cigarette smoking in causation of hepatocellular carcinoma: a case-control study in Fukuoka, Japan. *Jap J Cancer Res.* 1988;79:1075–1082.
31. Tsukuma H, Hiyama T, Oshima A, et al. A case-control study of hepatocellular carcinoma in Osaka, Japan. *Int J Cancer.* 1990;45:231–236.
32. Yu MC, Tong MJ, Coursaget P, et al. Prevalence of hepatitis B and C viral markers in black and white patients with hepatocellular carcinoma in the United States. *J Natl Cancer Inst.* 1990;82:1038–1041.
33. Kaklamani E, Trichopoulos D, Tzonou A, et al. Hepatitis B and C viruses and their interaction in the origin of hepatocellular carcinoma. *JAMA.* 1991;265:1974–1976.

34. Srivatanakul P, Parkin DM, Khlat M, et al. Liver cancer in Thailand. II. A case-control study of hepatocellular carcinoma. *Int J Cancer.* 1991;48:329–332.

35. Stroffolini T, Chiaramonte M, Tiribelli C, et al. Hepatitis C virus infection, HBsAg carrier state and hepatocellular carcinoma: relative risk and population attributable risk from a case-control study in Italy. *J Hepatol.* 1992;16:360–363.

36. Zavitsanos X, Hatzakis A, Kaklamani E, et al. Association between hepatitis C virus and hepatocellular carcinoma using assays based on structural and nonstructural hepatitis C virus peptides. *Cancer Res.* 1992;52:5364–5367.

37. Tanaka K, Hirohata T, Takeshita S, et al. Hepatitis B virus, cigarette smoking and alcohol consumption in the development of hepatocellular carcinoma: a case-control study in Fukuoka, Japan. *Int J Cancer.* 1992;51:509–514.

38. Chang CC, Yu MW, Lu CF, et al. A nested case-control study on association between hepatitis C virus antibodies and primary liver cancer in a cohort of 9,775 men in Taiwan. *J Med Virol.* 1994;43:276–280.

39. Pyong SJ, Tsukuma H, Hiyama T. Case-control study of hepatocellular carcinoma among Koreans living in Osaka, Japan. *Jpn J Cancer Res.* 1994;85:674–679.

40. Tanaka K, Hirohata T, Fukuda K, et al. Risk factors for hepatocellular carcinoma among Japanese women. *Cancer Causes Control.* 1995;6:91–98.

41. Hadziyannis S, Tabor E, Kaklamani E, et al. A case-control study of hepatitis B and C virus infections in the etiology of hepatocellular carcinoma. *Int J Cancer.* 1995;60:627–631.

42. Nomura A, Stemmermann GN, Chyou PH, Tabor E. Hepatitis B and C virus serologies among Japanese Americans with hepatocellular carcinoma. *J Infect Dis.* 1996;173:1474–1476.

43. Silini E, Bottelli R, Asti M, et al. Hepatitis C virus genotypes and risk of hepatocellular carcinoma in cirrhosis: a case-control study. *Gastroenterology.* 1996;111:199–205.

44. Sun CA, Farzadegan H, You SL, et al. Mutual confounding and interactive effects between hepatitis C and hepatitis B viral infections in hepatocellular carcinogenesis: a population-based case-control study in Taiwan. *Cancer Epidemiol Biomarkers Prev.* 1996;5:173–178.

45. Beasley RP, Hwang L-Y, Lin C-C, Chen C-S. Hepatocellular carcinoma and hepatitis B virus: a prospective study of 22,707 men in Taiwan. *Lancet.*1981;2:1129–1133.

46. Iijma T, Saitoh N, Nobutomo K, et al. A prospective cohort study of hepatitis B surface antigen carriers in a working population. *Gann.* 1984;75:571–573.

47. Oshima A, Tsukuma H, Hiyama T, et al. Follow-up study of HBsAg-positive blood donors with special reference to effect of drinking and smoking on development of liver cancer. *Int J Cancer.* 1984;34:775–779.

48. Tu JT, Gao RN, Zhang DH, Gu BC. Hepatitis B virus and primary liver cancer on Chongming Island, People's Republic of China. *Natl Cancer Inst Monogr.* 1985;69:213–215.

49. Tokudome S, Ikeda M, Matsushita K, et al. Hepatocellular carcinoma among female Japanese hepatitis B virus carriers. *Hepatogastroenterology.* 1987;34:246–248.

50. Tokudome S, Ikeda M, Matsushita K, et al. Hepatocellular carcinoma among HBsAg positive blood donors in Fukuoka, Japan. *Eur J Cancer Clin Oncol.* 1988;24:235–239.

51. Tsukuma H, Hiyama T, Tanaka S, et al. Risk factors for hepatocellular carcinoma among patients with chronic liver disease. *N Engl J Med.* 1993;328:1797–1801.

52. Norman JE, Beebe GW, Hoofnagle JH, Seeff LB. Mortality follow-up of the 1942 epidemic of hepatitis B in the US Army. *Hepatology.* 1993;18:790–797.

53. Chang M-H, Chen C-J, Lai M-S, et al. Universal hepatitis B vaccination in Taiwan and the incidence of hepatocellular carcinoma in children. *N Engl J Med.* 1997;336:1855–1859.

54. Summers J. Three recently described animal virus models for human hepatitis B virus. *Hepatology.* 1981;1:79–83.

55. Marion PL, Oshiro LS, Regnery DC, et al. A virus in Beechey ground squirrels that is related to hepatitis B virus of humans. *Proc Natl Acad Sci USA.* 1980;77:2941–2945.

56. Marion PL, Robinson WS. Hepadna viruses: hepatitis B and related viruses. *Curr Top Microbiol Immunol.* 1983;105:99–121.

57. Marion PL, Knight SS, Salazar FH, et al. Ground squirrel hepatitis virus infection. *Hepatology.* 1983;3:519–527.

58. Mason WS, Seal G, Summers J. Virus of Pekin ducks with structural and biological relatedness to human hepatitis B virus. *J Virol.* 1980;36:829–836.

59. Marion PL, Knight SS, Ho BK, et al. Liver disease associated with duck hepatitis B virus infection of domestic ducks. *Proc Natl Acad Sci USA.* 1984;81:898–902.

60. Cova L, Wild CP, Mehrotra R, et al. Contribution of aflatoxin B1 and hepatitis B virus infection in the induction of liver tumors in ducks. *Cancer Res.* 1990;50:2156–2163.

61. Summers J, Smolec JM, Snyder R. A virus similar to human hepatitis B virus associated with hepatitis and hepatoma in woodchucks. *Proc Natl Acad Sci USA*.1978;75:4533–4537.

62. Popper H, Roth L, Purcell RH, et al. Hepatocarcinogenicity of the woodchuck hepatitis virus. *Proc Natl Acad Sci USA*. 1987;84:866–870.

63. Gerin JL. Experimental WHV infection of woodchucks: an animal model of hepadnavirus-induced liver cancer. *Gastroenterol Jpn*. 1990;25(suppl 2):38–42.

64. Ponzetto A, Forzani B. Animal models of hepatocellular carcinoma: hepadnavirus-induced liver cancer in woodchucks. *Ital J Gastroenterol.* 1991;23:491–493.

65. Moss B, Smith GL, Gerin JL, Purcell RH. Live recombinant vaccinia virus protects chimpanzees against hepatitis B. *Nature.* 1984;311:67–69.

66. Prince AM, Brotman B, Purcell RH, Gerin JL. A final report on safety and immunogenicity of a bivalent aqueous subunit HBV vaccine. *J Med Virol.* 1985;15:399–419.

67. Cote PJ, Shapiro M, Engle RE, et al. Protection of chimpanzees from type B hepatitis by immunization with woodchuck hepatitis virus surface antigen. *J Virol.* 1986;60:895–901.

68. Gouillat C, Manganas D, Zoulim F, et al. Woodchuck hepatitis virus–induced carcinoma as a relevant natural model for therapy of human hepatoma. *J Hepatol.* 1997;26:1324–1330.

69. Pasek M, Goto T, Gilbert W, et al. Hepatitis B virus genes and their expression in E. coli. *Nature.* 1979;282:575–579.

70. Brechot C, Pourcel C, Louise A, et al. Presence of integrated hepatitis B virus DNA sequences in cellular DNA of human hepatocellular carcinoma. *Nature.* 1980;286:533–535.

71. Brechot C, Pourcel C, Louise A, et al. Detection of hepatitis B virus DNA sequences in human hepatocellular carcinoma in an integrated form. *Prog Med Virol.* 1981;27:99–102.

72. Shafritz DA, Kew MC. Identification of integrated hepatitis B virus DNA sequences in human hepatocellular carcinomas. *Hepatology.* 1981;1:1–8.

73. Shafritz DA, Shouval D, Sherman HI, et al. Integration of hepatitis B virus DNA into the genome of liver cells in chronic liver disease and hepatocellular carcinoma: studies in percutaneous liver biopsies and post-mortem tissue specimens. *N Engl J Med.* 1981;305:1067–1073.

74. Hino O, Shows TB, Rogler CE. Hepatitis B virus integration site in hepatocellular carcinoma at chromosome 17;18 translocation. *Proc Natl Acad Sci USA*. 1986;83:8338–8342.

75. Zhou Y-Z, Donehower LA, Slagle BL, et al. Hepatitis B virus DNA integration in chromosome 17p near the human p53 gene in hepatocellular carcinoma. In: *Abstracts of the Conference on Hepatitis B Viruses.* Cold Spring Harbor, NY: Cold Spring Harbor Laboratory; 1987:123.

76. Feitelson MA, Zhu M, Duan LX, London WT. Hepatitis B x antigen and p53 are associated in vitro and in liver tissues from patients with primary hepatocellular carcinoma. *Oncogene.* 1993;8:1109–1117.

77. Kennedy SM, Macgeogh C, Jaffe R, Spurr NK. Overexpression of the oncoprotein p53 in primary hepatic tumors of childhood does not correlate with gene mutations. *Hum Path.* 1994;25:438–442.

78. Ueda H, Ullrich SJ, Gangemi JD, et al. Functional inactivation but not structural mutation of p53 causes liver cancer. *Nat Genet.* 1995;9:41–47.

79. Butel JS, Lee TH, Slagle BL. Viral co-factors in liver cancer: lesions from hepatitis B virus. *Princess Takamatsu Symposia.* 1995;25:185–198.

80. Schiffman MH, Brinton LA. The epidemiology of cervical carcinogenesis. *Cancer.* 1995;76(suppl 10):1888–1901.

81. Schiffman MH. New epidemiology of human papillomavirus infection and cervical neoplasia. *J Natl Cancer Inst.* 1995;87:1345–1347.

82. Bosch FX, Munoz N, de Sanjose S. Human papillomavirus and other risk factors for cervical cancer. *Biomed Pharmacother.* 1997;51:268–275.

83. IARC Working Group on the Evaluation of Carcinogenic Risks to Humans. *Human Papillomaviruses.* Lyon, France: International Agency for Research on Cancer; 1995. Monographs on the Evaluation of Carcinogenic Risks to Humans, No. 64.

84. Strickler HD, Schiffman MH. Is human papillomavirus an infectious cause of non-cervical anogenital tract cancers? *BMJ.* 1997;315:620–621.

85. Franceschi S, Munoz N, Bosch XF, et al. Human papillomavirus and cancers of the upper aerodigestive tract: a review of epidemiological and experimental evidence. *Cancer Epidemiol Biomarkers Prev.* 1996;5:567–575.
86. Zur Hausen H. Viruses in human cancers. *Science.* 1991;254:1167–1173.
87. McCance DJ, Kopan R, Fuchs E, Laimins LA. Human papillomavirus type 16 alters human epithelial cell differentiation in vitro. *Proc Natl Acad Sci USA.* 1988;85:7169–7173.
88. Howley PM. Role of the human papillomaviruses in human cancer. *Cancer Res.* 1991;1(suppl):5019s–5022s.
89. Melnick JL, Rawls WE, Adam E. Cervical cancer. In: Evans AS, ed. *Viral Infections of Humans: Epidemiology and Control.* 3rd ed. New York: Plenum Medical Book Co; 1989:687–711.
90. Franco EL. The sexually transmitted disease model for cervical cancer: incoherent epidemiologic findings and the role of misclassification of human papillomavirus infection. *Epidemiology.* 1991;2:98–106.
91. Franco EL. Measurement errors in epidemiological studies of human papillomavirus and cervical cancer. *IARC Sci Publ.* 1992;119:181–197.
92. Schiffman MH. Schatzkin A. Test reliability is critically important to molecular epidemiology: an example from studies of human papillomavirus infection and cervical neoplasia. *Cancer Res.* 1994;54(suppl):1944s–1947s.
93. Guerrero E, Daniel RW, Bosch FX, et al. Comparison of ViraPap, Southern hybridization, and polymerase chain reaction methods for human papillomavirus identification in an epidemiological investigation of cervical cancer. *J Clin Microbiol.* 1992;30:2951–2959.
94. Kato I, Santamaria M, De Ruiz PA, et al. Inter-observer variation in cytological and histological diagnoses of cervical neoplasia and its epidemiologic implication. *J Clin Epidemiol.* 1995;48:1167–1174.
95. Schiffman MH, Bauer HM, Hoover RN, et al. Epidemiologic evidence showing that human papillomavirus infection causes most cervical intraepithelial neoplasia. *J Natl Cancer Inst.* 1993;85:958–964.
96. Bosch FX, Munoz N, de Sanjose S, et al. Human papillomavirus and cervical intraepithelial neoplasia grade III/carcinoma in situ: a case-control study in Spain and Colombia. *Cancer Epidemiol Biomarkers Prev.* 1993;2:415–422.
97. Sun Y, Eluf-Neto J, Bosch FX, et al. Human papillomavirus-related serological markers of invasive cervical carcinoma in Brazil. *Cancer Epidemiol Biomarkers Prev.* 1994;3:341–347.
98. Eluf-Neto J, Booth M, Munoz N, et al. Human papillomavirus and invasive cervical cancer in Brazil. *Br J Cancer.* 1994;69:114–119.
99. Wideroff L, Schiffman MH, Nonnenmacher B, et al. Evaluation of seroreactivity to human papillomavirus type 16 virus-like particles in an incident case-control study of cervical neoplasia. *J Infect Dis.* 1995;172:1425–1430.
100. Liaw KL, Hsing AW, Chen CJ, et al. Human papillomavirus and cervical neoplasia: a case-control study in Taiwan. *Int J Cancer.* 1995;62:565–571.
101. Nonnenmacher B, Hubbert NL, Kirnbauer R, et al. Serologic response to human papillomavirus type 16 (HPV-16) virus-like particles in HPV-16 DNA-positive invasive cervical cancer and cervical intraepithelial neoplasia grade III patients and controls from Colombia and Spain. *J Infect Dis.* 1995;172:19–24.
102. De Sanjose S, Bosch FX, Munoz N, et al. Socioeconomic differences in cervical cancer: two case-control studies in Colombia and Spain. *Am J Public Health.* 1996;86:1532–1538.
103. De Sanjose S, Hamsikova E, Munoz N, et al. Serological response to HPV16 in CIN-III and cervical cancer patients: case-control studies in Spain and Colombia. *Int J Cancer.* 1996;66:70–74.
104. Bosch FX, Castellsague X, Munoz N, et al. Male sexual behavior and human papillomavirus DNA: key risk factors for cervical cancer in Spain. *J Natl Cancer Inst.* 1996;88:1060–1067.
105. Munoz N, Castellsague X, Bosch FX, et al. Difficulty in elucidating the male role in cervical cancer in Colombia, a high-risk area for the disease. *J Natl Cancer Inst.*1996;88:1068–1075.
106. Castellsague X, Ghaffari A, Daniel RW, et al. Prevalence of penile human papillomavirus DNA in husbands of women with and without cervical neoplasia: a study in Spain and Colombia. *J Infect Dis.* 1997;176:353–361.
107. Burk RD, Ho GY, Beardsley L, et al. Sexual behavior and partner characteristics are the predominant risk factors for genital human papillomavirus infection in young women. *J Infect Dis.* 1996;174:679–689.
108. Bosch FX, Manos MM, Munoz N, et al. Prevalence of human papillomavirus in cervical cancer: a worldwide perspective: International Biological Study on Cervical Cancer (IBSCC) Study Group. *J Natl Cancer Inst.* 1995;87:796–802.
109. Jha PK, Beral V, Peto J, et al. Antibodies to human papillomavirus and to other genital infectious agents and invasive cervical cancer risk. *Lancet.* 1993;341:1116–1118.

110. Caussy D, Goedert JJ, Palefsky J, et al. Interaction of human immunodeficiency and papilloma viruses: association with anal epithelial abnormality in homosexual men. *Int J Cancer.* 1990;46:214–219.

111. Wright TC Jr, Sun XW. Anogenital papillomavirus infection and neoplasia in immunodeficient women. *Obstet Gynecol Clin North Am.* 1996;23:861–893.

112. Hillemanns P, Ellerbrock TV, McPhillips S, et al. Prevalence of anal human papillomavirus infection and anal cytologic abnormalities in HIV-seropositive women. *AIDS.* 1996;10:1641–1647.

113. Sun XW, Kuhn L, Ellerbrock TV, et al. Human papillomavirus infection in women infected with the human immunodeficiency virus. *N Engl J Med.* 1997;337:1343–1349.

114. Holly EA. Cervical intraepithelial neoplasia, cervical cancer, and HPV. *Annu Rev Public Health.* 1996;17:60–84.

115. Koutsky L. Epidemiology of genital human papillomavirus infection. *Am J Med.* 1997;102:3–8.

116. Brinton LA, Reeves WC, Brenes MM, et al. Oral contraceptive use and risk of invasive cervical cancer. *Int J Epidemiol.* 1990;19:4–11.

117. Lorincz AT, Schiffman MH, Jaffurs WJ, et al. Temporal associations of human papillomavirus infection with cervical cytologic abnormalities. *Am J Obstet Gynecol.* 1990;162:645–51.

118. Koutsky LA, Holmes KK, Critchlow CW, et al. A cohort study of the risk of cervical intraepithelial neoplasia grade 2 or 3 in relation to papillomavirus infection. *N Engl J Med.* 1992;327:1272–1278.

119. Eluf-Neto J, Booth M, Munoz N, et al. Human papillomavirus and invasive cervical cancer in Brazil. *Br J Cancer.* 1994;69:114–119.

120. Potischman N, Brinton LA. Nutrition and cervical neoplasia. *Cancer Causes Control.* 1996;7:113–126.

121. Butterworth CE Jr, Hatch KD, Macaluso M, et al. Folate deficiency and cervical neoplasia. *JAMA.* 1992;267:528–533.

122. Potischman N, Brinton LA, Laiming VA, et al. A case-control study of serum folate levels and invasive cervical cancer. *Cancer Res.* 1991;51:4785–4789.

123. Kiviat NB, Koutsky LA. Specific human papillomavirus types as the causal agents of most cervical intraepithelial neoplasia: implications for current views and treatment. *J Natl Cancer Inst.* 1993;85:934–935.

124. Ho GY, Burk RD, Klein S, et al. Persistent genital human papillomavirus infection as a risk factor for persistent cervical dysplasia. *J Natl Cancer Inst.* 1995;87:1365–1371.

125. Coker AL, Jenkins GR, Busnardo MS, et al. Human papillomaviruses and cervical neoplasia in South Carolina. *Cancer Epidemiol Biomarkers Prev.* 1993;2:207–212.

126. Herrero R, Schiffman MH, Bratti C, et al. Design and methods of a population-based natural history study of cervical neoplasia in a rural province of Costa Rica: the Guanacaste Project. *Revista Panamer de Salud Publica.* 1997;1:362–375.

127. Daling JR, Weiss NS, Hislop TG, et al. Sexual practices, sexually transmitted diseases, and the incidence of anal cancer. *N Engl J Med.* 1987;317:973–977.

128. Holmes F, Borek D, Owen-Kummer M, et al. Anal cancer in women. *Gastroenterology.* 1988;95:107–111.

129. Holly EA, Whittemore AS, Aston DA, et al . Anal cancer incidence: genital warts, anal fissure or fistula, hemorrhoids, and smoking. *J Natl Cancer Inst.* 1989;81:1726–1731.

130. Frisch M, Glimelius B, van den Brule AJ, et al. Sexually transmitted infection as a cause of anal cancer. *N Engl J Med.* 1997;337:1350–1358.

131. Sherman ME, Schiffman MH, Strickler H, Hildesheim A. Prospects for a prophylactic HPV vaccine: rationale and future implications for cervical cancer screening. *Diagn Cytopathol.* 1998;18:5–9.

132. Mueller N. An epidemiologist's view of the new molecular biology findings in Hodgkin's disease. *Ann Oncol.* 1991;2:23–28.

133. Merlino C, Giacchino F, Tognarelli G, et al. Epstein-Barr virus infection and lymphoproliferative disorders in patients after renal transplantation. *Minerva Urol Nefrol.* 1996;48:139–143.

134. Crawford DH, Edwards JMB, Sweny P, et al. Studies on long-term cell-mediated immunity to Epstein-Barr virus in immunosuppressed renal allograft recipients. *Int J Cancer.* 1981;28:705–709.

135. Hanto DW, Frizzera G, Purtilo DT, et al. Clinical spectrum of lymphoproliferative disorders in renal transplant recipients and evidence for the role of Epstein-Barr virus. *Cancer Res.* 1981;41:4253–4261.

136. Frizzara G, Hanto DW, Gajl-Peczalska KJ, et al. Polymorphic diffuse B-cell hyperplasias and lymphomas in renal transplant recipients. *Cancer Res.* 1981;41:4262–4279.

137. Cinque P, Brytting M, Vargo L, et al. Epstein-Barr virus in cerebrospinal fluid from patients with AIDS-related primary lymphoma of the central nervous system. *Lancet.* 1993;342:398–401.

138. Waterhouse J, Muir CS, Correa P, Powell G, eds. *Cancer Incidence in Five Continents, III.* Lyon, France: International Agency for Research on Cancer; 1976. IARC Scientific Publications, No. 15.

139. Henle W, Henle G, Ho H-C, et al. Antibodies to Epstein-Barr virus in nasopharyngeal carcinomas, other head and neck neoplasms, and control groups. *J Natl Cancer Inst.* 1970;44:225–231.

140. Zeng Y, Zhang LG, Wu LC, et al. Prospective studies on nasopharyngeal carcinomas in Epstein-Barr virus IgA/VCA antibody-positive persons in Wuzhou City, China. *Int J Cancer.* 1985;36:545–547.

141. Desgranges C, Wolf H, de-The G, et al. Nasopharyngeal carcinoma. X. Presence of Epstein-Barr genomes in separated epithelial cells of tumors in patients from Singapore, Tunisia, and Kenya. *Int J Cancer.* 1975;16:7–15.

142. Raab-Traub N, Flynn K, Pearson G, et al. The differentiated form of nasopharyngeal carcinoma contains Epstein-Barr virus DNA. *Int J Cancer.* 1987;39:25–29.

143. Pathmanathan R, Prasad U, Sadler R, et al. Clonal proliferation of cells infected with Epstein-Barr virus in preinvasive lesions related to nasopharyngeal carcinoma. *N Engl J Med.* 1995;333:693–698.

144. Kieff E. Epstein-Barr virus: increasing evidence of a link to carcinoma. *N Engl J Med.* 1995;333:724–726.

145. Hildesheim A, Levine PH. Etiology of nasopharyngeal carcinoma: a review. *Epidemiol Rev.* 1993;15:466–485.

146. Yu MC. Nasopharyngeal carcinoma: epidemiology and dietary factors. *IARC Sci Publ.* 1991;105:39–47.

147. Evans AS, de-The G. Burkitt lymphoma. In: Evans AS, ed. *Viral Infections of Humans: Epidemiology and Control.* 3rd ed. New York: Plenum Medical Book Co; 1989:713–735.

148. Burkitt DP. A sarcoma involving the jaws in African children. *Br J Surg.* 1958:46:218–223.

149. O'Conor GT, Davies JNP. Malignant tumors in African children with special reference to malignant lymphoma. *J Pediatr.*1960;56:526–535.

150. Burkitt DP. Determining the climatic limitations of a children's tumor common in Africa. *BMJ.* 1962;2:1019–1023.

151. Burkitt DP, Wright DH. Geographical and tribal distribution of the African lymphoma in Uganda. *BMJ.* 1966;5487:569–573.

152. Kafuko GW, Burkitt DP. Burkitt's lymphoma and malaria. *Int J Cancer.* 1970;6:1–9.

153. Epstein MA, Barr YM. Cultivation in vitro of human lymphoblasts from Burkitt's malignant lymphoma. *Lancet.* 1964;1:252–253.

154. Pulvertaft RJV. Cytology of Burkitt's tumor (African lymphoma). *Lancet.* 1964;1:238–240.

155. Epstein MA, Barr YM. Virus particles in cultured lymphoblasts from Burkitt's lymphoma. *Lancet.* 1964;1:702–703.

156. Henle G, Henle W. Immunofluorescence in cells derived from Burkitt's lymphoma. *J Bacteriol.* 1966;91:1248–1256.

157. Henle G, Henle W, Clifford P, et al. Antibodies to Epstein-Barr virus in Burkitt's lymphoma and control groups. *J Natl Cancer Inst.* 1969;43:1147–1157.

158. Zur Hausen H, Schulte-Holthausen H, Klein G, et al. EB-virus DNA in biopsies of Burkitt's tumors and anaplastic carcinomas of the nasopharynx. *Nature.* 1970;228:1056–1057.

159. Epstein MA, Hunt RD, Rabin H. Pilot experiments with EB virus in owl monkeys (*Aotus trivirgatus*). I. Reticuloproliferative disease in an inoculated animal. *Int J Cancer.* 1973;12:309–318.

160. Shope R, DeChairo D, Miller G. Malignant lymphoma in cotton-top marmosets following inoculation of Epstein-Barr virus. *Proc Natl Acad Sci USA.* 1973;70:2487–2491.

161. de-The G, Geser A, Day NE, et al. Epidemiological evidence for causal relationship between Epstein-Barr virus and Burkitt's lymphoma from Ugandan prospective study. *Nature.* 1978;274:756–761.

162. Manilov G, Manilov Y. A marker band on one chromosome no. 14 in Burkitt's lymphoma. *Heriditas.* 1971;68:300.

163. Zech L, Haglund AN, Nilsson K, Klein G. Characteristic chromosomal abnormalities in biopsies and lymphoid cell lines from patients with Burkitt's lymphoma. *Int J Cancer.* 1976;17:47–56.

164. Yunis JJ, Oken MM, Kaplan ME, et al. Distinctive chromosomal abnormalities in histologic sub-types of non-Hodgkin's lymphoma. *N Engl J Med.* 1982;307:1231–1236.

165. Anwar N, Kingma DW, Bloch AR, et al. The investigation of Epstein-Barr viral sequences in 41 cases of Burkitt's lymphoma from Egypt: epidemiologic correlations. *Cancer.* 1995;76:1245–1252.

166. Chao TY, Wang TY, Lee WH. Association between Epstein-Barr virus and Burkitt's lymphoma in Taiwan. *Cancer.* 1997;80:121–128.

167. Chan JK, Tsang WY, Ng CS, et al. A study of the association of Epstein-Barr virus with Burkitt's lymphoma occurring in a Chinese population. *Histopathology.* 1995;26:239–245.

168. Araujo I, Foss HD, Bittencourt A, et al. Expression of Epstein-Barr virus gene products in Burkitt's lymphoma in Northeast Brazil. *Blood.* 1996;87:5279–5286.

169. Bacchi MM, Bacchi CE, Alvarenga M, et al. Burkitt's lymphoma in Brazil: strong association with Epstein-Barr virus. *Mod Pathol.* 1996;9:63–67.

170. Sandlund JT, Fonseca T, Leimig T, et al. Predominance and characteristics of Burkitt lymphoma among children with non-Hodgkin lymphoma in northeastern Brazil. *Leukemia.* 1997;11:743–746.

171. Ertem U, Duru F, Pamir A, et al. Burkitt's lymphoma in 63 Turkish children diagnosed over a 10 year period. *Pediatr Hematol Oncol.* 1996;13:123–134.

172. Quintanilla-Martinez L, Lome-Maldonado C, Ott G, et al. Primary non-Hodgkin's lymphoma of the intestine: high prevalence of Epstein-Barr virus in Mexican lymphomas as compared with European cases. *Blood.* 997;89:644–651.

173. Klein G. Epstein-Barr virus, malaria, and Burkitt's lymphoma. *Scand J Infect Dis Suppl.* 1982:36:15–23.

174. Morrow RH Jr. Epidemiological evidence for a role of falciparum malaria in the pathogenesis of Burkitt's lymphoma. In: Lenoir GM, O'Conor GT, Olweny CLM, eds. *Burkitt's Lymphoma: A Human Cancer Model.* Lyon, France: International Agency for Research on Cancer; 1985:177–186.

175. de-The G. The etiology of Burkitt's lymphoma and the history of the shaken dogmas. *Blood Cells.* 1993;19:667–673.

176. Farrell PJ, Cludts I, Stuhler A. Epstein-Barr virus genes and cancer cells. *Biomed Pharmacother.* 1997;51:258–267.

177. Jox A, Rohen C, Belge G, et al. Integration of Epstein-Barr virus in Burkitt's lymphoma cells leads to a region of enhanced chromosome instability. *Ann Oncol.* 1997;8(suppl 2):131–135.

178. MacMahon B. The epidemiologic evidence on the nature of Hodgkin's disease. *Cancer.* 1957;10:1045–1054.

179. Gutensohn N, Cole P. Childhood social environment and Hodgkin's disease. *N Eng J Med.* 1981;304:135–140.

180. Gutensohn NM. Social class and age at diagnosis of Hodgkin's disease: new epidemiologic evidence on the two disease hypothesis. *Cancer Treat Rep.* 1982;66:689–695.

181. Mueller N, Evans A, Harris NL, et al. Hodgkin's disease and Epstein-Barr virus: altered antibody pattern before diagnosis. *N Eng J Med.* 1989;320:696–701.

182. Jarrett AF, Armstrong AA, Alexander E. Epidemiology of EBV and Hodgkin's lymphoma. *Ann Oncol.* 1996; 7(suppl 4):5–10.

183. Medeiros LJ, Greiner TC. Hodgkin's disease. *Cancer.* 1995;75(suppl):357–369.

184. Glaser SL, Lin RJ, Stewart SL, et al. Epstein-Barr virus-associated Hodgkin's disease: epidemiologic characteristics in international data. *Int J Cancer.* 1997;70:375–382.

185. Glaser SL, Jarrett RF. The epidemiology of Hodgkin's disease. *Baillieres Clin Haematol.* 1996;9:401–416.

186. Takatsuki K, Uchiyama T, Sagawa K, Yodoi J. Adult T-cell leukemia in Japan. In: Seno S, Takaku F, Irino S, eds. *Topics in Hematology.* New York: Elsevier Science; 1978:73–77.

187. Yamaguchi K, Nishimura H, Kohrogi H, et al. A proposal for smoldering adult T-cell leukemia: a clinicopathologic study of five cases. *Blood.* 1983;62:758–766.

188. Kinoshita K, Amagasaki T, Ikeda S, et al. Preleukemic state of adult T cell leukemia: abnormal T lymphocytosis induced by human adult T cell leukemia-lymphoma virus. *Blood.* 1985;66:120–127.

189. Levine PH, Cleghorn F, Manns A, et al. Adult T-cell leukemia/lymphoma: a working point-score classification for epidemiological studies. *Int J Cancer.* 1994;59:491–493.

190. Poiesz BJ, Ruscetti FW, Gazdar AF, et al. Detection and isolation of type C retrovirus particles from fresh and cultured lymphocytes of a patient with cutaneous T-cell lymphoma. *Proc Natl Acad Sci USA.* 1980;77:7415–7419.

191. Tajima K, Tominaga S, Suchi T, et al. Epidemiological analysis of the distribution of antibody to adult T-cell leukemia-virus-associated antigen: possible horizontal transmission of adult T-cell leukemia virus. *Gann.* 1982;73:893–901.

192. Takezaki T, Tajima K, Ito M, et al. Short-term breast-feeding may reduce the risk of vertical transmission of HTLV-I: The Tsushima ATL Study Group. *Leukemia.* 1997;11(suppl 3):60–62.

193. Takezaki T, Tajima K, Komoda H, Imai J. Incidence of human T lymphotropic virus type I seroconversion after age 40 among Japanese residents in an area where the virus is endemic. *J Infect Dis.* 1995;171:559–565.

194. Kinoshita T, Imamura J, Nagai H, et al. Absence of HTLV-I infection among seronegative subjects in an endemic area of Japan. *Int J Cancer.* 1993;54:16–19.

195. Tajima K, Tominaga S, Suchi T. Malignant lymphomas in Japan: epidemiological analysis on adult T-cell leukemia/lymphoma. *Hematol Oncol.* 1986;4:31–44.

196. Tajima K, The T- and B-Cell Malignancy Study Group, and co-authors. The 4th nation-wide study of adult T-cell leukemia/lymphoma (ATL) in Japan: estimates of risk of ATL and its geographical and clinical features. *Int J Cancer.* 1990;45:237–243.

197. Takezaki T, Hirose K, Hamajima N, et al. Estimation of adult T-cell leukemia incidence in Kyushu District from vital statistics Japan between 1983 and 1982: comparison with a nationwide survey. *Jpn J Clin Oncol.* 1997;27:140–145.

198. Tajima K, Tominaga S, Suchi T, et al. HTLV-I carriers among migrants from an ATL endemic area to ATL non-endemic metropolitan areas in Japan. *Int J Cancer.* 198;37:383–387.

199. Tajima K, Cartier L. Epidemiological features of HTLV-I and adult T cell leukemia. *Intervirology.* 1995;38:238–246.

200. Levine PH, Manns A, Jaffe ES, et al. The effect of ethnic differences on the pattern of HTLV-I-associated T-cell leukemia/lymphoma (HATL) in the United States. *Int J Cancer.* 1994;56:177–181.

201. Dosik H, Goldstein MF, Poiesz BJ, et al. Seroprevalence of human T-lymphotropic virus in blacks from a selected central Brooklyn population. *Cancer Invest.* 1994;12:289–295.

202. Welles SL, Levine PH, Joseph EM, et al. An enhanced surveillance program for adult T-cell leukemia in central Brooklyn. *Leukemia.* 1994;8(suppl 1):S111–S115.

203. Chen Y-G, Lin H-C, Chou P. A population-based epidemiological study of human t-cell leukemia virus type 1 infection in Kin-Hu, Kinmen. *Int J Cancer.* 1996;65:569–573.

204. Kaplan MH. Human retrovirus and neoplastic disease. *Clin Infect Dis.* 1993;17(suppl):S400–S406.

205. Weiss RA. Retroviruses and human cancer. *Semin Cancer Biol.* 1992;3:321–328.

206. Morris JDH, Eddleston ALWF, Crook T. Viral infection and cancer. *Lancet.* 1995;346:754–758.

Chapter 13

Immunity and Cancer Risk

Philip C. Nasca

The role that immunity plays in cancer etiology has received increased attention from epidemiologists in recent years, largely because of the increased risk of certain cancers among patients with various immunodeficiency disorders. This chapter provides an overview of the inborn immunodeficiency disorders associated with an unusually high risk of non-Hodgkin's lymphomas as well as an overview of the spectrum of cancers that occur with unusual frequency among patients who receive high doses of immunosuppressive drugs for organ transplantation or as therapies for specific diseases. It also discusses the unusually high risk of certain cancers among patients diagnosed with AIDS, along with the biological mechanisms underlying this high cancer risk and the various cofactors, including other viruses, that may act to increase the risk. It then presents the epidemiological study designs that have been used to examine the relationship between causes of immunodeficiency and selected cancers and discusses the effects that thymectomy, splenectomy, and tonsillectomy can have on cancer risk. Finally, it considers the role of immunostimulation as a possible protective mechanism against cancer.

A vast body of evidence supports the claim that impairment of the immune system increases the risk of developing a number of malignant tumors, most notably Kaposi's sarcoma (KS) and non-Hodgkin's lymphoma (NHL). An excess of risk has been observed among patients with inborn disorders of the immune system and among patients with induced immunosuppression resulting from treatment with immunosuppressive drugs for organ transplantation or for specific medical disorders such as rheumatoid arthritis. The AIDS epidemic provided evidence that viral attacks on the immune system could also lead to the development of a similar array of cancers. Table 13–1 summarizes the types of cancers that have been found to occur with excess frequency in patients with various inborn immunodeficiency disorders or with acquired immunodeficiency.

INBORN IMMUNODEFICIENCY DISORDERS

A number of inherited immunodeficiency disorders have been found to be associated with an increased risk of NHL. Risk estimates have been derived from several registries specifically designed to gather information on patients with these rare disorders. Case reports are sent by physicians in various parts of the world on a voluntary basis. Reported cases of inherited immunodeficiency disorders cannot be related to a defined population at risk, eliminating any possibility of calculating person-years at risk, numbers of expected cancers, and accompanying standardized mortality or morbidity ratios. Instead, the observed proportions of various cancer types among patients with these dis-

Table 13–1 Inherited and Acquired Immune Deficiency and Increased Cancer Risk

Cause of Immune Deficiency	*Associated Cancers*	*Remarks*
Inherited immune disorders: (e.g. ataxia-telangiectasia, Wiskott-Aldrich syndrome, severe combined immunodeficiency disorder, common variable immunodeficiency)	Non-Hodgkin's lymphomas (NHL)	Approximately 50% of cancer patients with these rare genetic disorders are diagnosed with NHL; tumors have a predilection for the brain.
Organ transplant recipients	Non-Hodgkin's lymphomas	Non-Hodgkin's lymphomas (kidney, liver, heart); increased risk observed in under a year to 4 years following transplant; 50-fold increased risk observed in transplant patients; predilection for the brain.
	Vulva and uterine cervix	Increased risk may be due to human papillomavirus (HPV).
	Liver	20 to 40-fold increased risk in transplant patients.
	Kaposi's sarcoma (KS)	Rare in the general population, risk may be increased a 1,000-fold in transplant patients.
	Skin	Most skin cancers in the general population are of the basal-cell type but more often of the squamous-cell type; also increased risk for malignant melanomas.
Acquired immune deficiency syndrome (AIDS)	Kaposi's sarcoma	Has occurred primarily in gay males infected with the human immunodeficiency virus (HIV); unlike the classical form of the disease, AIDS-related KS affects wide areas of the body, including mucous membranes, the gastrointestinal tract, lymph nodes, and other organs.
	Non-Hodgkin's lymphoma	40-fold increased risk in AIDS patients; predilection for the brain; occurs with equal frequency in various AIDS risk groups.
	Anus	40- to 80-fold increased risk in AIDS patients.

orders are compared to the "expected" distribution of these cancers calculated using data from population-based cancer registries.[1]

Data from these registries show that NHL accounts for more than 50% of the cancers diagnosed among patients with various inherited immunodeficiency disorders. This proportion is far in excess of the NHL frequency observed in the general population. The predominance of NHL is most striking among patients diagnosed with Wiskott-Aldrich syndrome, 74.5% of whose cancers are classified as NHL.[2] One study estimated more than a hundredfold increased risk of NHL among patients with Wiskott-Aldrich syndrome.[3] In some of these inherited disorders, NHL tends to show a predilection for the brain, a rare site of occurrence in the general population.

INDUCED IMMUNOSUPPRESSION

Immunosuppressive Drugs for Organ Transplantation

The first evidence that induced immunosuppression might cause an increased cancer risk came as a result of case reports of non-Hodgkin's lymphomas occurring among the growing number of patients undergoing kidney transplantation for end-stage renal disease. These patients received large doses of immunosuppressive drugs to help prevent rejection of the donated kidney. Because of these clinical reports, a number of surveillance systems were created to record and measure systematically the various outcomes of kidney transplantation, including increased risks for various cancers.[4–6]

Cohort studies showed 10- to 49-fold increases in NHL risk among renal transplant patients.[4, 6,7] Their tumors were also unusual in that they occurred in the central nervous system at a much higher rate than is seen in the general population. The induction period for these tumors was as short as 6 months, a finding in sharp contrast to the long induction periods usually associated with environmentally induced cancers.[8] Increased risks have also been observed for melanoma and nonmelanoma skin cancers, vulvar and cervical cancers, liver cancers, and Kaposi's sarcomas. There is a suggestion of some increased risk for cancers of the colon and lung, but the increased risk is of a much lower magnitude than for cancers of the lymphatic system. The excess cancers of the colon and lung, which are common cancers, only begin to emerge after 5 to 7 years following transplantation. Although some of the increase might be attributed to closer medical surveillance and earlier detection of cancer in transplant patients, long-term follow-up suggests that at least some of the increased risk is the result of immunosuppression.[8] Note that immunosuppressed patients have not been found to be at increased risk for developing other common tumor types.

These risk patterns have also been observed in patients receiving immunosuppressive therapy for cardiac,[9] liver,[10,11] and bone marrow[12–14] transplants. A recent study of patients receiving bone marrow transplants showed these patients to be at a higher risk for solid tumors than the general population (observed cases 80; ratio of observed to expected cancer cases 2:7; $p < 0.001$).[14] An eightfold increased risk was observed among patients surviving 10 or more years after transplantation. Significantly elevated risk ratios were observed for malignant melanomas and cancers of the oral cavity, liver, brain and central nervous system, thyroid, bone, and connective tissue. Risk was higher for younger recipients and those receiving higher doses of whole-body radiation.

The magnitude of the NHL risk also decreased over time as new immunosuppressive therapy was introduced for organ transplantation. As physicians gained experience in dealing with organ rejection, the intensity of immunosuppressive drug therapy was significantly reduced, with accompanying declines in NHL. Conversely, the introduction of potent immunosuppressive drugs for cardiac transplants was accompanied by significant increases in NHL incidence rates among recipients. These facts suggest that the excess risk is related to the immunosuppressive therapy and not to the underlying medical condition.[8]

Immunosuppressive Drug Therapy for Selected Medical Conditions

Autoimmune diseases treated with immunosuppressive therapy provide further evidence that impairment of the immune system through drug therapy can lead to increased cancer risk. Cohort studies have shown a 2.5 relative risk of NHL among patients with rheumatoid arthritis not treated with immunosuppressive drugs but a 9.7 relative risk among rheumatoid arthritis patients who are treated with immunosuppressive drugs, such as azathioprine or cyclophosphamide. Although an underlying autoimmune disease such as rheumatoid arthritis may increase NHL risk, the addition of immunosuppressive drug therapy clearly enhances the risk. The enhancement of risk has also been reported for patients with Sjögren's syndrome, an autoimmune condition. One study showed a 35-fold increased risk of NHL in patients not treated with immunosuppressive drugs but a nearly 100-fold increase in patients treated with the drug azathioprine. These findings need to be interpreted with caution given the small number of NHL cases used to calculate the risks. However, the results are in accordance with those observed for rheumatoid arthritis. The tendency of patients under immunosuppressive therapy to develop central nervous system NHL has also been noted.[15]

AIDS and Cancer

Approximately 40% of AIDS patients develop some form of cancer.[16] The first cancer to be recognized as a sequelae of HIV infection was Kaposi's sarcoma (KS). The classical form of KS was first described by Moritz Kaposi in 1872 as a localized, nodular, blue-to-purple tumor appearing on the lower extremities of persons over 50 years of age, with male cases markedly predominating over female cases. Those of Eastern European Jewish or Mediterranean background are at relatively high risk for the classic form of KS. This form rarely metastasizes and tends to be responsive to therapy.[17] Patients with AIDS tend to develop KS at a much younger age than patients with the classic form and to develop a much more aggressive form of KS than the classic form. Among AIDS patients, KS lesions are not limited to the extremities but can be found on almost any part of the body, including the respiratory system and viscera.[18] The disease can also progress very rapidly, and the median survival time for patients with other symptoms is 14 months.[19]

Several years following the initial recognition of increased KS incidence among AIDS patients, a number of case reports[18–21] on a possible relationship between AIDS and NHL appeared in the literature. Patients with AIDS were more likely than patients without AIDS to be diagnosed with aggressive histological subtypes of NHL: high-grade (small noncleaved cell, large cell, immunoblastic) and intermediate-grade (diffuse or large cell) B-cell lymphomas. The clinical course of these lymphomas was also more aggressive, and the median survival times ranged from 4 to 11 months. Involvement of extranodal sites, such as the central nervous system, bone marrow, and gastrointestinal tract, also was observed with greater frequency in AIDS patients.[22]

The epidemiological approaches used to document associations between AIDS and various cancers are summarized in Table 13–2. Stimulated by early case reports of a possible excess risk of NHL among HIV-infected individuals, a number of epidemiological approaches were developed to confirm this risk and search for associations between AIDS and other cancers.[23–41] These methods were particularly useful prior to the

Table 13–2 Epidemiological Study Designs Used To Determine Cancer Patterns among Patients with Inherited and Acquired Immune Deficiency Disorders

Source of Immune Suppression	*Study Design and Type of Comparison*
Inherited disorders	Registries based on physician reports of patients diagnosed with rare inherited immune deficiency disorders; no established denominator; frequency distribution of cancer types among patients with inherited immune deficiency disorders compared with the expected frequency distribution based on data from population-based cancer registries.
Organ transplants	Registries of patients receiving immunosuppressive therapy for kidney, heart, and liver transplants; the observed frequency of various cancers among transplant recipients compared with the number of expected cancers based on site-, sex-, and age- specific cancer rates derived from population-based cancer registries.
AIDS patients	Registries of patients diagnosed with AIDS; Kaposi's sarcomas diagnosed far more frequently in AIDS patients when compared with the number expected based on rates from population-based cancer registries.
	Comparison of time trends for cancers already known to be related to AIDS to time trends for cancers suspected to be occurring more frequently in AIDS patients based on data from population-based cancer registries.
	Ecological correlation of AIDS mortality rates in various geographical areas with incidence and mortality rates for cancers suspected to be occurring more frequently in AIDS patients based on data from population-based cancer registries.
	Studies involving the computer linkage of patient records from population-based cancer registries and AIDS patient registries.

availability of data from long-term follow-up of AIDS patients or cohorts of HIV-infected individuals.

Kristal et al[23] developed an ecological analysis of NHL incidence and mortality rates derived from the New York State Cancer Registry and of AIDS mortality rates derived from vital statistics data. The authors divided the city of New York into three geographic regions based on high, medium, and low cumulative AIDS mortality rates per 100,000 population. The NHL incidence and mortality rates for the years 1980 through 1984 were calculated for each area. Comparisons between AIDS and NHL disease rates were made for women, men currently or formerly married, and single men aged 25–54 years. At this point in the AIDS epidemic, AIDS was significantly more common among men than women, and early case reports had been confined to NHL in gay men. It was reasonable to suspect that the NHL increases might be more evident in men than women. Marital status was used as a surrogate measure for sexual preference, a variable not routinely collected on cancer registry reports or death certificates. The use of marital status as a surrogate variable was probably reasonable given that the range of AIDS cumulative mortality per 100,000 residents across the three regions ranged from less than 10 to more than 25 for women, less than 35 to more than 75 for ever-married men, and less than 250 to more than 600 for single men. The data showed no relation between the geographic distribution of AIDS mortality and NHL incidence or mortality among women or ever-married men. The data also failed to show any secular trends for NHL incidence or mortality in women or ever-married men within each of the three risk areas. For single men, the relation between NHL incidence and mortality was quite striking (Figure 13–1). The data clearly show that NHL incidence and mortality rates in-

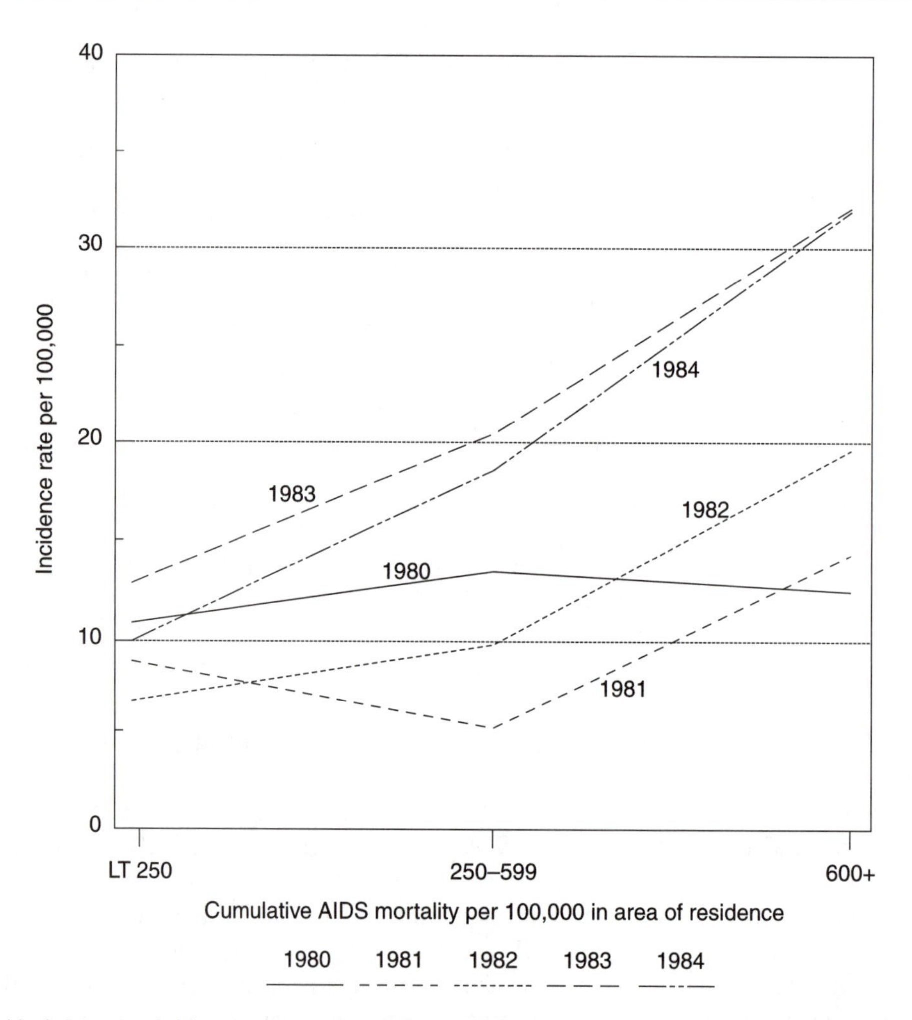

Figure 13–1 Non-Hodgkin's lymphoma age-adjusted incidence per 100,000 per year among never-married males, aged 25–54 years, by AIDS mortality in area of residence. *Source:* from A.R. Kristal, et al., Changes in the Epidemiology of Non-Hodgkin's Lymphoma Associated with the Epidemic of Human Immunodeficiency Virus (HIV) Infection, *American Journal of Epidemiology*, Vol. 128, pp. 711–718, © 1988. Reproduced by permission of Oxford University Press.

crease as the AIDS mortality rate increases. The relation between these two diseases also became more pronounced as the AIDS epidemic progressed. Strong secular trends for NHL were observed for single men residing in the highest AIDS mortality area.

Population-based cancer registry data have also been used to conduct proportional incidence studies of secular tends among single and married men.[24–27] This method was used instead of the usual standardized morbidity ratio (SMR) approach owing to the absence of reliable population estimates for each marital status group prior to the 1990 census. In this method, an odds ratio (OR) is able to be calculated by defining the AIDS epidemic time period as the "exposure" period and the pre-AIDS period as the unexposed time period. A 2 x 2 table is prepared for each cancer, with the number of cancer cases of interest shown in the A and B cells and the number of "control" cancer cases shown in the C and D cells for each time period. The control cancer group consists of all cancer types minus the cancer sites thought to be related to AIDS. The calculations showed not only the expected dramatic rise in Kaposi's sarcomas between the years 1973 and 1976 (the pre-AIDS period) but a statistically significant increase in NHL over this same time period. In the New York study, the NHL incidence rate in Manhattan increased from a rate of 5.5 per 100,000 single men in 1973–1976 to 44.0 per 100,000 in 1985.[26] The 1990 US Census data provided denominator data by marital status that could be used to calculate cancer rates for single men in defined geographic areas. One study was conducted using the geographic areas covered by the National Cancer Institute's Surveillance, Epidemiology, and End Results (SEER) program.[28] The SEER program covers nine population-based cancer registries located in various sections of the United States. Results from these analyses confirmed findings from the ecological correlation and proportional incidence studies. Incidence rates for KS and NHL rose dramatically among single men between the periods 1973–1979 and 1988–1990.

Cancer of the uterine cervix has been added to the Centers for Disease Control and Prevention's list of conditions associated with AIDS. An association between HIV infection and cancer of the uterine cervix is supported by the observation of increased risk of both vulvar and cervical cancer in patients receiving organ transplants.[42] Cervical dysplasia, a precursor of invasive cervical carcinoma, appears to occur with greater frequency and intensity in patients with HIV-related immunosuppression.[43,44] HIV infection also appears to enhance the replication of the human papillomavirus, an agent thought to be etiologically related to cancer of the uterine cervix.[45] In addition, cancer of the uterine cervix appears to be more aggressive in the presence of HIV, demonstrating poorer response to therapy and an increased tendency toward relapse.[46–48] However, the epidemiological data linking HIV infection to cervical cancer is not totally supportive. In New York City, an area with a high prevalence of HIV infection, both African American and Caucasian women showed a trend toward increased incidence of KS. African American women also showed higher NHL rates but Caucasian women did not. The incidence rates for Hodgkin's disease remained stable over time in both racial groups. Both invasive and in situ cancers of the uterine cervix declined over the same period among African American women residing in New York City, the remainder of New York State, and northern New Jersey, and the incidence of invasive and in situ lesions among Caucasian women tended to be stable in all three geographic areas.[36]

More recently, record linkage studies[37–41] in which computer algorithms are used to match individual records from population-based cancer and AIDS registries have been developed. Rabkin and Yellin[28] pointed out the strengths and weaknesses of this approach. Record linkage is particularly useful for detecting associations in populations with a low HIV prevalence, where changes in cancer incidence patterns might be obscured when the small number of AIDS-related cases are mixed with the large number of unrelated cases. The authors also pointed out that the period of risk prior to the AIDS diagnosis is uncertain, making it impossible to estimate a reasonable denominator and associated incidence rates for this period. Nonetheless, the record linkage studies showed the expected relation between KS, NHL, and AIDS. Reynolds et al[39] reported higher than expected numbers of Hodgkin's disease; rare nonmelanoma skin cancers; and cancers of the rectum, anus, and nasal cavity. Melbye et al[41] reported an increased risk of anal cancer in AIDS patients. However, these authors noted that homosexual men in the study were at an increased risk prior to the AIDS epidemic, and the nature of the association between anal cancer and AIDS is unclear.

The possible emergence of multiple cancers in AIDS patients has been investigated. Biggar et al[49] conducted a follow-up study of 4,946 cases of KS for the years 1980–1990. The risk of developing NHL was 198 times greater among AIDS patients than among the general population, but the risk of developing other cancers was only marginally increased (OR = 1.5, 95% CI = 0.95-2.3). Among the subgroup of patients without AIDS-associated KS, the odds ratio for developing any second primary cancer was 0.9 and the odds ratio for developing a second primary cancer that was an NHL was only 0.6.

POSSIBLE BIOLOGIC MECHANISMS

In malignancies associated with organ transplantation, the short induction period and the high rate of viral infections in transplant patients suggest a biological mechanism whereby the immunosuppression might activate viral DNA already present in the host genome.[8,50] The Epstein-Barr virus (EBV) has been identified as the most likely candidate. In studies from South Africa[51] and Italy[52] all patients had serologic evidence of EBV antibodies prior to transplantation, demonstrating the ubiquity of the virus. In the Italian study, 54% of the patients showed evidence of viral reactivation, whereas almost all of the South African patients showed reactivation. Studies have found EBV to be present in the malignant cells of all affected patients tested[53,54] and have demonstrated the ability of immunosuppression to reactivate EBV and to produce polyclonal B-cell proliferation.[55] EBV is also suspected to be etiologically related to lymphomas in AIDS patients, and most AIDS patients test positive for EBV.[56] In addition, EBV DNA has been found in the cerebral spinal fluid of all 17 patients with primary central nervous system lymphomas but in only one of 68 patients without a CNS lymphoma.[57] The predilection for KS to occur in male homosexuals is particularly striking. This has raised the possibility that a cofactor acts in conjunction with HIV infection to cause KS in these men. Although a specific cofactor has not been identified, several possibilities have been suggested, including a hormonal basis and a sexually transmitted agent.[56]

OTHER CANCERS

To date, inherited immunodeficiency or immunosuppression caused by drugs or viral agents has been linked primarily to NHL and KS. As indicated previously, the increased risk for these cancers is probably related to the activation of latent EBV, with yet-to-be-identified cofactors involved in tumor promotion. Among patients diagnosed with inherited immunodeficiency syndromes, no increased risk of common malignancies, such as breast or colon cancers, has been observed. Similarly, no increased incidence rates have been observed for common cancers among patients diagnosed with AIDS or patients given large doses of immunosuppressive drugs. The role of the immune system in providing protection against the development of cancerous cells is still unclear. The discovery of natural killer lymphocytes (NKLs) has prompted the theory that these lymphocytes have the ability to identify and eliminate a variety of tumor cells. However, it appears that tumor cells have the ability to reduce the expression of their surface antigens and to thus hide from the NKLs. The absence of an increased incidence of common cancers in the presence of severe forms of immunodeficiency suggest that the body's ability to maintain effective immunosurveillance over cancerous cells may be limited.[58]

THYMECTOMY, SPLENECTOMY, AND TONSILLECTOMY

Given that inherited immunodeficiency or immunosuppression by drugs or viral agents is associated with an increased risk of various forms of cancer, it seems natural to consider the possible etiologic role of thymectomy,[59–61] splenectomy,[62–64] and tonsillectomy.[65–80] Epidemiological studies that have examined the relation between thymectomy, splenectomy, and cancer risk are listed in Table 13–3. A number of experimental models show that neonatal thymectomy severely depresses the immune system and causes an increase in cancer incidence. However, neonatal thymectomy is rare in humans, and most epidemiological studies have focused on older children and adults.[8]

Papatestas et al,[59] in a study of 789 patients who had undergone thymectomy for myasthenia gravis, calculated the risk of cancer for the time period after the initial diagnosis but prior to the thymectomy and for the period following the operative procedure. Data from the Connecticut Cancer Registry were used to calculate the expected number of cancers in each study period. The authors reported that myasthenia gravis was associated with an increased risk of cancer but that thymectomy prevented the development of malignancies. Vessey et al[60] suggested that the apparent protective effect of thymectomy in the study by Papatestas et al[59] may be the result of a survival bias. If we only include patients who live long enough to be included in the thymectomy group, then individuals who die of cancer prior to the operation are excluded, possibly leading to an underestimation of the true cancer risk.

Vessey et al[60] followed 419 patients with an initial diagnosis of myasthenia gravis. The observed number of extra-thymic tumors was not in excess of the number expected to occur in this group of patients. In a more recent study, Masaoka et al[61] followed 390 patients who had received a thymectomy for myasthenia gravis, 102 of whom had a thymoma and 288 of whom were not diagnosed with a thymoma. Ten malignancies developed in the thymoma group, against an expectation of 2.63. In the patients without a thymoma, only 1 cancer was observed, as compared with 2.65 expected. The authors concluded that the presence of a thymoma increases the risk of developing a cancer and that a thymectomy does not enhance cancer risk but may actually be protective. The number of cancers observed in this study was small. Of the 10 cancers observed, 2 were thymic carcinoids and 4 had already been diagnosed at the time of the diagnosis of myas-

Table 13–3 Studies of Thymectomy and Splenectomy and Subsequent Cancer

Authors (Year)	*Population Studied*	*Results*
Thymectomy		
Papatestas et al. (1977)[59]	Observed cancer cases in 789 patients treated with thymectomy for myasthenia gravis compared with number of expected cancers based on incidence rates from the Connecticut Cancer Registry	No increased risk from extrathymic cancers
Vessey et al. (1979)[60]	Observed cancer deaths in 381 patients treated with thymectomy for myasthenia gravis compared with number of expected cancers based on death rates for England and Wales	No increased risk from extrathymic cancers
Masaoka et al. (1994)[61]	Observed cancer cases in 288 patients without thymoma treated with thymectomy compared with number of expected cancers based on incidence rates from the Osaka Prefecture Regional Cancer Registry	No increased risk from extrathymic cancers
Splenectomy		
Robinette and Fraumeni (1977)[62]	740 American servicemen splenectomized for trauma during 1939–1945	No increased cancer risk
Mellemkjoer et al (1995)[63]	Observed number of cancer cases in 1,103 patients treated with splenectomy for traumatic rupture of the spleen and 5,212 patients treated with splenectomy for nontraumatic indications compared with number of expected cases based on incidence rates from the Danish National Cancer Registry	No increased cancer risk among posttraumatic patients; increased risk for leukemia, Hodgkin's and non-Hodgkin's lymphoma, and lung cancer in non-traumatized patients; no control for treatments prior to splenectomy or previous lifestyle factors such as cigarette smoking
Linet et al. (1996)[64]	Observed number of cancer cases in 1,295 patients treated with splenectomy for traumatic rupture of the spleen and 985 patients treated with splenectomy for nontraumatic indications compared with number of expected cases based on incidence rates from the Swedish National Cancer Registry	No increased cancer risk among posttraumatic patients; increased risk for lung and ovarian cancers; cannot exclude diseases for which splenectomy performed, treatments prior to splenectomy, or previous lifestyle factors such as cigarette smoking

thenia gravis. None of the cancers was a NHL or KS, two tumor types already associated with immunosuppression.

Robinette and Fraumeni found no excess cancer among US veterans of World War II who had received a splenectomy.[62] Two large follow-up studies of patients receiving a splenectomy were conducted in Denmark[63] and Sweden.[64] In both studies, patients were divided into two groups, one in which the patients received a splenectomy because of trauma and the other in which they received a splenectomy for nontraumatic indications, primarily hematological conditions, including hematopoietic cancers, polycythemia and myelofibrosis, and other benign hematological disorders. In both studies, no significant increased cancer risk was observed among posttraumatic patients treated with a splenectomy. The Danish study showed an increased risk of lung and nonmelanoma skin cancers in the patients initially treated for hematological conditions, while the Swedish data showed an excess risk of cancers of the lung and ovary in these patients. The authors of both reports noted that they were unable to exclude the possibility that the excess cancers might have been due to the original condition for which the splenectomy was performed, other treatments given for the initial condition, or known risk factors for these cancers, such as cigarette smoking.

In 1971, Vianna et al[65] reported a risk of Hodgkin's disease 2.9 higher among subjects with a prior tonsillectomy than among those without a prior tonsillectomy. The authors hypothesized that surgical ablation of the tonsils removed a lymphoid barrier to external agents, possibly facilitating the development of Hodgkin's disease. This report stirred much interest and was followed by many additional studies.[66–80] The results of these studies are summarized in Figure 13–2. The studies are divided into four groups based on the source of the control subjects used in the study. The source of controls was a major methodological issue. Tonsillectomy rates in the general population have been shown to be higher in upper socioeconomic groups and to decrease with increasing family size and birth order. Higher social class and lower birth order have been shown to be risk factors for Hodgkin's disease.[78] It was therefore critical to tightly control for the potential confounding effects of these variables. Several studies used siblings to help control for these factors, while other studies used neighbors, classmates, and spouses. The data presented in Figure 13–2 show a lack of a consistent association between tonsillectomy status and Hodgkin's disease risk within each of the control groups.

IMMUNOSTIMULATION

If immunosuppression can increase the risk of developing various cancers, researchers reasoned that stimulating the immune system might actually provide protection against these cancers. Immunostimulation by means of vaccination with the bacille Calmette-Guérin (BCG) tuberculosis vaccine has received much attention. In 1971, researchers in Canada[81] matched death certificates of children dying from leukemia with a central record file of children vaccinated with BCG. The investigators reported that the leukemia death rate was reduced by 50% in children immunized with BCG. However, a number of methodological problems were discovered, and possible matching procedure inadequacies and the use of inappropriate denominators cast doubt on the findings. Ecologic studies in Canada and other parts of the world also failed to support the hypothesis.[8] Most important, data from the actual BCG clinical trials failed to confirm a protective role for the BCG vaccine.[82–86] In the Puerto Rican trial,[82] a significant excess of NHL cases was observed in the group receiving BCG, and in New Zealand,[86] an excess of NHL deaths (but not cases) was observed.

Allergies are another form of immunostimulation that have been studied in relation to cancer risk.[87–97] In 1986, Vena et al[87] published a paper summarizing the results of 16

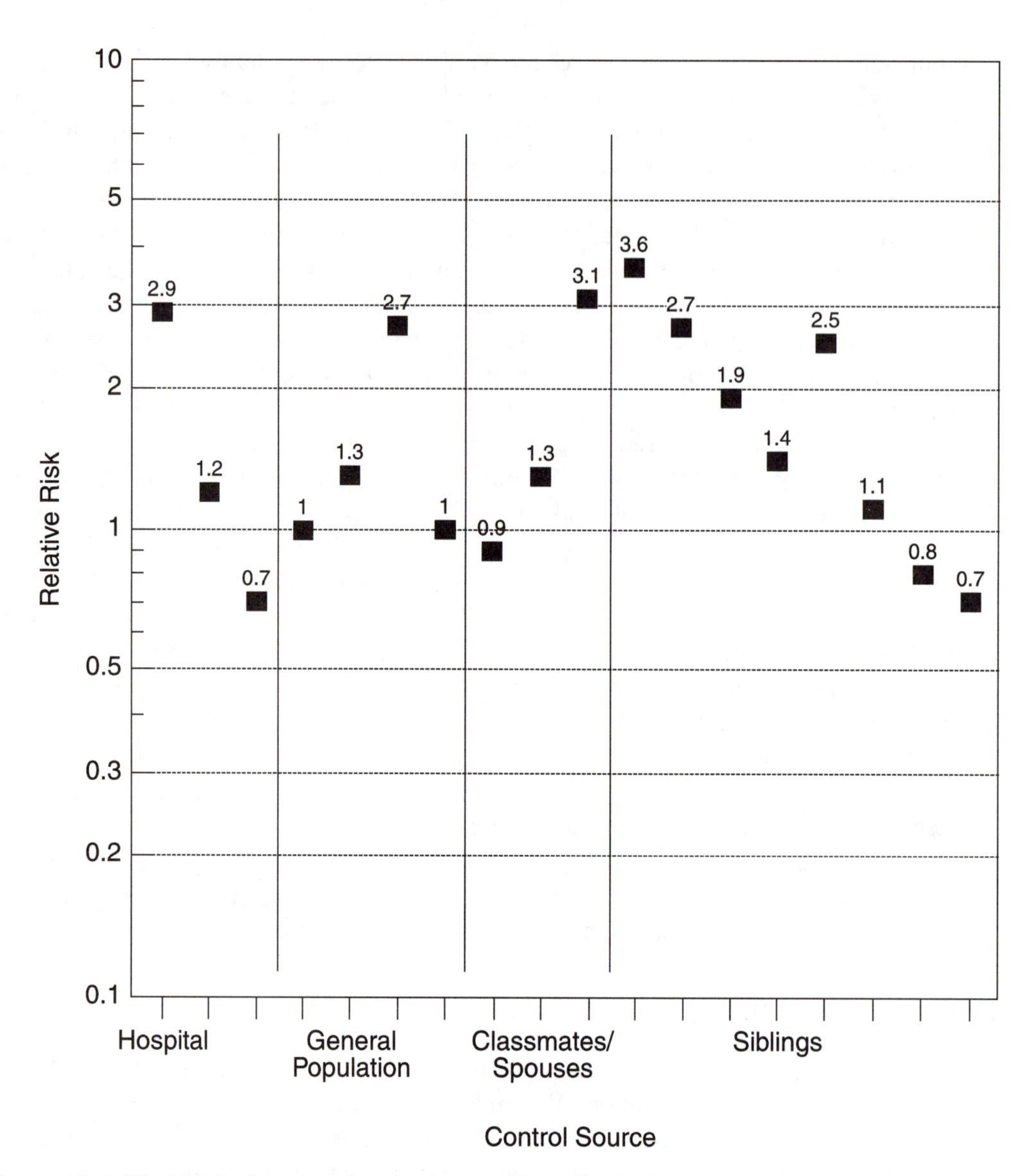

Figure 13–2 Hodgkin's disease risk and prior tonsillectomy by source of control subjects.

---

previous studies reported in the literature. Eleven of these studies showed a decreased risk for all cancers combined or for selected cancers in patients reporting various allergic disorders. Vena et al[87] pointed out a number of methodological issues, including the variability in allergic conditions and cancer outcomes investigated from study to study, the small sample sizes, and the general failure to control for potentially important confounders, such as age, gender, and smoking status. Kinlen[8] raised the possibility that the results of the studies might have been affected by differential recall bias, with interviewers probing more deeply in the case of the healthy control subjects. One study[98] compared findings derived from a questionnaire administered by interviewers who were aware of the interviewees' case or control status with findings derived from blinded interviews. The unblinded interviews showed a decreased risk associated with prior allergy, whereas the blinded interviews showed no differences in reported allergy prevalence between cases and controls.

The data shown in Table 13-4 summarize the findings of studies of allergies and cancer conducted from 1986 to the present. These more recent studies also tend to show that allergic conditions have a protective effect with regard to several specific cancer

Table 13–4 The Relation between Allergy-related Disorders and Subsequent Cancer Risk

First Author (Year)	*Study Type*	*Allergies*	*Results*	*Confounders*
Vena (1985)[87]	Case-control; 13,665 cancer patients, 4,079 nonneoplastic controls	Asthma, hay fever, hives, eczema	(–) Various cancers (hives)	Age, smoking
Linet (1987)[88]	Case-control; 100 multiple myeloma cases, 100 hospital controls	Allergy disorders, autoimmune disorders	(0)	Age, hospital, sex, year of diagnosis
McWhorter (1988)[89]	Cohort; 6,913 adults NHANESI	Asthma, hay fever, hives, food allergy	(+) Various cancers (hives, food allergy)	Age, sex, race, smoking
Severson (1989)[90]	Case-control; 98 cases acute myelocytic leukemia, 133 random digit dialing controls	Asthma, eczema, hives	(–) Asthma, eczema, hives	Age, smoking
La Vecchia (1990)[91]	Case-control; 247 cases pancreatic cancer, 1,089 hospital controls	Drug allergy	(0)	Age, sex
La Vecchia (1990)[92]	Case-control; 242 cases liver cancer, 1,169 hospital controls	Drug allergy	(–)	Age, sex, residence, education, smoking, alcohol

continues

Table 13–4 continued

First Author (Year)	*Study Type*	*Allergies*	*Results*	*Confounders*
La Vecchia (1991)[93]	Case-control; 673 cases colon cancer 405 cases rectal cancer 1501 hospital controls	Drug allergy	(–) Colon (–) Rectum	Age, sex, residence, education, body mass, diet
Mills (1992)[94]	Cohort; 34,198 Seventh-Day Adventists	Asthma, hay fever, drug allergy, bee sting, chemical or plant allergy	(+) Prostate (+) Breast (+) Lymphatic (+) Hematopoietic (–) Ovarian	Age, smoking time since last physician visit
Bernstein (1992)[95]	Case-control; 619 non-Hodgkin's lymphoma cases, 619 neighborhood controls	Asthma, hay fever, eczema	(–) Eczema, allergy to nuts and berries, insect bites and stings	Age, sex, residence
Mesquita (1992)[96]	Case-control; 176 pancreatic cancer cases, 487 population controls	Asthma, hay fever and allergies grouped as "other" allergies, and eczema	(–) Eczema (–) "Other" allergies	Age, gender, smoking
Dai (1995)[97]	Case-control; 108 pancreatic cancer cases, 275 population controls	Food allergies, contact dermatitis, urticaria, asthma, allergic rhinitis, drug allergies	(–) For all allergy types except drug allergies	Age, gender, smoking, income

sites. Although the allergic conditions included are variable, the studies were restricted to specific cancer sites and achieved better control of potential confounding factors, such as age, gender, socioeconomic status, residence, and smoking, than earlier studies.

SUMMARY

Various clinical and epidemiological research studies conducted over the past two decades have clearly demonstrated that suppression of the immune system can lead to a significant increase in the incidence of several cancers, including NHL and KS. In patients receiving immunosuppressive drugs to prevent rejection of transplanted organs or as treatment for autoimmune diseases, the increased cancer incidence appears to be related to the treatments and not the underlying condition. The studies have also shown that these cancers tend to exhibit unusual clinical patterns, including the involvement of anatomic sites not usually associated with these cancers. Cancers occurring in immunosuppressed patients also tend to be more clinically aggressive than the more classic forms of these neoplasms. The distributional and clinical patterns appear to occur in cases of inherited and acquired immunosuppression. The biological mechanisms responsible for the increased risks are not entirely understood, but the evidence strongly suggests that the immunosuppression may activate latent viral DNA, which then proceeds to transform the infected cell. Epstein-Barr virus is likely to be the source of the latent viral DNA given the high level of reactivation noted in immunosuppressed patients. The exact cofactor that might be acting with HIV infection to cause the extremely high incidence of KS in men diagnosed with AIDS has yet to be identified. No convincing evidence exists to link cancer risk with thymectomy, splenectomy, or tonsillectomy. The role of allergies in reducing cancer risk through immunostimulation remains controversial. The findings of the majority of studies suggest a decreased cancer risk among patients reporting treatment for various allergic conditions. However, a number of potential methodological problems necessitate caution in interpreting the data. Finally, the relation of immunosuppression to the more commonly occurring cancers is unclear, and long-term follow-up studies and record linkages studies will be needed to shed more light on the role of immunosuppression in cancer etiology.

Discussion Questions

1. Describe the various epidemiological research designs that have been used to assess whether etiological relationships between various forms of immunodeficiency and selected cancers exist.
2. Discuss the strengths and weaknesses of these epidemiological research designs.
3. Discuss the biological mechanisms that may explain the high incidence of certain cancers among patients diagnosed with AIDS.
4. Discuss the strengths and weaknesses of past epidemiological studies of thymectomy and cancer and of splenectomy and cancer.
5. Discuss the confounding variables that might have had a substantial effect on the findings of past studies of tonsillectomy and Hodgkin's disease. How did investigators deal with these confounding variables?
6. Discuss the strengths and weaknesses of past epidemiological studies of immunostimulation and cancer. Suggest a study design that would help avoid the major limitations of past studies.

References

1. Kinlen LJ. Immunosuppression and cancer. In: Vainio H, Magee PN, McGregor DB, McMichael AJ, eds. *Mechanisms of Carcinogenesis in Risk Identification.* Lyon, France: International Agency for Research on Cancer; 1992:237–253.
2. Filipovich AH, Heinitz KJ, Robison LL, Frizzera G. The immunodeficiency cancer registry: a research resource. *Am J Pediatr Hematol Oncol.* 1987;9:183–184.

3. Perry GS, Spector BD, Shuman LM, Mandel JS. The Wiskott-Aldrich syndrome in the United States and Canada (1892–1979). *J Pediatr.* 1980;97:72–78.
4. Hoover R, Fraumeni JF Jr. Risk of cancer in renal transplant recipients. *Lancet.* 1973;2:55–57.
5. Hoover R. Effects of drugs: Immunosuppression. In: Hiatt H, Watson JD, Winsten JA, eds. *Origins of Human Cancer.* Cold Spring Harbor, NY: Cold Spring Harbor Laboratory; 1977:369–379.
6. Kinlen LJ, Sheh AGR, Peto J, Doll R. A collaborative UK-Australasian study of cancer in patients treated with immunosuppressive drugs. *BMJ.* 1979;2:1461–1466.
7. Birkeland SA, Storm HH, Lamm LU, et al. Cancer risk after renal transplantation in the Nordic countries, 1964–1986. *Int J Cancer.* 1995;60:183–189.
8. Kinlen LJ. Immunologic factors, including AIDS. In: Schottenfeld D, Fraumeni JF Jr, eds. *Cancer Epidemiology and Prevention.* Philadelphia: WB Saunders Co; 1997:532–545.
9. Anderson JL, Bieber CP, Fowles RE, Stinson EB. Idiopathic cardiomyopathy, age and suppressor-cell dysfunction as risk determinants of lymphoma after cardiac transplantation. *Lancet.* 1978;2:1174–1177.
10. Polson RJ, Neuberger J, Forman D, et al. De novo malignancies after liver transplantation. *Transplant Proc.* 1988;20:94–97.
11. Tan-Shalaby J, Tempero M. Malignancies after liver transplantation: a comparative review. *Semin Liver Dis.* 1995;15:156–164.
12. Forman SJ, Sullivan JL, Wright C, et al. Epstein-Barr virus related malignant B cell lymphoplasmacytic lymphoma following allogeneic bone marrow transplantation for aplastic anemia. *Transplantation.* 1987;44:244–249.
13. Shapiro RS, McClain K, Frizzera G, et al. Epstein-Barr virus associated B cell lymphoproliferative disorders following bone marrow transplantation. *Blood.* 1988;71:1234–1243.
14. Curtis RE, Rowlings PA, Deeg HJ, et al. Solid cancers after bone marrow transplantation. *N Engl J Med.* 1997;336:897–904.
15. Kinlen LJ. Malignancy in autoimmune diseases. *J Autoimmunity.* 1992;5(suppl A):363–371.
16. Levine AM. AIDS-related malignancies: the emerging epidemic. *J Natl Cancer Inst.* 1993;85:1382–1397.
17. Schwartz JJ, Dias BM, Safai B. HIV-related malignancies. *Dermatol Clin.* 1991;9:503–515.
18. Snider WD, Simpson DM, Aronyk EE, Nielsen SL. Primary lymphoma of the nervous system associated with acquired immunodeficiency syndrome. *N Engl J Med.* 1983;308:45. Letter.
19. Ziegler JL, Beckstead JA, Volberding PA, et al. Non-Hodgkin's lymphoma in 90 homosexual men: relation to generalized lymphadenopathy and the acquired immunodeficiency syndrome. *N Engl J Med.* 1984;311:565–570.
20. Doll DC, List AF. Burkitt's lymphoma in a homosexual man. *Lancet.* 1982;1:1026–1027.
21. Ziegler JL, Drew WL, Miner RC, et al. Outbreak of Burkitt's-like lymphoma in homosexual men. *Lancet.* 1982;2:631–633.
22. Chachoua A, Krigel RC, LaFleur F, et al. Prognostic factors and staging classification of patients with epidemic Kaposi's sarcoma. *J Clin Oncol.* 1989;7:774–780.
23. Kristal AR, Nasca PC, Burnett WS, Mikl J. Changes in the epidemiology of non-Hodgkin's lymphoma associated with the epidemic of human immunodeficiency virus (HIV) infection. *Am J Epidemiol.* 1988;128:711–718.
24. Biggar RJ, Horm J, Lubin JH, et al. Cancer trends in a population at risk of acquired immunodeficiency syndrome. *J Natl Cancer Inst.* 1985;74:793–797.
25. Biggar RJ, Horm J, Goedert JJ, Melbye M. Cancer in a group at risk of acquired immunodeficiency syndrome (AIDS) through 1984. *Am J Epidemiol.* 1987;174:578–586.
26. Biggar RJ, Burnett WS, Mikl J, Nasca PC. Cancer among New York men at risk of acquired immunodeficiency syndrome. *Int J Cancer.* 1989;43:979–985.
27. Biggar RJ, Nasca PC, Burnett WS. AIDS-related Kaposi's sarcoma in New York City in 1977. *N Engl J Med.* 1988;318:252. Letter.
28. Rabkin CS, Yellin F. Cancer incidence in a population with a high prevalence of infection with human immunodeficiency virus type 1. *J Natl Cancer Inst.* 1994;86:1711–1716.
29. Ross R, Dworsky R, Paganini-Hill A, et al. Non-Hodgkin's lymphomas in never married men in Los Angeles. *Br J Cancer.* 1985;52:785–787.
30. Harnly ME, Swan SH, Holly E, et al. Temporal trends in the incidence of non-Hodgkin's lymphoma and selected malignancies in a population with a high incidence of acquired immunodeficiency syndrome (AIDS). *Am J Epidemiol.* 1988;128:261–267.

31. Biggar RJ, Horm J, Fraumeni JF Jr, et al. Incidence of Kaposi's sarcoma and mycosis fungoides in the United States including Puerto Rico, 1973–1981. *J Natl Cancer Inst.* 1984;73:89–94.
32. Horn PL, DeLorenze GN, Brown SR, et al. Re: Temporal trends in the incidence of non-Hodgkin's lymphoma and selected malignancies in a population with a high incidence of acquired immunodeficiency syndrome (AIDS). *Am J Epidemiol.* 1989;130:1069–1070. Letter.
33. Harnly ME, Swan SH, Kelter A. The authors reply. *Am J Epidemiol.* 1989;130:1070–1071. Letter.
34. Bernstein L, Levin D, Menck H, et al. AIDS-related secular trends in cancer in Los Angeles County men: a comparison by martial status. *Cancer Res.* 1989;49:466–470.
35. Rabkin CS, Biggar RJ, Horm JW. Increasing incidence of cancers associated with the human immunodeficiency virus epidemic. *Int J Cancer.* 1991;47:692–696.
36. Rabkin CS, Biggar RJ, Baptiste MS, et al. Cancer incidence trends in women at high risk of human immunodeficiency virus (HIV) infection. *Int J Cancer.* 1993;55:208–212.
37. Holtzman D, Trapido EJ, MacKinnon JA, et al. AIDS and cancer: findings from a statewide registry match. Paper presented at the Fourth International Conference on AIDS; June 12–16, 1988; Stockholm, Sweden.
38. Cote TR, Howe HL, Anderson SP, et al. A systematic consideration of the neoplastic spectrum of AIDS: registry linkage in Illinois. *AIDS.* 1991;5:49–53.
39. Reynolds P, Saunders LD, Layefsky ME, Lemp GF. The spectrum of acquired immunodeficiency syndrome (AIDS)–associated malignancies in San Francisco, 1980–1987. *Am J Epidemiol.* 1993;137:19–30.
40. Cote TR, Manns A, Hardy CR, et al. Epidemiology of brain lymphoma among people with or without acquired immunodeficiency syndrome: AIDS/Cancer Study Group. *J Natl Cancer Inst.* 1996;88:675–679.
41. Melbye M, Cote TR, Kessler L, et al. High incidence of anal cancer among AIDS patients: The AIDS/Cancer Working Group. *Lancet.* 1994;343:636–639.
42. Penn I. Cancers of the anogenital region in renal transplant recipients: analysis of 65 cases. *Cancer.* 1986;58:611–616.
43. Feingold AR, Vermund SH, Burk RD, et al. Cervical cytologic abnormalities and papillomavirus in women infected with human immunodeficiency virus. *J AIDS.* 1990;3:896–903.
44. Schafer A, Friedmann W, Mielke M, et al. The increased frequency of cervical dysplasia-neoplasia in women infected with human immunodeficiency virus is related to the degree of immunosuppression. *Am J Obstet Gynecol.* 1991;164:593–599.
45. Vermund SH, Kelly KF, Klein RS, et al. High risk of human papillomavirus infection and cervical squamous intraepithelial lesions among women with symptomatic human immunodeficiency virus infection. *Am J Obstet Gynecol.* 1991;165:392–400.
46. Giorda G, Vaccher E, Volpe R, et al. An unusual presentation of vulvar carcinoma in an HIV patient. *Gynecol Oncol.* 1992;44:191–194.
47. Maiman M, Fruchter RG, Serur E, et al. Human immunodeficiency virus and cervical neoplasia. *Gynecol Oncol.* 1990;38:377–382.
48. Matorras R, Ariceta JM, Corral J, et al. Human immunodeficiency virus-induced immunosuppression: a risk factor for human papillomavirus infection. *Am J Obstet Gynecol.* 1991;164:42–44.
49. Biggar RJ, Curtis RE, Cote TR, et al. Risk of other cancers following Kaposi's sarcoma: relation to acquired immunodeficiency syndrome. *Am J Epidemol.* 1994;139:362–368.
50. Boubenider S, Hiesse C, Goupy C, et al. Incidence and consequences of post-transplantation lymphoproliferative disorders. *J Nephrol.* 1997;10:136–145.
51. Hallett AF, Bestbier A, Ford BM, Mohrcken SI. Epstein-Barr virus reactivation in renal transplant recipients. *S Afr Med J.* 1987;71:347–351.
52. Merlino C, Giacchino F, Tognarelli G, et al. Epstein-Barr virus infection and lymphoproliferative disorders in patients after renal transplantation. *Minerva Urol Nefrol.* 1996;48:139–143.
53. Crawford DH, Edwards JMB, Sweny P, et al. Studies on long-term T-cell mediated immunity to Epstein-Barr virus in immunosuppressed renal allograft recipients. *Int J Cancer.* 1981;28:705–709.
54. Hanto DW, Frizzera G, Purtilo DT, et al. Clinical spectrum of lymphoproliferative disorders in renal transplant recipients and evidence for the role of Epstein-Barr virus. *Cancer Res.* 1981;41:4253–4261.
55. Frizzera G, Hanto DW, Gajl-Peczalska KJ, et al. Polymorphic diffuse B-cell hyperplasias and lymphomas in renal transplant recipients. *Cancer Res.* 1981;41:4262–4279.
56. Rabkin CS. Epidemiology of AIDS-related malignancies. *Curr Opinion Oncol.* 1994;6:492–496.

57. Cinque P, Brytting M, Vargo L, et al. Epstein-Barr virus in cerebrospinal fluid from patients with AIDS-related primary lymphoma of the central nervous system. *Lancet.* 1993;342:398–401.
58. Varmus H, Weinberg RA. *Genes and the Biology of Cancer.* New York: Scientific American Library; 1993.
59. Papatestas AE, Kark AE, Genkins G, Aufses AH. Protective effects of thymectomy in a high cancer risk population. In: *Prevention and Detection of Cancer.* Nieburgs HE, ed. New York: Marcel Dekker; 1977.
60. Vessey MP, Doll R, Norman-Smith B, Hill ID. Thymectomy and cancer: a further report. *Br J Cancer.* 1979;39:193–195.
61. Masaoka A, Yamakawa Y, Niwa H, et al. Thymectomy and malignancy. *Eur J Cardiothorac Surg.* 1994;8:251–253.
62. Robinette CD, Fraumeni JF Jr. Splenectomy and subsequent mortality in veterans of the 1939–1945 war. *Lancet.* 1977;2:127–129.
63. Mellemkjoer L, Olsen JH, Linet MS, et al. Cancer risk after splenectomy. *Cancer.* 1995;75:577–583.
64. Linet MS, Nyren O, Gridley G, et al. Risk of cancer following splenectomy. *Int J Cancer.* 1996;66:611–616.
65. Vianna NJ, Greenwald P, Davies JNP. Tonsillectomy and Hodgkin's disease: the lymphoid tissue barrier. *Lancet.* 1971;1:431–432.
66. Ruuskanen C, Vanha-Perttula T, Kouvailanen K. Tonsillectomy, appendectomy and Hodgkin's disease. *Lancet.* 1971;1:1127–1128.
67. Johnson SK, Johnson RE. Tonsillectomy history in Hodgkin's disease. *N Engl J Med.* 1972;287:1122–1125.
68. Newell G, Rawlings W, Kinnera B, Correa P. Case-control study of Hodgkin's disease. I. Results of the interview questionnaire. *J Natl Cancer Inst.* 1973;51:1437–1441.
69. Vianna NJ, Greenwald P, Polan A, et al. Tonsillectomy and Hodgkin's disease. *Lancet.* 1974;2:168–169.
70. Gutensohn N, Frederick SM, Johnson RE, Cole P. Hodgkin's disease, tonsillectomy and family size. *N Engl J Med.* 1975;292:22–25.
71. Paffenbarger RS Jr, Wing AL, Hyde RT. Characteristics in youth indicative of adult-onset of Hodgkin's disease. *J Natl Cancer Inst.* 1977;58:1489–1491.
72. Abramson JH, Pridan H, Sachs MI, et al. A case-control study of Hodgkin's disease in Israel. *J Natl Cancer Inst.* 1978;61:307–314.
73. Andersen E, Isager H. Pre-morbid factors in Hodgkin's disease. II. BCG-vaccination status, tuberculosis, infectious diseases, tonsillectomy, and appendectomy. *Scand J Haematol.* 1978;21:273–277.
74. Henderson BE, Dworsky R, Pike MC, et al. Risk factors for nodular sclerosis and other types of Hodgkin's disease. *Cancer Res.* 1979;39:4507–4511.
75. Vianna NJ, Lawrence CE, Davies JNP, et al. Tonsillectomy and childhood Hodgkin's disease. *Lancet.* 1980;2:338–340.
76. Kirchhoff LV, Evans AS, McClelland KE, et al. A case-control study of Hodgkin's disease in Brazil. I. Epidemiologic aspects. *Am J Epidemiol.* 1980;112:595–608.
77. Hardell L, Bengtsson NO. Epidemiological study of socioeconomic factors and clinical findings in Hodgkin's disease, and reanalysis of previous data regarding chemical exposure. *Br J Cancer.* 1983;48:217–225.
78. Mueller N, Swanson GM, Hsieh CC, Cole P. Tonsillectomy and Hodgkin's disease: results from comparison population-based studies. *J Natl Cancer Inst.* 1987;78:1–5.
79. Bonelli L, Vitale V, Bistolfi F, et al. Hodgkin's disease in adults: association with social factors and age at tonsillectomy: a case-control study. *Int J Cancer.* 1990;45:423–427.
80. Gledovic Z, Radovanovic Z. History of tonsillectomy and appendectomy in Hodgkin's disease. *Eur J Epidemiol.* 1991;7:612–615.
81. Davignon L, Lemonde P, St-Pierre J, et al. BCG vaccination and leukemia mortality. *Lancet.* 1971;1:80–81.
82. Comstock GW, Martinez I, Livesay BT. Efficacy of BCG vaccination in the prevention of cancer. *J Natl Cancer Inst.* 1975;54:834–839.
83. Snider DE, Comstock GW, Martinez I, Caras GJ. Efficacy of BCG vaccination in prevention of cancer: an update. *J Natl Cancer Inst.* 1978;60:785–788.
84. Kendrick MA, Comstock GW. BCG vaccination and the subsequent development of cancer in humans. *J Natl Cancer Inst.* 1981;66:431–437.
85. Sutherland I. BCG and vole bacillus vaccination in adolescence and mortality from leukemia. *Stat Med.* 1982;1:329–335.

86. Skegg DCG. BCG vaccination and the incidence of lymphoma and leukemia. *Int J Cancer.* 1978;21:18–21.
87. Vena JE, Bona JR, Byers TE, et al. Allergy-related diseases and cancer: an inverse association. *Am J Epidemiol.* 1985;122:66–74.
88. Linet MS, Harlow SD, McLaughlin JK. A case-control study of multiple myeloma in whites: chronic antigenic stimulation, occupation, and drug use. *Cancer Res.* 1987;47:2978–2981.
89. McWhorter WP. Allergy and risk of cancer: a prospective study using NHANES I follow-up data. *Cancer.* 1988;62:451–455.
90. Severson RK, Davis S, Thomas DB, et al. Acute myelocytic leukemia and prior allergies. *J Clin Epidemiol.* 1989;42:995–1001.
91. La Vecchia C, Negri E, D'Avanzo B, et al. Medical history, diet, and pancreatic cancer. *Oncology.* 1990;47:463–466.
92. La Vecchia C, Negri E, D'Avanzo B, et al. Medical history and primary liver cancer. *Cancer Res.* 1990;50:6274–6277.
93. La Vecchia C, D'Avanzo B, Negri E, Franceschi S. History of selected diseases and the risk of colorectal cancer. *Eur J Cancer.* 1991;27:582–586.
94. Mills PK, Beeson L, Fraser GE, Phillips RL. Allergy and cancer: organ site-specific results from the Adventist Health Study. *Am J Epidemiol.* 1992;136:287–295.
95. Bernstein L, Ross RK. Prior medication use and health history as risk factors for non-Hodgkin's lymphoma: preliminary results from a case-control study in Los Angeles County. *Cancer Res.* 1992;52:5510–5515.
96. Bueno de Mesquita HB, Maisonneuve P, Moerman CJ, Walker AM. Aspects of medical history and exocrine carcinoma of the pancreas: a population-based case-control study in the Netherlands. *Int J Cancer.* 1992;52:17–23.
97. Dai Q, Zheng W, Ji B-T, et al. Prior immunity-related medical conditions and pancreatic-cancer risk in Shanghai. *Int J Cancer.* 1995;63:337–340.
98. Chilvers C, Johnson B, Leach S, et al. The common cold, allergy, and cancer. *Br J Cancer.* 1986;54:123–126.

Chapter 14

Epidemiology of Endogenous Hormones and Cancer

Lisa Chasan-Taber

The chapter begins with a review of the risk factors for and environmental causes of breast cancer, including reproductive practices, diet, and physical activity, and, as part of the review, summarizes the evidence from the major epidemiological studies. It then discusses the etiologic association between hormones and breast cancer, the methods of hormone measurement, and the determinants and biological markers of endogenous hormones. Personal susceptibility factors, such as family history and genetically determined susceptibilities, are also considered. The second half of the chapter covers the role that endogenous hormones play in the development of prostate, endometrial, ovarian, and cervical cancers.

A substantial body of experimental, clinical, and epidemiological evidence indicates that endogenous hormones play a major role in the etiology of several human cancers,[1] and epidemiological hypotheses regarding cancers of the breast, endometrium, prostate, ovary, and testis have been formulated and tested.[2,3] As a result, estrogen, for example, has been identified as a critical factor in breast cancer etiology. The purpose of the chapter is not to present an exhaustive review of hormones and cancer risk but instead to provide a generalizable lesson about cancer etiology and prevention through focusing on the role of hormonal factors in the development of breast cancer.

BREAST CANCER

Risk Factors

Descriptive Epidemiology

The incidence of breast cancer among women increases steadily with age, and the most rapid rise occurs between the ages of 40 and 55. After menopause, the increase in incidence continues but is attenuated. Although the age-adjusted mortality rate has been relatively constant since 1930, the age-adjusted incidence rate has risen over the past several decades (Figure 14–1). For most of that period the rise was slow, but between 1980 and 1987 the incidence rate increased by 32%. Until 1980, most of the long-term increase was seen in women aged 50 and over, but from 1980 to 1987 the incidence rate for younger women also increased. The extent to which the apparent increase in the overall incidence rate is attributable to early case-finding through screening programs and to the detection and removal of lesions that were not previously called cancer is uncertain.[4]

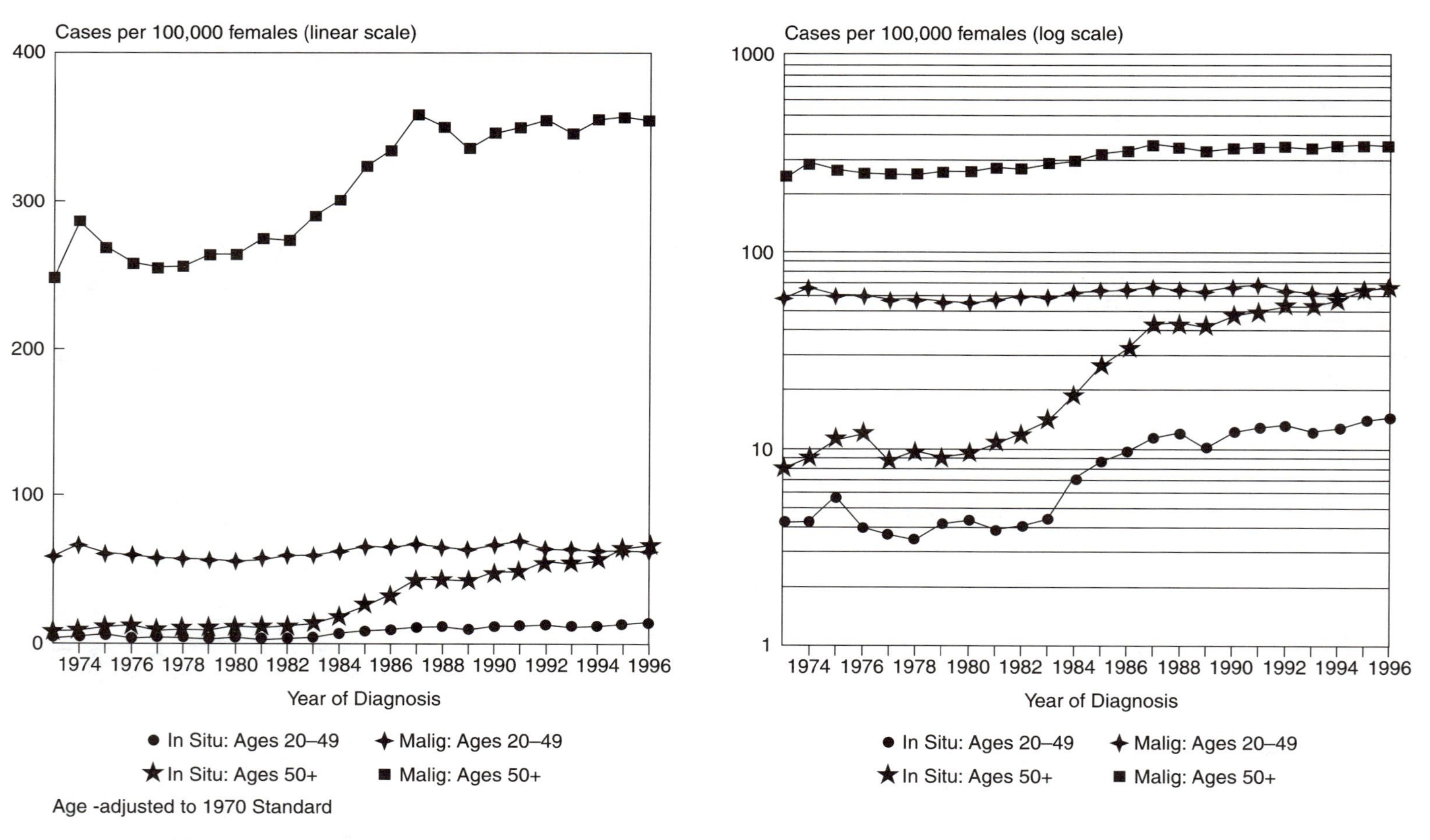

Figure 14–1 Breast cancer incidence rates, 1973–1996, by age, in situ versus malignant, all races, female. *Source:* Reprinted from L.A.G. Ries, et al., eds., *SEER Cancer Statistics Review, 1973–1996*, National Cancer Institute, 1999.

In addition to the dramatic increase in breast cancer incidence in the last two decades, there exists a wide disparity in rates between geographic regions. Underdeveloped countries have traditionally low incidence rates,[5] and the difference between the rates of undeveloped and developed countries may reach upwards of tenfold.[6]

Migrant studies have demonstrated that, as women move from a low-risk to a high-risk country, their breast cancer incidence rate changes. For example, first-generation Japanese migrants to the United States have a breast cancer incidence rate similar to the rate for women in Japan, whereas the incidence rates for second- and third-generation migrants approach the rate for American-born Caucasian women.[7] The speed with which the incidence of breast cancer among migrants and their offspring reaches the overall incidence in their adopted country varies across studies and ethnic groups. Polish immigrants appear to adopt US Caucasian incidence rates within one generation, while Chinese, Japanese, and Mexican women require two or more generations and even then do not fully reach the higher rates of American-born Caucasian women.[8,9] These differences suggest that behavioral practices characteristic of the Asian and Mexican cultures are protective against breast cancer and may be carried over into the second generation. Alternatively, some risk factors for breast cancer, possibly dietary factors or reproductive behaviors, may be avoided by migrant parents as well as by their offspring.

A study of Japanese and Hispanic immigrants to Los Angeles found that age of immigration was important in determining breast cancer risk. Those who migrated later in life had a breast cancer rate that, although higher than the rate in their country of birth, was still substantially lower than the rate for those who migrated at a younger age.[10] The slower change in risk among women who migrate during adulthood indicates that environmental factors operating early in life may affect future breast cancer risk.

Reproductive Factors

Differences in reproductive factors between countries may partially explain geographic differences in breast cancer incidence rates as well. Similarly, to some degree, changes in breast cancer incidence over time parallel trends in reproductive behavior believed to be associated with breast cancer risk (eg, smaller family size and later age at first birth).

The younger a woman's age at menarche, the higher her risk of breast cancer.[11–15] One large study[16] found that for each 2-year delay in onset of menstruation, breast cancer risk was reduced by about 10%. Another study found that women with onset of menstruation at or after age 15 years had a 23% lower risk than those with an age at menarche of 12 years or younger.[17] The later a woman's age at menopause, the higher her risk of breast cancer. For every 5-year difference in age at menopause, the risk of breast cancer changes by approximately 17%.[16] Bilateral oophorectomy before menopause also brings about a reduction in risk that appears to last into older ages,[4] probably after a latency period of 10–20 years. Bilateral oophorectomy before age 40, for instance, is associated with a lifetime decrease in risk of about 50%.[17,18]

The majority of studies have found that, on average, the younger a woman is when she has her first full-term pregnancy, the lower her risk of breast cancer[4] (the decrease in risk perhaps starts about 10 years after the pregnancy).[19] Most studies find this association to be independent of parity and other breast cancer risk factors. Nulliparous women experience a greater risk of breast cancer than parous women, with estimates of relative risk ranging from about 1.2 to 1.7.[4]

In short, early age at menarche, late age at menopause, late age at first full-term pregnancy, and nulliparity are associated with modest increases in breast cancer risk. Oophorectomy before menopause protects against the development of breast cancer. Less clear are the etiologic roles of spacing of births, spontaneous and induced abortion, infertility, breast feeding, multiple births, and hypertension during pregnancy.

Environmental Factors

The large international differences in the rates of breast cancer and the striking increases among populations migrating from low- to high-incidence areas suggest that environmental factors have a strong influence on the occurrence of breast cancer. One example is diet. Correlational studies demonstrated a high correlation between per capita fat consumption and breast cancer incidence. The findings of these studies, together with data from laboratory and animal experiments, suggested that a high intake of dietary fat may be an important risk factor for breast cancer. Most cohort studies did not corroborate this association, but they were criticized for small numbers of cases, homogenous fat intake, and measurement errors in estimates of fat intake. In a recent pooled study of the primary data from seven major cohort studies of dietary fat and breast cancer, there was no evidence of a positive association between total dietary fat intake and the risk of breast cancer. There was no reduction in risk even among women whose energy intake from fat was less than 20% of total energy intake.[20] The observational data, taken together, suggest that modification of dietary fat intake among adult women is unlikely to reduce the risk of breast cancer.

Additional light will be shed on this issue by the Women's Health Initiative, a randomized clinical trial that was initiated in 1992, is currently underway, and has a planned completion date of 2007. Postmenopausal women ranging in age from 50 to 79 are enrolled at one of 40 Women's Health Initiative clinical centers nationwide into a clinical trial that will include about 64,500 women randomized to three distinct interventions—a low-fat eating pattern, hormone replacement therapy, and calcium and vitamin D supplementation—with an average follow-up of approximately 9 years.

Alternatively, a large body of evidence suggests that even moderate alcohol consumption can increase breast cancer risk. In a recent meta-analysis, Longnecker[21] found that women who consumed an average of two drinks per day had an increased risk of 25%. A detailed discussion of this association is found in Chapter 10.

It is plausible that environmental pesticides and industrial chemicals associated with a westernized lifestyle may be related to breast cancer risk. The hypothesis that, among these pollutants, organochlorine chemicals may be especially responsible for increasing breast cancer risk has garnered wide attention. The most abundant organochlorine contaminants are the pesticide DDT (2,2-bis(*p*-chlorophenyl)-1,1,1-trichloroethane) and certain polychlorinated biphenyls (PCBs). Many of these compounds accumulate in adipose tissue because of their lipid solubility and resistance to metabolism. They are also present in breast milk.[22] Only limited epidemiological data, however, are available to assess possible associations. The majority of previous studies included relatively small number of patients with breast cancer. In a recent case-control study conducted in Europe, concentrations of DDE [1,1-dichloro-2,2-bis(*p*-chlorophenyl)ethylene, the main metabolite of DDT] in adipose tissue were lower in patients with breast cancer than in controls.[23] Data on PCBs were not available. A prospective study of 58 breast cancer cases found a significant increase in the risk of breast cancer associated with higher serum levels of DDE and a nonsignificant positive association between breast cancer and PCBs.[24] In the largest prospective study to date, Hunter et al[25] examined serum from 240 case patients and 240 controls from the Nurses' Health Study cohort. The authors did not observe any evidence of an increased risk of breast cancer among women with relatively high levels of plasma DDE or PCBs. The absence of an association, however, does not rule out the possibility that other pesticides and environmental contaminants may be associated with breast cancer.

Physical Activity

A number of recent epidemiological studies have suggested that physical activity is related to breast cancer risk. As reviewed by Friedenreich, 15 of the 21 most recent studies suggest that physical activity reduces risk, whereas 4 found no association and 2 found an increased risk.[26] Specific subgroups of women, specifically women who are lean, parous, and premenopausal, may experience an especially great decrease in breast cancer with increased levels of physical activity.[26] Lifetime activity may be more important than current activity. One case-control study limited to premenopausal women found a linear trend toward lower risk with increasing hours per week spent in physical exercise during a woman's reproductive life. Consistent participation in exercise lasting 4 or more hours per week was associated with a nearly 60% reduction in breast cancer risk. Exercise within 10 years after menarche provided similar or slightly diminished protection.[27]

While results have not been entirely consistent across studies, overall they indicate that physical activity protects against breast cancer. Many crucial questions remain, such as the level of activity required, whether there is a risk reduction for both pre- and postmenopausal women, and whether the risk reduction occurs primarily as a result of exercise during adolescence.[28]

Role of Endogenous Hormones

Some of the generally accepted reproductive risk factors for breast cancer—the timing of menarche, first birth, and menopause—strongly implicate ovarian hormones in the etiology of the disease. Further support is provided by the shape of the age-specific incidence curve for breast cancer, specifically the slowing of the rate of increase around the age of menopause. This age-incidence pattern is not seen in non-hormone-dependent cancers, such as lung cancer, which instead show a stable increase that continues past menopause. The decline in slope characteristic of breast incidence in women aged over 50 years is absent from the incidence pattern for men, further implicating hormones such as estrogen, which are present at high levels in the premenopausal years and then decrease sharply.

A hormone is a chemical messenger that is carried by the blood from the endocrine glands to responsive cells, where the hormone controls normal growth and function. A key element of the role of endogenous hormones in cancer risk is that neoplasia is the consequence of excessive hormonal stimulation of the particular target organ. Among all of the hormones associated with ovarian activity, endogenous estrogens, because of their effects on the growth of breast epithelium, have been most extensively studied. Endogenous estrogens are the principal regulators of growth and differentiation in normal breast tissue during puberty and pregnancy.

Association between Reproductive Factors and Endogenous Hormones

In premenopausal, nonpregnant women, nearly all estrogen is of ovarian origin,[29] and there is substantial epidemiological evidence that a positive relationship exists between breast cancer risk and the cumulative number of ovulatory menstrual cycles in a woman's life.[30] The existence of this relationship is supported by associations between breast cancer and factors that influence this number, such as age at menarche and menopause, menstrual cycle patterns, pregnancy, and years until cycle regularity.[4]

Since menarche at a young age is associated with earlier onset of regular menstrual cycles, early exposure to the hormonal environment characteristic of regular ovulatory menstrual cycles may be an important etiologic factor.[4] In addition, some studies have reported that women with early menarche have higher estrogen levels for several years after menarche and potentially throughout their reproductive lives.[31,32]

The increased risk of breast cancer associated with early age at menopause further supports the hypothesis that cyclic ovarian function is an important stimulus to or prerequisite for the malignant transformation of the breast.[33,34] Taken together, the increased risks associated with early age at menarche and late age at menopause suggest that the longer the exposure to sex hormones during the reproductive years, the higher the risk of breast cancer.[35] It is also possible that early age at menarche and late age at menopause are independent risk factors for breast cancer.[4]

As discussed above, pregnancy is associated with breast cancer risk. Prior to pregnancy, the mammary glands contain undifferentiated terminal ductal structures with high proliferative activity. The breast, therefore, is more susceptible to initiating carcinogens at this time. Subsequent exposure to elevated levels of estrogen brought on by a full-term pregnancy may promote the selective proliferation of already initiated breast cells prior to their terminal differentiation.[36] Thus, pregnancy might be followed for several years by an increased risk for breast cancer. Ultimately, however, a long-term reduction in breast cancer risk results from changes in the susceptibility of breast tissue. Pregnancy induces permanent structural changes in the mammary gland along with accompanying decreases in cell proliferation and carcinogen binding and increases in DNA repair capacity.[37] These permanent changes make the breast less susceptible to chemically induced carcinogenesis.[37]

The pattern of increasing risk with increasing age at first full-term pregnancy can be attributed to the extended duration of the interval of susceptibility prior to terminal differentiation. It has been hypothesized that the earlier the age at full-term pregnancy, the earlier this period of decreased susceptibility to initiation begins,[4] while a late first full-term pregnancy increases the time interval of susceptibility. Therefore, in addition to its potential role as an anti-initiator, pregnancy may also act as a promoter. A late first full-term pregnancy, which increases the interval of susceptibility to initiation, may then, via elevated levels of estrogen during pregnancy, promote the selective proliferation of already initiated breast cells prior to terminal differentiation.[37]

Association between Physical Activity, the Environment, and Endogenous Hormones

Factors that influence the cumulative number of ovulatory menstrual cycles in a woman's life, such as age at menarche and menopause, menstrual cycle patterns, and years until cycle regularity,[38] in turn may be influenced by physical activity.[39,40] Strenuous and competitive physical activity among premenarcheal girls has been associated with later age at menarche[41–43] and secondary amenorrhea after the onset of menses.[41,42,44–46] Sustained levels of moderate physical activity have been associated with greater frequency of anovulatory cycles than occur with little or no activity.[47] Thus, women who participate in vigorous training and moderate leisure-time activity may have lower risk of breast cancer due to a lower lifetime exposure to ovarian hormones.

After menopause, direct ovarian estrogen production ceases and most estrogen is derived from the aromatization of adrenal androgens to estrone, a form of estrogen. Obesity and fat stores provide the substrate for aromatization.[48–50] In turn, obesity (particularly abdominal obesity) and elevated concentrations of endogenous estrogens are associated with increased risk of postmenopausal breast cancer.[51–54] Physical activity may act on risk of postmenopausal breast cancer by reducing obesity and thereby reducing fat stores. Indeed, exercise has been shown in observational and experimental studies to preferentially reduce the highly metabolic stores of abdominal visceral and subcutaneous fat.[55]

As described in Chapter 10, alcohol may act on breast cancer risk by affecting the level of estradiol and other steroid hormones. Several studies have observed a short-term increase in serum estradiol and prolactin levels following alcohol consumption. The data on the long-term effect of alcohol on plasma hormone levels are mixed: one cross-sectional study found no association, a nested case-control study found an association between alcohol and estrone sulfate only, and a controlled trial found associations between alcohol and both the total estrogen level and the bioavailable estrogen level.[56–58]

Many pesticides and industrial chemicals have the potential to act as "environmental estrogens" and have been shown to affect wildlife adversely. In vitro assays demonstrate that DDE and certain PCB congeners exhibit estrogen-like activity.[59] Other PCB congeners and organochlorines exhibit antiestrogenic activity. This is of interest since estrogens are growth factors for tissues of the breast and uterus. In general, however, these compounds are very weak estrogens in in vitro assays, and concentrations of up to 100,000 times more than natural estrogen are required to achieve equivalent estrogenic activity.[59] Indeed, humans may be exposed to much larger amounts of naturally occurring estrogenic compounds in their diets than via environmental organochlorine estrogens.[60]

Nevertheless, given that organochlorines are fat soluble, persist in adipose tissue, and are excreted in breast milk,[61] ductal and other cells in the breast may be exposed to these compounds over a period of many decades. Such prolonged exposure may counterbalance the low estrogenic potency of organochlorines.[25] At lower doses, the aromatic organochlorines may serve as tumor promoters, increasing the rate at which a transformed cell grows into a clinically detectable tumor.

A recent review article on the association of organochlorines and breast cancer found conflicting evidence.[27] Note also that recent trends and international, racial, and socioeconomic patterns in breast cancer incidence do not match data on exposure to organochlorines.[62]

Association between Other Risk Factors and Endogenous Hormones

During the prenatal period, rapid breast cell proliferation occurs in the mother and reflects high estrogen levels, which, in turn can imprint susceptible fetal breast cells. It has been hypothesized that various perinatal indicators of high pregnancy estrogen levels (high birthweight, birth length, and placental weight) and indicators of low pregnancy estrogen levels (pre-eclampsia or eclampsia) may be associated with mammographic patterns. During adolescence, rapid proliferation can promote already initiated breast cells.[31]

Recent studies show that alcohol increases the levels of estrogens in the bloodstream,[27] which would be expected to increase breast cell division and increase cancer risk.

Measurement of Endogenous Hormones

Key and Pike[53] and more recently Bernstein[29] reviewed the epidemiological studies of hormones and breast cancer. Case-control studies of postmenopausal women fairly consistently demonstrate that breast cancer case subjects have higher levels of estrogen than control subjects.[53] However, case-control studies in this area of investigation face a variety of limitations. The cancer itself, the treatment for it, and the psychological stress associated with it may each affect plasma and urinary hormone concentrations.[29] Thus, if related to the latter two factors, observed differences in hormone concentrations between case and control subjects may not be etiologically meaningful. Alternatively, the timing of the sample may mask the true extent of the difference between case and control subjects. That is, the etiologic hormonal difference between case and control subjects may have existed some time prior to diagnosis but may not be as evident at the time of sampling.[29] Confounding is also a concern. If case subjects or control subjects are as a group heavier, for example, this could explain any observed difference in hormone levels between the two groups.

Cohort studies address many of the limitations of case-control studies but possess others. Three cohort studies that collected and stored hormone samples prior to diagnosis of breast cancer did not observe any relation between estrogen levels and risk of breast cancer among postmenopausal women.[63–65] However, hormones in storage over long periods of time undergo degradation.[66–68] Laboratory analysis of the hormone samples is also subject to error.

Case-control and cohort studies of endogenous hormones among premenopausal women are particularly challenging to design and conduct. Hormone levels substantially increase from the follicular to the luteal phases of the menstrual cycle. Therefore, multiple measurements may be required to characterize a subject adequately.[29] Case-control studies of premenopausal women do not provide consistent evidence of greater estrogen levels among case subjects.[53]

Personal Susceptibility Factors

Genetic Factors

The etiology of breast cancer involves a complex interplay of various factors, including genetic alterations. Any attempt to investigate breast cancer from an epidemiological standpoint must recognize the increasingly crucial role of molecular genetics in understanding correlations with established breast cancer risk factors. It may be possible to identify specific genes that are responsible for the estrogen-mediated proliferative activity of hormone-responsive breast cells. These genetic markers can then potentially be used to define specific breast cancer risk patterns.[36]

Because family history remains the strongest single predictor of breast cancer risk, attention has focused on the role of such genes in cancer-prone families. Five to ten percent of breast cancer cases, in particular those arising at a young age, are attributable to two highly penetrant autosomal dominant susceptibility genes, *BRCA1* and *BRCA2.* As discussed in Chapter 7, the risk of developing breast cancer among women who carry defective breast cancer susceptibility genes has been estimated at nearly 60% by age 50 and over 80% by age 70.[69,70]

During pregnancy, there is a large increase in *BRCA1* mRNA in mammary epithelial cells, suggesting that this increase parallels functional differentiation of the cells. Because high rates of breast cancer are associated with loss of *BRCA1* expression, it is possible that this gene provides an important growth regulatory function in these cells. Furthermore, there is evidence suggesting that *BRCA1* abnormalities may be involved in the pathogenesis of many sporadic breast cancers.[71]

Mutations in *BRCA2* account for approximately 40% of hereditary early onset breast cancer and confer a much higher risk of breast cancer among men than women. Loss of heterozygosity is also observed in tumors of the prostate, ovary, cervix, colon, male breast, and ureter. Almost all breast tumors or tumor cell lines that show loss of *BRCA2* also exhibit the simultaneous loss of *RB1* (at 13q14), suggesting that the genes may act in concert.

Although these mutant genes give rise to an extremely high risk of cancer, they are rare in the general population and thus have a low population attributable risk. Importantly, the fact that not all mutant gene carriers will develop cancer during their lifetime supports the notion that environmental factors and other genes may be involved in the development of cancer even among individuals with a very strong genetic predisposition.

Low-penetrance polymorphic genes confer only a moderately elevated risk of cancer and in many situations only give rise to an increased susceptibility to environmental carcinogens. The low-penetrance genes are usually common polymorphisms in the metabolism of endogenous or exogenous compounds. As discussed in Chapter 7, catechol-*O*-methyltransferase (COMT) catalyzes *O*-methylation of catechol estrogens and was recently reported to be associated with the risk of breast cancer.[72,73]

Other Personal Susceptibility Factors

The recognized risk factors for the development of breast cancer described in the chapter thus far are present in only about 25% of those who develop breast cancer.[74]

Because of the high incidence of the disease and the lack of definitive evidence regarding its etiology and pathogenesis, more specific and more sensitive markers for breast cancer risk need to be identified and validated. Previous clinical investigations[75,76] have shown that E_2 metabolism via the C16α-hydroxylation pathway is increased in patients who express one or more conventional risk factors for breast cancer or in patients with identifiable breast cancer. Because the three major oxidative pathways of E_2 biotransformation (C17-oxidation, C2-hydroxylation, and C16α-hydroxylation) are essentially unaltered with respect to age, menopausal status, or stage in the progression of the disease,[75,77] the pattern of E_2 metabolism may turn out to be an intrinsic endocrine biomarker for breast cancer risk.[78]

In addition to genetic biomarkers of estrogen exposure and breast cancer susceptibility, nipple aspiration and mammography show promise as biological markers for proliferative epithelium and breast cancer risk.[36] Women with atypical epithelial cells in their breast fluid have been shown to have a risk of breast cancer about three times greater than women with breast fluid having normal cytology.[79] Recent studies have suggested that mammographic pattern may be a strong predictor of breast cancer risk, with risks for women with severe duct prominence and dense parenchyma ranging from 3.7 to 5.5 times greater than for women with normal or minimal duct prominence.[80]

Summary of Endogenous Hormones and Breast Cancer

Current epidemiological data on breast cancer risk factors highlight the etiologic importance of the estrogen-related factors of length of exposure to cyclic hormones (represented by the woman's age at menopause minus her age at menarche) and, among postmenopausal women, obesity and exogenous hormone use. However, while there is a general consensus that estrogens are involved in the etiology of breast cancer,[29,53,81] there is no clear understanding of the precise estrogen environment that increases risk, nor of the causal role, if any, played by many reproductive factors. Consequently, studies of endogenous hormones in premenopausal women may face substantial complexity-of-design issues.

The reproductive factors believed to influence breast cancer risk suggest that the tumor-promoting effects of endogenous hormones continue to operate throughout a woman's reproductive life. The change in slope at the time of cessation of ovarian hormone secretion is consistent with a growth-enhancing effect of estrogen on already initiated breast tumors. At the same time, many of these reproductive factors appear to have their effect long before breast cancer becomes manifest. This suggests that estrogens may play a role in early tumor stages, including perhaps preinitiating stages.[33,82]

A comprehensive model that accommodates these factors together with the other epidemiological features of breast cancer is still lacking, and a precise differentiation of the independent effects of reproductive factors may be difficult to achieve given that changes in different factors often occur simultaneously.[83] Certain risk factors for breast cancer may be age-specific, and relationships between risk factors and cancer sometimes become evident when cases are stratified by age at diagnosis. Factors acting during early reproductive life may be significant risk factors only for younger women and may not influence the risk of developing breast cancer in older women, for whom risk factors are those occurring later in life.[84]

PROSTATE CANCER

Descriptive Epidemiology and Reproductive Risk Factors

Little is known about the etiology of prostate cancer despite its high incidence rate. In virtually all areas of the world for which data are available, an increase in the incidence rate of prostate cancer has been noted,[85] and in the United States the rate has increased dramatically in recent years (Figure 14–2). The increase in the survival rate

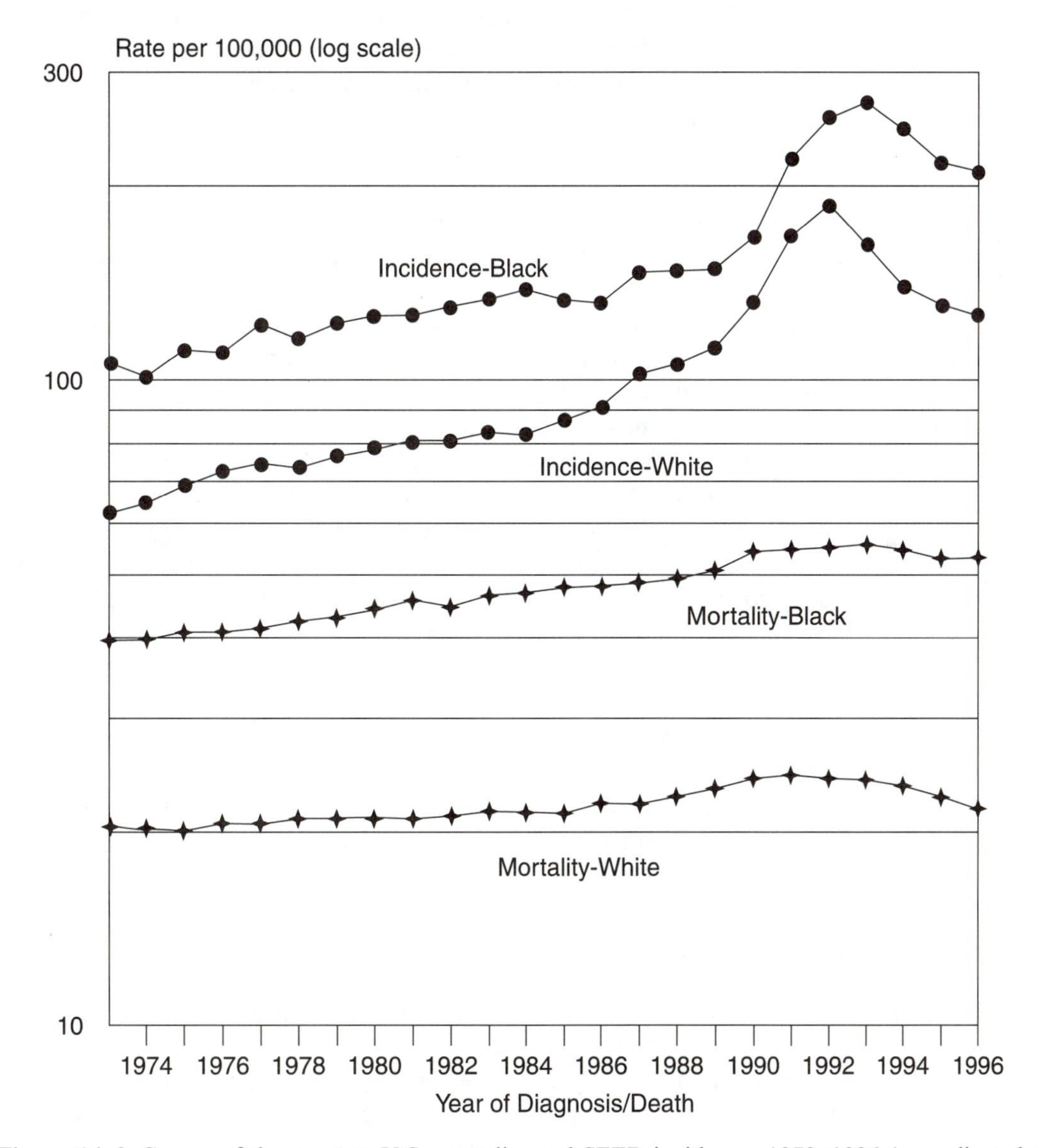

Figure 14–2 Cancer of the prostate U.S. mortality and SEER incidence, 1973–1996 (age-adjusted to 1970 standard). *Source:* Reprinted from L.A.G. Ries, et al., eds., *SEER Cancer Statistics Review, 1973–1996*, National Cancer Institute, 1999.

over the past 25 years suggests that part of the increase in incidence may be due to an increased use of medical services, especially for treatment of benign prostatic hypertrophy, another prostatic disorder. However, a simultaneous increase in the mortality rate suggests that some of the increase in the incidence rate is real. Prostate cancer is a disease that typically strikes older men; the incidence rate of prostate cancer rises exponentially with age faster than that of any other form of cancer.[86] Much of the increase appears to occur after age 50. However, with the growing incidence of prostate cancer, the peak has shifted to a younger age.

There is a striking international difference, as much as 50-fold, in prostate cancer incidence and mortality rates between highly developed countries and less developed countries. As in the case of breast cancer, studies of migrant populations suggest that environmental factors play a major role in prostate cancer. For example, immigrants from Poland and Japan, where the incidence is low, experience a substantial increase in risk upon coming to the United States. Trends toward higher levels of incidence among immigrants have been attributed to an increased prevalence of carcinogenic agents or a weaker effect of protective factors in the country of destination,[87–89] and the increase in incidence with age may be an indicator of accumulated exposure time and not a consequence of aging.

Prostate cancer can be considered as two general categories: small, latent tumors that have low likelihood of progression, and those that do progress. This variation in biological behavior complicates comparisons of incidence rates between countries because the likelihood of diagnosing latent tumors can vary among countries and over time. However, it appears from autopsy studies that the true prevalence of the small latent tumors does not differ substantially among countries and that the large differences in incidence are due principally to the clinically detected tumor.

Reproductive factors have been related to prostate cancer risk. Castrated men, men with no or undeveloped testes, and eunuchs whose testes have been removed or never developed have not been observed clinically with prostate cancer.[90] Mortality from prostate cancer has been observed to be higher among Catholic priests. Case-control studies comparing case and control subjects with regard to sexual factors have demonstrated that case subjects were sexually active at a younger age, had more sexual partners before marriage, higher fertility, higher rates of sexual transmitted disease, and lower circumcision rates than control subjects.[91,92] Vasectomy may also increase prostate cancer risk. Autopsy studies show that patients with cirrhosis of the liver have lower age-adjusted rates of prostate cancer than controls.[93]

Role of Endogenous Hormones

The biologic mechanisms that convert the latent form of prostate cancer to the more aggressive clinical forms have not yet been identified.[86] The similarity in the incidence rate of latent cancers internationally and the wide discrepancy between clinical prostate cancer suggests that cancer initiation may be more closely related to endogenous factors whereas promotion may be more strongly related to exogenous factors.

The prostate gland depends on androgens, both for development within the fetus and for growth, maintenance, and functioning in mature adults. Dihydrotestosterone (DHT) is the androgen highest in concentration in the prostate and appears to be the major intracellular androgenic hormone regulating its growth and function.[86,94] Sex hormones have been implicated in the pathogenesis of prostate cancer based on the dependence of the prostate gland on androgens and the fact that hormonal treatment of prostate cancer (specifically androgen ablation) provides a clear benefit. Furthermore, the increased sexual activity and fertility observed among prostate cancer cases may be a consequence of increased androgen levels. Alcohol depresses circulating testosterone levels, possibly explaining the lower incidence of the cancer among patients with cirrhosis of the liver.[95]

While extreme variations in endogenous hormone levels have long been related to risk of prostate cancer, normal variation in levels of androgens and estrogen may also affect risk.[96] Epidemiological studies in this area have compared circulating hormone levels in men with and without prostate cancer. Case-control studies of blood levels of sex hormones have been inconsistent and difficult to interpret[94]; the majority possessed several limitations. For example, hormone levels were often obtained from case patients after diagnosis of prostate cancer. Thus, these levels could have been due to the cancer.[94,97,98] Indeed, prostate cancer has a suppressive effect on androgen levels.[98–100] Additionally, studies tended to be of small size, and control subjects were typically not representative of the source population from which the cases arose.[98]

Prospective studies, including case-control studies nested within cohorts, avoid these biases but are subject to others.[99–101] Because intraindividual hormone levels are correlated, any observed association or lack of association between an individual hormone and cancer risk could be due to confounding by the other hormones. For example, sex hormone–binding globulin (SHBG) binds to testosterone, reducing the bioavailable amounts of this hormone. As the majority of prior studies evaluated the impact of each hormone individually, the true risk may have been masked.

In the largest study of prostate cancer and endogenous hormones, Gann et al[98] performed a nested case control study within the prospective Physicians' Health Study. The authors estimated the impact of differences in total testosterone on risk at any given level of SHBG and, conversely, the impact of differences in SHBG at any given level of total testosterone (Figure 14–3). Those whose plasma testosterone level fell in the highest quartile had two and one half times the risk of prostate cancer (95% CI = 1.34–5.02) possessed by those whose level fell in the lowest quartile. Men with the highest levels of SHBG had approximately a 50% lower risk than those with the lowest SHBG levels. It is interesting to note that these levels were all within normal endogenous ranges.

In summary, although the results of previous studies have been contradictory, recent findings suggest that long-term exposure to high levels of endogenous bioavailable testosterone promotes the development of prostate cancer. While the search for a common endogenous hormonal pattern among breast cancer patients continues, the picture for prostate cancer has become clearer.

ENDOMETRIAL CANCER

Descriptive Epidemiology and Risk Factors

Endometrial cancer shares many epidemiological features and risk factors with breast cancer.[102,103] Endometrial cancer incidence rises more steeply than breast cancer in

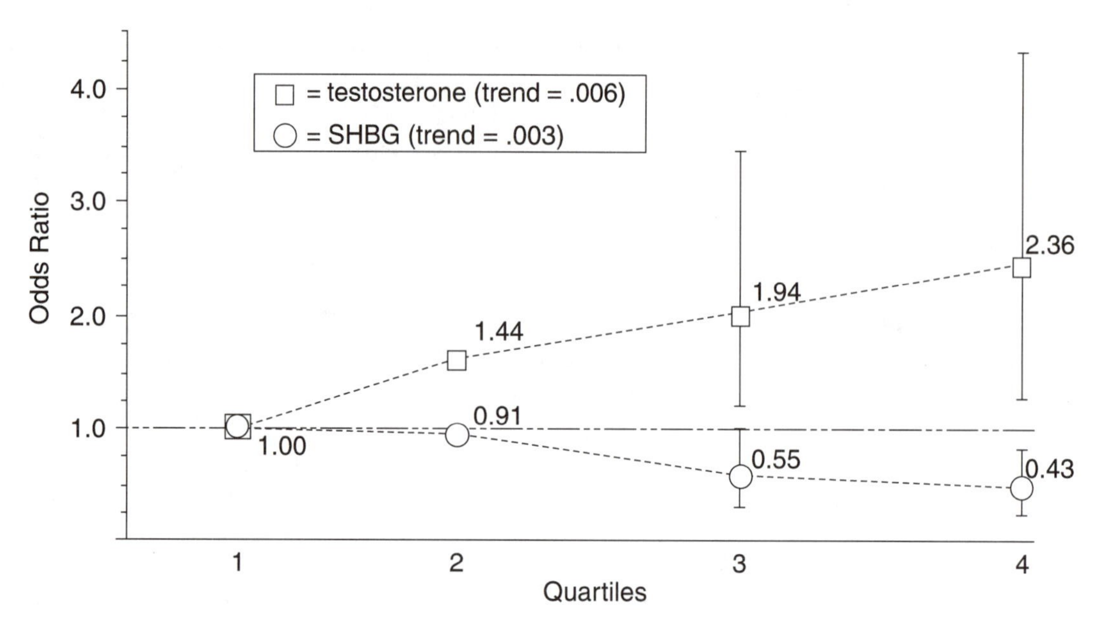

Figure 14–3 Prostate cancer odds ratios (ORs) by quartile levels of plasma testosterone and sex hormone–binding globulin (SHBG): simultaneous adjustment for testosterone, SHBG, and estradiol. Quartile cutpoints were defined by use of control subject values, with quartile 1 values representing the lowest plasma levels and quartile 4 values representing the highest. ORs (95% confidence intervals [CIs]) for successive estradiol quartiles are as follows: 1.00, 0.56 (0.35–0.90), 0.43 (0.25–0.73), and 0.65 (0.39–1.09) (p for trend = .08). Ninety-five percent CIs for testosterone quartile 2 and SHBG quartile 2 are not shown in the figure; these CIs are 0.85–2.43 and 0.54–1.51, respectively. *Source:* Reprinted from P.H. Gann, et al., Prospective Study of Sex Hormone Levels and Risk of Prostate Cancer, *Journal of the National Cancer Institute*, Vol. 88, pp. 1118–1126, 1996, National Cancer Institute.

women up to the age of 50 and thereafter increases at a much reduced rate. The suggestion that menopause has a strong protective effect is evident, and case-control studies have established late age at menopause as a risk factor. As with breast cancer, parity appears to lower the risk. An increased number of pregnancies provides an increased degree of protection, especially in young women[104]; however, there appears to be no association with age at first birth.[104] Obesity is a risk factor for endometrial cancer both after and before menopause.[103,105] Early age at menarche generally has been found to increase endometrial cancer risk, although whether this association is independent of obesity is unclear.[106]

Role of Endogenous Hormones

The incidence of endometrial cancer has been linked closely to unopposed estrogen (ie, estrogen in the absence of progesterone), which may explain the relation between the cancer and a number of reproductive variables.[107–109] It has been postulated that during the premenopausal period, the rate of increase in risk of endometrial cancer with increasing age depends on the accumulation of mitotic activity during the first half of the normal menstrual cycle, when estrogens are unopposed by progesterone.[103] Late age at menopause is associated positively with this disease, presumably owing to the longer period of exposure to high premenopausal estrogen levels. With loss of ovarian function at menopause, the incidence of endometrial cancer depends entirely on estrogen formation in adipose tissue[104] and the use of estrogen replacement therapy. Obesity is a risk factor because it can lead to anovulation and ensuing progesterone deficiency.[103]

OVARIAN CANCER

Descriptive Epidemiology and Risk Factors

Ovarian cancer shares some risk factors with breast and endometrial cancer. The age-specific curve for ovarian cancer, like the curve for endometrial cancer, rises up to the age at menopause and then tends to flatten off. This curve can be described in mathematical models as a function of the number of years of regular cycles.[102] Indeed, epidemiological studies show with relative consistency that factors associated with the suppression of ovulation, such as pregnancy, are protective.[110] A number of authors have shown that ovarian cancer risk increases with the number of ovulatory years, which is computed as the number of years between menarche and menopause (or diagnosis, if the woman is premenopausal) minus the number of years in which the woman was either pregnant or taking oral contraceptives.

By far the most consistent finding in epidemiological studies has been the inverse association between ovarian cancer and parity.[111] A collaborative analysis of 12 US case-control studies involving 2,197 white ovarian cancer patients and 8,893 white control subjects conducted from 1956 to 1986 found a trend of decreasing risk with increasing number of pregnancies (regardless of outcome).[112] Parous women had a lower ovarian cancer risk than nulliparous women (OR = 0.76, 95% CI = 0.63–0.93 for hospital studies; OR = 0.47, 95% CI = 0.40–0.56 for population studies). In general, women who have had three or more children have a 30% to 50% lower risk of ovarian cancer than nulliparous women.

Results showing the relationship between ovarian cancer and age at first birth, age at menarche, age at menopause, or lactation have been much less consistent.[104,106] The collaborative analysis found only weak trends of decreasing risk with delayed menarche and increasing age at menarche.[112]

Role of Endogenous Hormones

Most ovarian cancers arise from epithelial cells that make up the external surface of the ovary. Ovulation may increase ovarian cancer risk by subjecting these epithelial cells to repeated minor trauma (occurring when the ovum breaks through the surface epithelium during ovulation), increased cellular division (associated with repair of the surface epithelium after each ovulation), or exposure to hormone-rich fluid that surrounds the ovum.[113] This theory suggests that factors, such as parity, that decrease the number of ovulations would decrease ovarian cancer risk. High levels of gonadotropins, hormones secreted by the pituitary gland, also have been hypothesized to increase ovarian cancer risk. Since pregnancy decreases gonadotropin levels and a late age at menopause postpones exposure to high postmenopausal gonadotropin levels, each of these factors would be expected to reduce ovarian cancer risk according to this hypothesis.

SUMMARY

A substantial body of experimental, clinical, and epidemiological evidence indicates that endogenous hormones play a major role in the etiology of several human cancers. Generally accepted reproductive risk factors for breast cancer, such as the timing of menarche, first birth, and menopause, strongly implicate ovarian hormones in the etiology of the disease. Further support is provided by the shape of the age-specific incidence curve for breast cancer, especially the slowing of the rate of increase around the age of menopause. This age-incidence pattern is not seen in non-hormone-dependent cancers.

Factors that influence the cumulative number of ovulatory menstrual cycles in a woman's life, such as age at menarche and menopause, menstrual cycle patterns, and years until cycle regularity, may be influenced by environmental factors, such as diet, physical activity, and alcohol. Indeed, the fact that breast cancer rates vary across the world implies that there may be something about the American or Western lifestyle that affects risk. On the other hand, breast cancer has long been known to occur more frequently in some families. Thus, breast cancer is a complex disease that may be the consequence of a combination of genetic predisposition, lifestyle characteristics, and environmental exposures.

Observational data suggest that modification of dietary fat intake among adult women is unlikely to reduce the risk of breast cancer. While results have not been entirely consistent across studies, overall they suggest a protective role for physical activity in the prevention of breast cancer. Alternatively, a large body of evidence suggests that even moderate alcohol consumption can increase breast cancer risk. It is plausible that environmental pesticides and industrial chemicals may be related to breast cancer risk.

While there is general consensus that estrogens are involved in the etiology of breast cancer,[29,53,81] there is no clear understanding of how the precise estrogen environment affects risk. Case-control studies of postmenopausal women show with fair consistency that breast cancer patients have higher levels of estrogen than control subjects.[53] However, case-control studies in this area of investigation are subject to a variety of limitations. Cohort studies address many of the limitations of case-control studies but possess others, such as degradation of samples during long periods of storage and laboratory error. In general, studies of endogenous hormones in premenopausal women face challenging complexity-of-design issues.

Studies show that the association between reproductive factors and cancer vary by cancer type. For instance, nulliparity, late age at first birth, early age at menarche, and late age at menopause are consistently associated with increased breast cancer risk. Similarly, ovarian and endometrial cancer are consistently associated with nulliparity. In some cases, reproductive factors are associated with a twofold increase in cancer risk, but in general the elevated risk is somewhat lower.[106] In contrast, there is no solid evidence of an association between reproductive factors and colon cancer.

Given that most of the established risk factors for breast cancer confer only weak or moderate elevations in risk and few offer feasible prospects for primary intervention,[114] the identification of causal agents acting during the prenatal and adolescent periods is critical. Future research should try to identify factors that affect endogenous hormone levels, particularly factors that increase the likelihood of prolonged exposure to endogenous hormones.

Discussion Questions

1. Describe the epidemiological evidence indicating that endogenous hormones play a role in the etiology of breast cancer.
2. There is substantial epidemiological evidence that a positive relationship exists between breast cancer risk and the cumulative number of ovulatory menstrual cycles in a woman's life. Explain how observed associations between breast cancer and reproductive factors, such as age at menarche and menopause, support the hypothesis that such a relationship exists.
3. Compare and contrast the risk factors for breast cancer with those for ovarian cancer.
4. As in the case of breast cancer, studies of migrant populations suggest that environmental factors play a major role in prostate cancer. Describe the findings of these studies and their implications for the etiology of these cancers.
5. Discuss the challenges associated with measuring endogenous hormones. Explain how and why these challenges differ between premenopausal women and postmenopausal women.

References

1. Bernstein L, Henderson BE. Exogenous hormones. In: Schottenfeld D, Fraumeni JF Jr, eds. *Cancer Epidemiology and Prevention.* 2nd ed. New York: Oxford University Press; 1996:462–489.
2. Henderson BE, Ross RK, Bernstein L. Estrogens as a cause of human cancer: The Richard and Hinda Rosenthal Foundation award lecture. *Cancer Res.* 1988;48:246–253.
3. Henderson BE, Ross RK, Pike MC, Casagrande JT. Endogenous hormones as a major factor in human cancer. *Cancer Res.* 1982;43:3232–3239.
4. Kelsey JL, Gammon MD, John EM. Reproductive factors and breast cancer. *Epidemiol Rev.* 1993;15:36–47.
5. Boyle P, Leake R. Progress in understanding breast cancer: epidemiological and biological interactions. *Breast Cancer Res Treat.* 1988;11:91–112.
6. Willett W. The search for the causes of breast and colon cancer. *Nature.* 1989;338:389–394.
7. Buell P. Changing incidence of breast cancer in Japanese-American women. *J Natl Cancer Inst.* 1973;51:1479–1483.
8. Thomas DB, Karagas MR. Cancer in first and second generation Americans. *Cancer Res.* 1987;47:5771–5776.
9. Yu H, Harris RE, Gao Y-T, et al. Comparative epidemiology of cancers of the colon, rectum, prostate and breast in Shanghai, China, versus the United States. *Int J Epidemiol.* 1991;20:76–81.
10. Schimizu H, Ross RK, Bernstein L, et al. Cancers of the prostate and breast among Japanese and White immigrants in Los Angeles County. *Br J Cancer.* 1991;63:963–966.
11. Kelsey JL, Hildreth NG. *Breast and Gynecologic Cancer Epidemiology.* Boca Raton, FL: CRC Press; 1983.
12. Kvale G, Heuch I. Menstrual factors and breast cancer risk. *Cancer.* 1988;62:1525–1531.
13. Brinton LA, Schairer C, Hoover RN, et al. Menstrual factors and risk of breast cancer. *Cancer Invest.* 1988;6:245–254.
14. Negri E, La Vecchia C, Bruzzi P, et al. Risk factors for breast cancer: pooled results from three Italian case-control studies. *Am J Epidemiology.* 1988;128:1207–1215.

15. Tao S-C, Yu MC, Ross RK, et al. Risk factors for breast cancer in Chinese women of Beijing. *Int J Cancer.* 1988;42:495–498.
16. Hsieh C-C, Trichopoulos D, Katsouyanni K, et al. Age at menarche, age at menopause, height and obesity as risk factors for breast cancer: associations and interactions in an international case-control study. *Int J Cancer.* 1990;46:796–800.
17. Brinton LA, Schairer C, Hoover RN, et al. Menstrual factors and risk of breast cancer. *Cancer Invest.* 1988;6:245–254.
18. Irwin KL, Lee NC, Peterson HB, et al. Hysterectomy, tubal sterilization, and the risk of breast cancer. *Am J Epidemiol.* 1988;127:1192–1201.
19. Bruzzi P, Negri E, La Vecchia C, et al. Short term increase in risk of breast cancer after full term pregnancy. *BMJ.* 1988;297:1096–1098.
20. Hunter DJ, Spiegelman D, Adami HO, et al. Cohort studies of fat intake and the risk of breast cancer: a pooled analysis. *N Engl J Med.* 1996;334:356–361.
21. Longnecker MP. Alcoholic beverage consumption in relation to breast cancer: meta-analysis and review. *Cancer Causes Control.* 1994;5:73–82.
22. Rogan WJ, Gladen BC, McKinney JD, et al. Polychlorinated biphenyls (PCBs) and dichlorodiphenyl dichloroethene (DDE) in human milk: effects on growth, morbidity, and duration of lactation. *Am J Public Health.* 1987;77:1294–1297.
23. van't Veer P, Lobbezoo IE, Martin-Moreno JM, et al. DDT (dicophane) and postmenopausal breast cancer in Europe: case-control study. *BMJ.* 1997;315:81–85.
24. Wolff MS, Toniolo PG, Lee EW, Rivera M, Dubin N. Blood levels of organochlorine residues and risk of breast cancer. *J Natl Cancer Inst.* 1993;85:648–652.
25. Hunter DJ, Hankinson SE, Laden F, et al. Plasma organochlorine levels and the risk of breast cancer. *N Engl J Med.* 1997;337:1253–1258.
26. Friedenreich CM, Thune I, Brinton LA, Albanes D. Epidemiologic issues related to the association between physical activity and breast cancer. *Cancer.* 1998;83:600–610.
27. Reichman ME, Judd JT, Longcope C, et al. Effects of alcohol consumption on plasma and urinary hormone concentrations in premenopausal women. *J Natl Cancer Inst.* 1993;75:722–727.
28. Harvard Center for Cancer Prevention. Causes of human cancer. Exercise. *Cancer Causes Control.* 1996;7(suppl 1):S15–S18.
29. Bernstein L, Ross RK. Endogenous hormones and breast cancer risk. *Epidemiologic Reviews.* 1993;15:48–65.
30. Bernstein L, Ross RK, Henderson BE. Prospects for the primary prevention of breast cancer. *Am J Epidemiol.* 1992;135:142–152.
31. MacMahon B, Trichopoulos D, Brown J, et al. Age at menarche, urine estrogens and breast cancer risk. *Int J Cancer.* 1982;30:427–431.
32. Apter D, Reinila M, Vihko R. Some endocrine characteristics of early menarche, a risk factor for breast cancer, are preserved into adulthood. *Int J Cancer.* 1989;44:783–787.
33. Kelsey TJA, Pike MC. The role of oestrogens and progestagens in the epidemiology and prevention of breast cancer. *Eur J Cancer Clin Oncol.* 1988;24:29–34.
34. Adami HO, Adams G, Boyle P, et al. Breast cancer etiology. *Int J Cancer.* 1990;5(suppl):22–39.
35. Henderson BE, Ross RK, Judd HL, et al. Do regular ovulatory cycles increase breast cancer risk? *Cancer.* 1985;56:1206–1208.
36. Lipworth L. Epidemiology of breast cancer. *Eur J Cancer Prev.* 1995;4:7–30.
37. Russo J, Russo IH. Toward a physiological approach to breast cancer prevention. *Cancer Epidemiol Biomarkers Prev.* 1994;3:353–364.
38. Kelsey JL, Gammon MD, John EM. Reproductive factors and breast cancer. *Epidemiol Rev.* 1993;15:36–47.
39. Friedenreich CM, Rohan TE. A review of physical activity and breast cancer. *Epidemiology.* 1995;6:311–317.
40. Gammon MD, John EM. Recent etiologic hypotheses concerning breast cancer. *Epidemiol Rev.* 1993;15:163–168.
41. Frisch RE, Wyshak G, Vincent L. Delayed menarche and amenorrhea in ballet dancers. *N Engl J Med.* 1980;303:17–19.
42. Frisch RE, Gotz-Welbergen AV, McArthur JW, et al. Delayed menarche and amenorrhea of college athletes in relation to age at onset of training. *JAMA.* 1981;246:1559–1563.

43. Moisan J, Meyer F, Gingras S. A nested case-control study of the correlates of early menarche. *Am J Epidemiol.* 1990;132:953–961.

44. Feicht CB, Johnson TS, Martic BJ, et al. Secondary amenorrhea in athletes. *Lancet.* 1978;2:1145–1146.

45. Wakat DK, Sweeney KA, Rogol AD. Reproductive system function in women cross-country runners. *Med Sci Sports Exerc.* 1982;14:263–269.

46. Russel JB, Mitchell D, Mussey PL, et al. The relationship of exercise to anovulatory cycles in female athletes: hormonal and physical characteristics. *Obstet Gynecol.* 1984;63:452–456.

47. Bernstein L, Ross RK, Henderson BE. Prospects for the primary prevention of breast cancer. *Am J Epidemiol.* 1992;135:142–152.

48. McTiernan A. Exercise and breast cancer: time to get moving? *N Engl J Med.* 1197;336:1311–1312. Editorial.

49. Cauley JA, Gutai JP, Kuller LH, LeDonne D, Powell JG. The epidemiology of serum sex hormones in postmenopausal women. *Am J Epidemiol.* 1989;129:1120–1131.

50. Siiteri PK. Adipose tissue as a source of hormones. *Am J Clin Nutr.* 1987;45:277–282.

51. Sellers TA, Gapstur SM, Potter JD, Kushi LH, Bostick RM, Folsum AR. Association of body fat distribution and family histories of breast and ovarian cancer with risk of postmenopausal breast cancer. *Am J Epidemiol.* 1993;138:799–803.

52. Toniolo PG, Levitz M, Zeleniuch-Jacquotte A, et al. A prospective study of endogenous estrogens and breast cancer in postmenopausal women. *J Natl Cancer Inst.* 1995;87:190–197.

53. Key TJA, Pike MC. The role of oestrogens and progestagens in the epidemiology and prevention of breast cancer. *Eur J Cancer Clin Oncol.* 1988;24:29–43.

54. Tretli S, Haldorsen T, Ottestad L. The effect of premorbid height and weight on the survival of breast cancer patients. *Br J Cancer.* 1990;62:299–303.

55. Kohrt WM, Obert KA, Hollowszy JO. Exercise training improves fat distribution in 60- to 70-year-old men and women. *J Gerontol.* 1992;47:M99–M105.

56. Dorgan JF, Reichman ME, Judd JT, et al. The relation of reported alcohol ingestion to plasma levels of estrogens and androgens in premenopausal women (Maryland, United States) *Cancer Causes Control.* 1994;5:53–60.

57. Hankinson SE, Willett WC, Manson JE, et al. Alcohol, weight and adiposity in relation to estrogen and prolactin levels in postmenopausal women. *J Natl Cancer Inst.* 1995;87:1297–1302.

58. Reichman ME, Judd JT, Longcope C, et al. Effects of alcohol consumption on plasma and urinary hormone concentrations in premenopausal women. *J Natl Cancer Inst.* 1993;85:722–727.

59. Soto AM, Sonnenschein C, Chung KL, Fernandez MF, Olea N, Serrano FO. The E-SCREEN assay as a tool to identify estrogens: an update on estrogenic environmental pollutants. *Environ Health Perspect.* 1995;103(suppl 7):113–122.

60. Safe SH. Environmental and dietary estrogens and human health: is there a problem? *Environ Health Perspect.* 1995;103:346–351.

61. Rogan WJ, Gladen BC, McKinney JD, et al. Polychlorinated biphenyls (PCBs) and dichlorodiphenyl dichloroethene (DDE) in human milk: effects of maternal factors and previous lactation. *Am J Public Health.* 1986;76:172–177.

62. Harvard Center for Cancer Prevention. Causes of human cancer. Environmental pollution. *Cancer Causes Control.* 1996;7(suppl 1):S37–S39.

63. Wysowski DK, Comstock GW, Helsing KJ, et al. Sex hormone levels in serum in relation to the development of breast cancer. *Am J Epidemiol.* 1987;125:791–799.

64. Garland CF, Friedlander NJ, Barrett-Connor E, et al. Sex hormones and postmenopausal breast cancer: a prospective study in an adult community. *Am J Epidemiol.* 1992;135:1220–1230.

65. Bulbrook RD, Moore JW, Clark GMG, et al. Relation between risk of breast cancer and biological availability of estradiol in the blood: prospective study in Guernsey. *Ann NY Acad Sci.* 1986;464:378–388.

66. Moore JW, Key TJA, Bulbrook RD, et al. Sex hormone binding globulin and risk factors for breast cancer in a population of normal women who had never used exogenous sex hormones. *Br J Cancer.* 1987;56:661–666.

67. Langley MS, Hammond GL, Bardsley A, et al. Serum steroid binding proteins and the bioavailability of estradiol in relation to breast diseases. *J Natl Cancer Inst.* 1985;75:823–829.

68. Phillips GB, Yano K, Stemmermann GN. Serum sex hormone levels and myocardial infarction in the Honolulu Heart Program: pitfalls in prospective studies on sex hormones. *J Clin Epidemiol.* 1988;41:1151–1156.

69. DeMichele A, Weber BL. Recent advances in breast cancer biology. *Curr Opin Oncol.* 1997;9:499–504.

70. Yang X, Lippman ME. *BRCA1* and *BRCA2* in breast cancer. *Breast Cancer Res Treat.* 1999;54:1–10.
71. Teich NM. Oncogenes and cancer. In: Franks LM, Teich NM, eds. *Introduction to the Cellular and Molecular Biology of Cancer.* Oxford: Oxford University Press; 1997:169–201.
72. Lavigne JA, Helzlsouer KJ, Huang HY, et al. An association between the allele coding for a low activity variant of catechol-*O*-methyltransferase and the risk for breast cancer. *Cancer Res.* 1997;57:5493–5497.
73. Thompson PA, Shields PG, Freudenheim JL, et al. Genetic polymorphisms in catechol-*O*-methyltransferase, menopausal status, and breast cancer risk. *Cancer Res.* 1998;58:2107–2110.
74. Harris J, Lipman ME, Veronesi U, et al. Breast cancer. *N Engl J Med.* 1992;327:319–328.
75. Bradlow HL, Hershcopf RJ, Martucci CP, et al. 16?-Hydroxylation of estradiol: a possible risk marker for breast cancer. *Ann NY Acad Sci.* 1989;464;138–151.
76. Osborne MP, Karmali RA, Bradlow HL, et al. Omega-3 fatty acids: modulation of estrogen metabolism and potential for breast cancer prevention. *Cancer Invest.* 1988;6:629–631.
77. Schneider J, Kinne D, Fracchia A, et al. Abnormal oxidative metabolism of estradiol in women with breast cancer. *Proc Natl Acad Sci USA.* 1982;79:3047–3051.
78. Nebert DW. Elevated estrogen 16?-hydroxylase activity: is this a genotoxic or nongenotoxic biomarker in human breast cancer risk? *J Natl Cancer Inst.* 1993;85:1888–1920. Editorial.
79. Petrakis NL. Nipple aspirate fluid in epidemiologic studies of breast disease. Epidemiol Rev. 1993;15:188–195.
80. Brisson J, Verrault R, Morrison AS, et al. Diet, mammographic features of breast tissue, and breast cancer risk. *Am J Epdemiol.* 1989;130:14–24.
81. Kelsey JL, Hildreth NG. Breast and gynecologic cancer epidemiology. Boca Raton, FL: CRC Press; 1983.
82. Ponton J, Holmberg L, Trichopoulos D, et al. Biology and natural history of breast cancer. *Int J Cancer.* 1990;5(suppl):5–21.
83. Rosero-Bixby L, Oberle MW, Lee NC. Reproductive history and breast cancer in a population of high fertility. *Int J. Cancer.* 1987;40:747–754.
84. Segala C, Gerber M, Richardson S. The pattern of risk factors for breast cancer in a southern France population: interest for a stratified analysis by age at diagnosis. *Br J Cancer.* 1991;38:919–925.
85. Doll R, Payne P, Waterhouse J, eds. *Cancer Incidence in Five Continents.* Lyon, France: International Agency for Research on Cancer; 1985. IARC Scientific Publications, No. 88.
86. National Cancer Institute roundtable on prostate cancer: future research directions. *Cancer Res.* 1991;51:2498–2505.
87. Mandel JS, Schuman LM. Epidemiology of cancer of the prostate. In: Lilienfeld AM, ed. *Reviews in Cancer Epidemiology.* Vol 1. New York: Elsevier/North Holland Publishing Co; 1980;1–83.
88. Cook PJ, Doll R, Fellingham SA. A mathematical model for the age distribution of cancer in man. *Int J Cancer.* 1968;4:93–112.
89. Hirayama, T. Epidemiology of cancer of the stomach with special reference to its recent decrease in Japan. *Cancer Res.* 1975;35:3460–3463.
90. Huggins C, Hodges CV. Studies on prostate cancer: effect of castration, of estrogen, and of androgen injection on serum phosphatase in metastatic carcinoma of the prostate. *Cancer Res.* 1941;1:291–293.
91. Honda GD, Bernstein L, Ross RK, et al. Vasectomy, cigarette smoking, and age at first sexual intercourse as risk factors for prostate cancer in middle-aged men. *Br J Cancer.* 1988;57:326–331.
92. Ross RK, Shimizu H, Paganini-Hill A, et al. Case-control studies of prostate cancer in blacks and whites in Southern California. *J Natl Cancer Inst.* 1987;78:869–874.
93. Glantz GM. Cirrhosis and carcinoma of the prostate gland. *J Urol.* 1964;91:291–293.
94. Nomura AM, Kolonel LN. Prostate cancer: a current perspective. *Epidemiol Rev.* 1991;13:200–227.
95. Gordon GG, Altman K, Southern AL, Rubin E, Lieber CS. Effect of alcohol (ethanol) administration on sex-hormone metabolism in normal men. *N Engl J Med.* 1976;295:793–797.
96. Henderson BE, Ross RF, Pike MC, Casagrande JT. Endogenous hormones as a major factor in human cancer. *Cancer Res.* 1982;42:3232–3239.
97. Meikle AW, Smith JA Jr. Epidemiology of prostate cancer. *Urol Clin North Am.* 1990;17:709–718.
98. Gann PH, Hennekens CH, Ma J, Longcope C, Stampfer MJ. Prospective study of sex hormone levels and risk of prostate cancer. *J Natl Cancer Inst.* 1996;88:1118–1126.

99. Barrett-Connor E, Garland C, McPhillips JB, Khaw KT, Wingard DL. A prospective, population-based study of androstenedione, estrogens, and prostatic cancer. *Cancer Res.* 1990;50:169–173.
100. Nomura A, Heilbrun LK, Stemmermann GN, Judd HL. Prediagnostic serum hormones and the risk of prostate cancer. *Cancer Res.* 1988;48:3515–3517.
101. Hsing AW, Comstock GW. Serological precursors of cancer: serum hormones and risk of subsequent prostate cancer. *Cancer Epidemiol Biomarkers Prev.* 1993;2:27–32.
102. Pike MC. Age-related factors in cancers of the breast, ovary, and endometrium. *J Chronic Dis.* 1987;40(suppl 2):59S–69S.
103. Henderson BE, Casagrande JT, Pike MC, Mack T, Rosario I, Duke A. The epidemiology of endometrial cancer in young women. *Br J Cancer.* 1983;47:749–756.
104. International Agency for Research on Cancer. Endogenous hormones, reproductive factors and sexual behavior. In: Tomatis L, ed. *Cancer: Causes, Occurrence and Control.* Lyon, France: International Agency for Research on Cancer; 1990: 240–247.
105. La Vecchia C, Franceschi S, DeCarli A, Gallus G, Tognoni G. Risk factors for endometrial cancer at different ages. *J Natl Cancer Inst.* 1984;73:667–671.
106. Harvard Center for Cancer Prevention. Causes of human cancer. Reproductive factors. *Cancer Causes Control.* 1996;7(suppl 1):S29–S32.
107. Parazzini F, La Vecchia C, Bociolone L, Franceschi S. The epidemiology of endometrial cancer. *Gynecol Oncol.* 1991;41:1–16.
108. Koumantaki Y, Tzonou A, Koumantakis E, Kaklamani E, Aravantinos D, Trichopoulos D. A case-control study of cancer of endometrium in Athens. *Int J Cancer.* 1989;43:795–799.
109. Elwood JM, Cole P, Rothman KJ, Kaplan SD. Epidemiology of endometrial cancer. *J Natl Cancer Inst.* 1977;59:1055–1060.
110. Centers for Disease Control Cancer and Steroid Hormone Study. Oral contraceptive use and the risk of ovarian cancer. *JAMA.* 1983;249:1596–1599.
111. Hankinson SE, Colditz GA, Hunter DJ, et al. A prospective study of reproductive factors and risk of epithelial ovarian cancer. *Cancer.* 1995;76:284–290.
112. Whittemore AS, Harris R, Itnyre J, Collaborative Ovarian Cancer Group. Characteristics relating to ovarian cancer risk: collaborative analysis of 12 US case-control studies. II. Invasive epithelial ovarian cancers in white women. *Am J Epidemiol.* 1992;136:1184–1203.
113. Whittemore AS, Harris R, Itnyre J, Collaborative Ovarian Cancer Group. Characteristics relating to ovarian cancer risk: collaborative analysis of 12 US case-control studies. IV. The pathogenesis of epithelial ovarian cancer. *Am J Epidemiol.* 1992;136:1212–1220.
114. MacMahon B. Risk factors for breast cancer. *Adv Oncol.* 1994;10:3–9.

Chapter 15

Epidemiology of Exogenous Hormones and Cancer

Lisa Chasan-Taber

As shown in Chapter 14, endogenous hormones can increase the risk of specific human cancers. Since the same or closely related hormones are administered for therapeutic purposes, it is reasonable to worry that they may similarly increase cancer risk. In fact, studies show that exogenous hormones and hormone antagonists appear to increase the risk of some cancers while decreasing the risk of others.

Combined oral contraceptives and postmenopausal hormones may be the most important sources of exogenous estrogen for women today. Similarly, hormonal treatment for breast cancer, in particular, the use of tamoxifen, is accepted and widespread. In the past, synthetic hormones were widely prescribed for the prevention of miscarriage. This chapter describes the effect of these exogenous hormones on cancer risk. As exposure to exogenous hormones is potentially under the control of individual women and thus modifiable, use of these hormones is particularly important from a public health perspective. Furthermore, unlike some exposures, exposure to exogenous hormones may often span months or years.

The vast majority of pharmaceutical drugs are not carcinogenic. Of the drugs that have been associated with cancer, only in a few cases have the cancer-related risks been as large as the risks posed by the diseases that the drugs are intended to treat. Historically, the association between a drug and risk of cancer was observed on a case-by-case basis. However, only very rare cancers or those that are somehow unusual (eg, occurring at an unusual anatomic site or age of onset) are likely to be detected in this manner. In addition, case series lack a control group and cannot account for confounding factors, such as diet, smoking, and occupation, which must be carefully measured and controlled for.

Case-control studies are able to address many of the limitations of case series. The rarity of many cancers and the low prevalence of usage for most drugs also point to the case-control study design as the one of choice. However, the possibility of recall bias (the tendency of case subjects to overreport prior drug use) must be considered when interpreting study findings.

The recent introduction of computerized databases linking drug prescription data with subsequent medical records in large populations is a boon for epidemiological investigation, since the prospective nature of the data collection rules out the threat of recall bias. Drug exposure data are obtained prior to diagnosis and therefore cannot be influenced by disease status. The database also provides the means for ascertainment of those with the disease.

Prospective studies in this area, however, have several disadvantages. The process of cancer initiation and promotion can last 20 or more years before a cancer becomes clinically detectable.[1] Therefore, a long and potentially costly follow-up period would be necessary before negative findings could be considered definitive.[2] Studies must include subjects who have long durations of drug use or must follow subjects for a sufficient period of time after initial exposure. Only in this manner can a carcinogenic effect be adequately ruled out.[2] Overall, both case-control and prospective studies have strengths and limitations. However, the case-control study may remain one of the most feasible methods for testing hypotheses regarding the cancer risk posed by drug use.

Finally, drugs by their nature are generally given to people who already have an illness, and the illness itself, not the drug, may be related to any cancer that develops.[3] Similarly, preexisting malignancies may be the reason for treatment. The only way to disentangle these associations is to compare individuals receiving different kinds of therapies for the same condition. Furthermore, the time course of the proposed drug-cancer relation must be consistent with what is currently known about the biology of the cancer.[3]

COMBINED ORAL CONTRACEPTIVES

The formulation of combined oral contraceptives has changed dramatically over the past 30 years. Modern combined oral contraceptives have a quarter of the estrogen dose and a tenth of the progestogen dose. Because of the marked changes in formulation, the findings of early epidemiological studies on cancer risk may not be fully generalizable to today's preparations. In addition, the population of oral contraceptive users has changed over time. Women now begin use at younger ages and continue use for longer durations. A major concern regarding the impact of the pill on human health is whether steroid contraception causes cancer, particularly in the uterus, ovaries, and breast. Most cancers are uncommon in women in their twenties and thirties but not in older women.

Breast Cancer

Because combined oral contraceptives are widely used,[4] even a small effect on breast cancer risk will have an important impact on public health. A large number of epidemiological studies have been performed to address the association between oral contraceptives and breast cancer risk.[5]

Until fairly recently, review studies had concluded that there was no association between ever having used combined oral contraceptives and risk of breast cancer.[6] Previous studies, however, faced several limitations. The development of breast cancer may require prolonged exposure to combined oral contraceptives[7]; therefore, an extended follow-up period is necessary before any effect can be ruled out. Earlier studies, conducted shortly after the introduction of combined oral contraceptives, lacked long-term users. In addition, risk factors for breast cancer may differ according to menopausal status[5,8]; different proportions of premenopausal and postmenopausal women in different studies could obscure a potential relation. Age at use may also influence the carcinogenic process,[7,9] and recent trends toward decreasing age at first use could reduce comparability between study results.

Findings from the more recent studies suggest that certain subgroups of users may be particularly susceptible to breast cancer. For example, several studies suggest an excess risk of breast cancer at young ages associated with long-term oral contraceptive use.[10] In 1990, Romeiu et al[5] performed a meta-analysis of the studies on combined oral contraceptives. This type of analysis combines study results and weights them to derive an overall risk estimate. While the authors observed no overall increased risk of breast cancer for women who had ever used combined oral contraceptives, combined data from the case-control studies alone showed a positive trend ($p = 0.001$) in the risk of premenopausal breast cancer for women with longer durations of use.

A meta-analysis, however, has several limitations. Because chance alone makes some studies suggest one conclusion and others suggest another conclusion, biases may be produced by placing undue emphasis on particular studies with extreme results. Estimates of effect may be less stable in smaller studies. Studies may use different categorizations for oral contraceptive use, precluding a comparison of findings. Finally, studies may control for different confounding factors and be subject to different threats from selection and information bias.

In 1996, the Collaborative Group on Hormonal Factors in Breast Cancer brought together the majority of the data collected on this relationship (54 studies conducted in 25 countries) (Table 15–1).[8] The pooled data set included 53,297 women with breast cancer and 100,239 women without breast cancer. By "pooling" the raw data and re-analyzing it as one large data set, the limitations of the meta-analysis may be largely overcome. However, recategorization of oral contraceptive use is limited by the lowest common denominator—if one study collected information on duration in two-year groupings, the pooled analysis cannot present results for one-year increments in duration.

The collaborative group found a small increased risk of breast cancer among current oral contraceptive users that persisted for 10 years after discontinuation.[8] Once recency of use had been taken into account, duration of use, age at first use, and the dose and type of formulation had little additional effect on risk. Women who began use before age 20 had higher relative risks of breast cancer than those who began use at older ages, but breast cancer is rare in this age group. Figure 15–1 shows the cumulative number of breast cancers among users and nonusers in their twenties and thirties. The graphs not only demonstrate the rarity of breast cancer among young women but also the small excess number of cancers in current and recent users in relation to the cumulative risk of breast cancer.

In this pooled analysis, combined oral contraceptive users diagnosed with breast cancer had less advanced cancers, pointing toward better prognosis in this group than in nonusers with cancer. Detection bias may explain this finding. Users of oral contraceptives must visit a physician to renew their prescription and therefore may be more likely to undergo screening for breast cancer than nonusers. Cancers would therefore be diagnosed earlier in the development of the disease among users than nonusers. However, the relative excess of localized tumors was similar in current and past users and did not vary significantly with time since last use. Thus, any excess surveillance among users would have to have continued many years after use ceased.[11] An alternative explanation to one of bias is that oral contraceptives may affect the rate of growth of tumors and their tendency to metastasize.

The relationships observed in this study are unusual, since the risk increases soon after first exposure, does not increase with duration of exposure, and returns to normal

Table 15–1 Relative risk of breast cancer in ever users compared with never users of combined oral contraceptives.

Median Year of Diagnosis	Study	*Combined Oral Contraceptive Use* — *Ever Cases/ Controls*	*Never Cases/ Controls*	*Statistics* — *(O-E)*	*var(O-E)*	*Relative Risk of Breast Cancer In Ever Users versus Never Users* — *RR* & 99% CI*	*RR*±SD*
	PROSPECTIVE STUDIES						
1960	RCGP	198/728	128/576	13.0	55.6		1.26±0.151
1962	Oxford/FPA	96/437	101/342	–9.7	26.6		0.69±0.162
1985	Nurses Health	1105/4243	1656/6703	35.6	431.0		1.09±0.050
1985	CanadianNBSS	741/2905	594/2418	11.5	209.2		1.06±0.071
1987	AmerCancSoc	264/1091	907/3671	1.5	93.4		1.02±0.104
1988	Netherlands Cohort	105/406	348/1248	2.9	46.1		1.06±0.152
	Other	138/431	436/1576	2.5	25.4		1.10±0.206
	All prospective studies	2647/10243	4159/16534	57.3	887.3		1.07±0.035
	CASE-CONTROL STUDIES, WITH POPULATION CONTROLS						
1976	Brinton	714/781	2503/2764	14.0	193.7		1.07±0.075
1980	Bernstein/Pike	373/369	66/70	0.3	21.3		1.01±0.218
1981	Hislop	370/414	579/535	–5.0	51.5		0.91±0.133
1981	CASH	2815/2872	1879/1784	–27.9	394.7		0.93±0.049
1983	UKNational	684/673	71/82	5.9	31.2		1.20±0.197
1983	Baln/Siskind	197/424	343/671	–3.9	31.6		0.88±0.167
1983	Ewertz	479/458	1066/941	–4.0	80.8		0.95±0.109
1984	Melrik/Lund	289/338	133/189	8.7	42.0		1.23±0.171
1984	Long Island	266/230	914/950	13.8	57.2		1.27±0.149
1984	Clarke	257/543	350/669	–4.0	47.8		0.92±0.139
1985	Yu/Yuan/Wang	184/180	650/654	6.7	44.0		1.16±0.163
1985	Paul/Skegg	674/1521	217/343	4.5	69.2		1.07±0.124
1987	Daling	685/875	62/86	–0.0	26.5		1.00±0.194
1988	4StateStudy	2427/3726	4443/5793	8.9	416.6		1.02±0.050
1988	Rookus/van Leeuven	781/1782	137/136	2.5	40.0		1.07±0.163
1989	Yang/Gallagher	407/441	609/584	–15.3	55.1		0.76±0.118
1989	Primic-Zakelj	296/297	323/322	3.0	58.1		1.05±0.135
1991	WISH	1532/1597	334/412	20.5	119.8		1.19±0.100
	Other	1563/2029	1417/2141	16.3	168.5		1.10±0.081
	All case-control studies, with population controls	14993/18550	16096/19126	44.8	1949.6		1.02±0.023
	CASE-CONTROL STUDIES, WITH HOSPITAL CONTROLS						
1980	Vessey	963/972	1420/1419	8.5	193.4		1.04±0.074
1981	Ravnihar	161/460	370/1479	26.6	59.2		1.57±0.163
1983	WHO(developing)	525/5117	1180/9936	27.6	177.1		1.17±0.081
	WHO(developed)	667/1933	922/2116	10.9	157.6		1.07±0.082
1986	Claver	247/424	248/472	8.6	44.1		1.21±0.166
1987	LaVecchia	366/238	2897/2490	30.2	94.1		1.38±0.121
1992	Franceshi	382/314	2187/2274	25.3	104.7		1.27±0.111
	Other	616/1378	1879/3543	10.1	102.5		1.10±0.104
	All case control studies, with hospital controls	3927/10636	11103/23729	147.8	932.7		1.17±0.035
	All studies	21567/39629	31358/59389	249.8	3769.6		1.07±0.017

0.0 0.5 1.0 1.5 2.0

Test for heterogeneity between study designs: X^2 (2 df) = 11.6; p = 0.003

Test for heterogeneity between studies: X^2 (33 df) = 51.8; p = 0.02

*Relative risk (given with the 99% CI) is relative to never users, stratified by study, aged at diagnosis, parity, and, where appropriate, the age a woman was when her first child was born and the age she was when her risk of conception ceased.

Separate results are given for individual studies. Each relative risk and its 99% confidence interval (CI) is plotted as a black square and a line. The area of the square is proportional to the amount of statistical information (ie, to the inverse of the variance of the logarithm of the relative risk). Diamonds indicate 99% CIs for totals. The solid vertical line represents a relative risk of 1.0, and the broken vertical line indicates the overall relative risk estimate for all studies combined.

Source: Collaborative Group on Hormonal Factors in Breast Cancer, *Lancet*, Vol. 347, pp. 1713–1727, © by The Lancet Ltd. 1996.

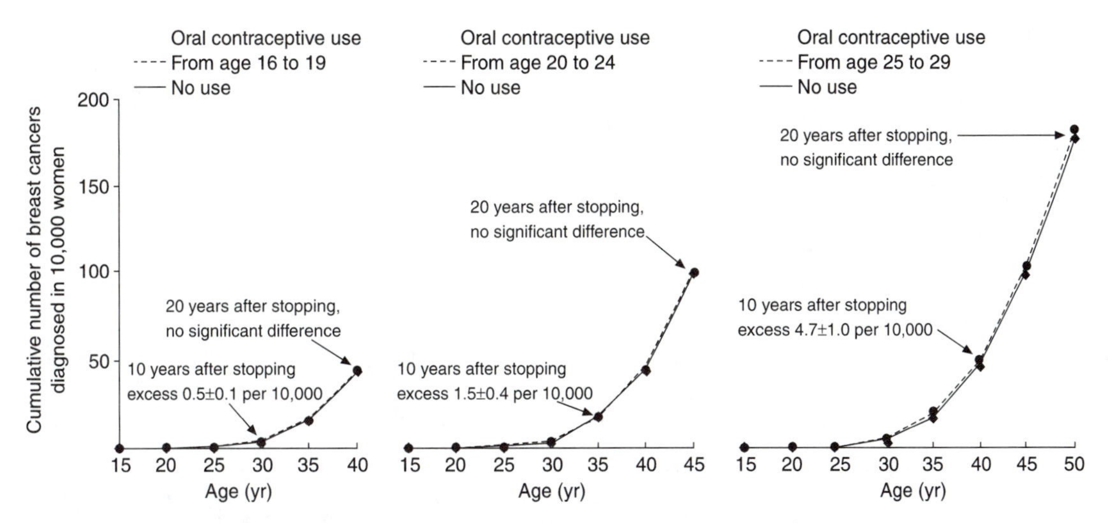

Figure 15–1 Estimated cumulative number of breast cancers diagnosed in never users and in women who used oral contraceptives at various ages. Estimated numbers for 10,000 women in Europe or North America. *Note:* the estimated numbers for ever users and never users are so similar in some age ranges that they overlap almost entirely. *Source:* Collaborative Group on Hormonal Factors in Breast Cancer, *Lancet*, Vol. 347, pp. 1713–1727, © by The Lancet Ltd. 1996.

10 years after. The collaborative group concluded that the pattern seems incompatible with a genotoxic effect.[8] An increased risk in recent users may be compatible with promotion of tumors that are already initiated. Further research is necessary in this area.

Endometrial and Ovarian Cancer

It is well-established that combined oral contraceptives (estrogen in combination with progestin) are strongly protective against endometrial[12] and epithelial ovarian cancer.[7] Case-control studies have consistently demonstrated that use of oral contraceptives decreases risk of endometrial cancer by approximately 50% (Table 15–2). Two large prospective studies, the Walnut Creek Contraceptive Drug Study[13] and the Royal College of General Practitioners' Study,[14] also demonstrated a similar decrease in risk.

A number of studies have examined the association between use of combined oral contraceptives and ovarian cancer (primarily epithelial cancer).[15] Whittemore et al[16] conducted a collaborative analysis of 12 US case-control studies involving 2,197 white ovarian cancer patients and 8,893 white control subjects conducted from 1956 to 1986. Women who had used oral contraceptives had a lower risk of invasive epithelial ovarian cancer than did nonusers (OR = 0.70, 95% CI = 0.52–0.94 in hospital studies; OR = 0.66, 95% CI = 0.55–0.78 in population studies). Among ever users, risk decreased with increasing years of use. There was little additional protection conferred by use beyond 6 years.

For both endometrial and epithelial ovarian cancer, the protection provided by oral contraceptives lasts for many years, perhaps even decades, after the use of oral contraceptives has stopped. The degree of protection seems likely to be related to duration of use.[3,17] However, because current findings are based on the effects of formulations of oral contraceptives as they were in the 1960s and 1970s, it is not clear that current low-dose formulations will carry the same degree of benefit.

Table 15–2 Case-Control Studies of Combination Oral Contraceptives and Endometrial Cancer

First Author and Year of Publication	*Age Range*	*Relative Risk**	*Number of Cases Using Oral Contraceptives*
Kaufman (1980)	59	0.5	16
Weiss (1980)	35–54	0.5	17
Hulka (1982)	59	0.4	5
Kelsey (1982)	45–74	0.6	6
Centers for Disease Control (CASH) (1983, 1987)	20–54	0.6	70
Henderson (1983)	45	0.5	43
WHO Collaborative Study (1988)	25–59	0.6	12
Stanford (1993)	20–74	0.4	78

*Ever versus never users of oral contraceptives.

Source: From CANCER EPIDEMIOLOGY AND PREVENTION, SECOND EDITION, edited by David Schottenfeld & J.F. Fraumeni. Copyright © 1996 by Oxford University Press, Inc. Used by permission of Oxford University Press, Inc.

Cervical Cancer

Combined oral contraceptive use is associated with an increased risk of invasive cervical cancer (cancer of the uterine cervix), with the risk increasing with longer duration of use.[14,18] Table 15–3 shows the duration-risk results from four recent studies. Recently, the World Health Organization (WHO) Collaborative Study of Neoplasia and Steroid Contraceptives conducted a large hospital-based case-control study among 10 participating hospitals in eight countries.[19,20] Risk for ever users was about 1.5 and was highest in recent and current users. A dose-response relationship was observed with increasing duration, and, after discontinuation, risk declined in line with time since cessation of use.

Table 15–3 Relative Risk Estimates from Four Studies of Invasive Adenomatous and Squamous Cervical Carcinomas by Duration of Oral Contraceptive Use

		Relative Risks			*Relative Risks*	
Study and Year	*Years of Use*	*Adenomatous*	*Squamous*	*Years of Use*	*Adenomatous*	*Squamous*
Latin America (1990)	5–9	1.7	1.3	10	1.8	1.4
Los Angeles (1994)	6–9	1.3	—	9–12	2.5	—
Multicenter US study (1986)	5–9	2.6	2.1	10	2.9	1.6
WHO collaborative study (1993)	5–8	1.4	1.5	8	2.2	2.2

Source: Reprinted with permission from D.B. Thomas and R.M. Ray, The World Health Organization Collaborative Study of Neoplasia and Steroid Contraceptives. Oral Contraceptives and Invasive Adenocarcinomas and Adenosquamous Carcinomas of the Cervix, *American Journal of Epidemiology*, Vol. 144, pp. 281–289, © 1996, The Johns Hopkins University School of Hygiene and Public Health.

In studies of contraceptive use and cervical cancer, design and analysis issues are complex and highlight several important sources of bias.[18–24] Women on combined oral contraceptives undergo greater medical surveillance than nonusers. They therefore have greater access to cervical cancer screening and are more likely to be diagnosed with this cancer. This could lead to the seeming identification of a relationship between combined oral contraceptive use and cervical cancer where none exists. One way to assess this potential bias is to compare the oral contraceptive–cervical cancer association between women with localized disease and women with advanced invasive disease. Women with more advanced disease have accompanying symptoms that lead them to come to screening regardless of combined oral contraceptive use. Routine screening, on the other hand, is more likely to pick up asymptomatic localized tumors. The WHO group observed no difference in association between those with localized and those with advanced invasive disease,[19,20] and no difference appeared after removing from the analysis women who did not present with symptoms (eg, vaginal bleeding) or controlling for the number of prior Pap smears as a proxy for medical utilization. This suggests that diagnostic bias did not play a major role in the study.

Questions also arise about potential confounding, particularly by sexual behavior, which is a major risk factor for cervical cancer. Certain human papillomaviruses (HPV) are sexually transmitted etiologic agents that have been implicated in the etiology of cervical cancer.[25] Combined oral contraceptives may act as a late-stage promoter, enhancing the risk associated with these agents.[18,26] Precise ascertainment of information on sexual behavior is necessary to avoid residual confounding by this factor. The WHO study addressed this potential source of bias by using serologic variables as indices of exposure to sexually transmitted agents and also by including the husband's sexual behavior in the analysis.[19,20] Table 15–4 shows the adjusted relative risks for women with and without various sexual risk factors. The relation of risk to duration of use was apparent in both groups but was greater, although not statistically so, in women with sexual risk factors. Further studies of oral contraceptive use and risk of cervical cancer in the presence and absence of HPV are necessary.[20]

POSTMENOPAUSAL HORMONES

Breast Cancer

The association between hormone replacement therapy and breast cancer is an ever more important public health issue because of the increasing size of the older female population. Although exogenous estrogens have long been suspected of increasing the risk of breast cancer, most prior studies, including several meta-analyses,[27–29] observed no relationship between hormones and risk. However, the majority of these studies focused on ever use without distinguishing between current and past use. Postmenopausal estrogen may act as a late-stage growth promoter for breast cancer, in which case the relationship between breast cancer risk and hormone use among current or recent-past users may differ from the relationship for women who discontinued use in the distant past.

A meta-analysis conducted in 1993 by Colditz et al[30] incorporated the results from 31 studies (Figure 15–2). The authors were able to address the roles of current, past, and

Table 15–4 Adjusted Relative Risks of Cervical Adenocarcinoma and Adenosquamous Carcinoma for Women Using Oral Contraceptives

	Months of Use				
Risk Factor	*None*	*12*	*13–60*	*61*	*p Value for Interaction*
No. of sexual partners					
1	1.0*	1.4†	1.3	1.5† (1.5)#	0.21
2–3	1.4	1.2	2.9†	3.6† (2.7)	
4	1.6	4.0	6.3†	1.5 (0.9)	
Vaginal discharge‡					
No	1.0*	1.2	1.3	1.6† (1.6)	0.62
Yes	1.4	2.0†	2.7†	3.5† (2.4)	
Sexually transmitted disease§					
No	1.0*	1.3	1.4	1.6† (1.6)	0.41
Yes	1.1	1.5	2.9†	4.1† (3.8)	
Induced abortion‖					
No	1.0*	1.4	1.6†	1.7† (1.7)	0.87
Yes	2.6§	2.7†	3.6†	5.6† (2.2)	
Any of these risk factors					
No	1.0*	1.1	1.1	1.2 (1.2)	0.08
Yes	1.2	1.9†	2.5†	3.1† (2.5)	

Note: Risk was adjusted for age, hospital, and year of entry into the study by the matching procedure and for number of live births, history of an induced abortion, number of prior Pap smears, and marital status. Excluded from all analyses were six cases with unknown duration of use and their 44 matched controls and 54 controls with unknown duration of use.

*Reference groups.

†95% confidence interval excludes 1.0.

‡Three cases with unknown history of vaginal discharge and their 20 matched controls and 14 controls with unknown history of vaginal discharge were excluded.

§Seven cases with unknown history of sexual transmitted disease and their 52 matched controls and 23 controls with unknown history of sexual transmitted disease were excluded.

‖Seven cases who were never pregnant and their 54 matched controls and 155 controls who were never pregnant were excluded.

#Relative risks compared with nonusers of oral contraceptives in the same strata are shown in parentheses.

Source: Reprinted with permission from D.B. Thomas and R.M. Ray, The World Health Organization Collaborative Study of Neoplasia and Steroid Contraceptives. Oral Contraceptives and Invasive Adenocarcinomas and Adenosquamous Carcinomas of the Cervix, *American Journal of Epidemiology*, Vol. 144, pp. 281–289, © 1996, The Johns Hopkins University School of Hygiene and Public Health.

ever use. Ever use was not associated with an increased risk (RR = 1.02, 95% CI = 0.93–1.12) even among those with a family history. Current users, however, had a 40% increased risk of breast cancer (95% CI = 1.20–1.63). Although no significant trend of increasing risk with increasing duration or dose was observed, those with very long durations of use (10 or more years) had a statistically significant 20% to 30% increase in risk. The addition of progestin to estrogen therapy did not affect the risk.

Several limitations should be considered. First, meta-analyses combine risk estimates from studies that may have adjusted for different risk factors. In this particular case, however, adjustment for risk factors in general did not affect the results, suggesting that confounding would not be a significant source of bias. Second, few studies have been able to evaluate very long-term use (20 years or more), which may itself be associ-

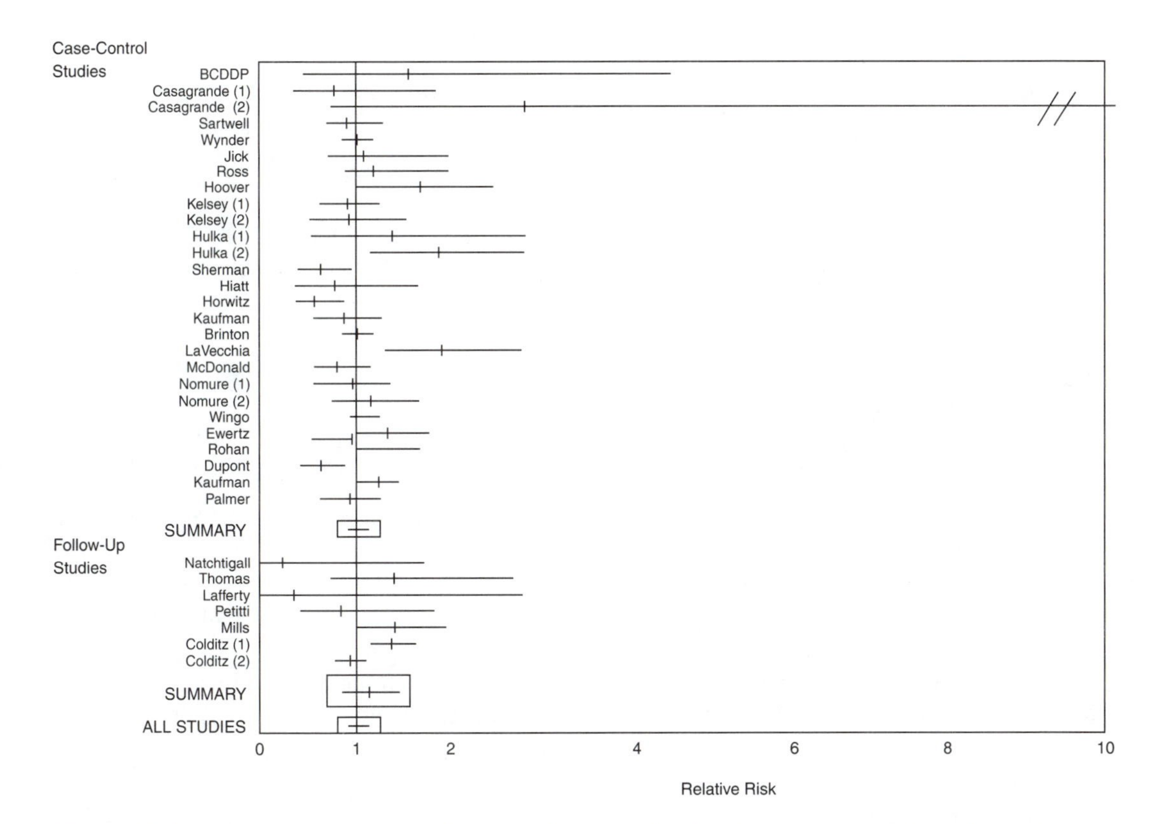

Figure 15–2 Ever use of hormone replacement therapy and risk of breast cancer in 29 studies included in meta-analysis. Studies with more than one set of results presented their findings for subgroups of women or separately for current and past users of hormone replacement therapy. Summary estimate confidence intervals are presented for random effects (open boxes) and fixed effects (lines). BCDDP = Breast Cancer Detection Demonstration Project. *Source:* Reprinted with permission from G.A. Colditz, K.M. Egan, and M.J. Stampfer, Hormone Replacement Therapy and Risk of Breast Cancer: Results from Epidemiologic Studies, *American Journal of Obstetrics and Gynecology*, Vol. 168, pp. 1473–1480, © 1993, Mosby, Inc.

ated with higher risk. On the other hand, the finding of increased risk among those with long duration of use may be caused by an increased proportion of current users in the long-duration categories.[30]

Recent findings from the large Nurses' Health Study[31,32] observed similar results for those with long duration of use. The authors followed participants for 16 years and found about a 50% increased risk of breast cancer among those with 5 to 10 or more years of use. Previous users, even those who had used postmenopausal hormones for 10 or more years, were not at increased risk.

Again, detection bias cannot be ruled out. Current users must see a physician to renew prescriptions and therefore are more likely to be screened for breast cancer. In fact, in the Nurse's Health Study,[33] current users had a 14% higher prevalence of mammography than never users. As earlier screening tends to lead to earlier diagnosis of breast cancer, data on survival can be used to evaluate this bias. Data from several studies[32,34,35] show improved survival and diagnosis of less advanced disease among cases diagnosed with breast cancer while using hormone replacement therapy, suggesting that detection bias may be present. Whether such a bias exists, however, is not conclusive, for there is evidence that postmenopausal hormones predispose women to low-risk breast tumors,[36] a possibility that also could account for the survival data.

In summary, although the results rule out a large effect of hormone therapy on breast cancer risk, some risk associated with current or long-term hormone replacement therapy may exist. Additional follow-up in this area is needed to clarify the influence of bias.

Endometrial Cancer

Epidemiological evidence consistently shows that administration of exogenous estrogen unopposed by progestin increases the risk of endometrial cancer.[37,38] The excess risk is evident within a few years of starting therapy and is observed 10 or more years after last use. The strength of the association is large and appears in all subgroups and with all patterns of hormone use. The reported size of the association tends to range from 2.9 for 1–4 years, 5.6 for 5–9 years, and 10 for 10+ years,[39] and it appears to decrease with increasing time since cessation of use.

Endometrial cancers caused by estrogen replacement therapy are on average better differentiated and have a better prognosis than other endometrial cancers. This finding does not appear to be explained wholly by detection bias.[37] Estrogens may stimulate early, well-differentiated, hormone-responsive cancers to grow faster and reach a size that can be diagnosed, preventing further damage. The large consistent risk ratio, the biologic plausibility of the association, and the consistency of epidemiological findings suggest a causal association. The observation in epidemiological studies that the risk ratio wanes with increasing time since cessation suggests that estrogen replacement therapy acts as a cancer promoter.

Current hormone replacement therapies include an opposing hormone, progestin, which inhibits endometrial growth. Although it is not yet certain that the combination therapy completely eliminates the risk of cancer, it is certain that it greatly reduces it.[3]

Colon Cancer

Male and female colon cancer incidence rates are almost equal, but during the past 30 years mortality from colon cancer has risen 16% in men and declined 21% in women. It has been suggested that part of this difference is due to the increased use of postmenopausal hormones over this time period.[40–42]

Epidemiological studies of large-bowel cancer epidemiology suggest that risk of this cancer may be related to exogenous hormone use. While earlier studies observed little or no association,[43–45] they were limited by modest size and small numbers of women using postmenopausal hormones. On the other hand, seven[12,46–51] of eleven[32,52–55] recent studies found a lower risk of colon cancer associated with postmenopausal hormones.

In the most recent study of this issue, Newcomb et al[51] performed a large population-based case-control study encompassing 694 case subjects and 1,622 control subjects. Women who had recently used postmenopausal hormones had approximately one-half the risk of large-bowel cancer that never users had (Table 15–5). This reduction in risk was maintained for about 10 years after discontinuation of use but was stronger with more recent exposure. Increasing duration of use was not associated with decreasing risk for colon cancer, suggesting that, for this disease, estrogen may act acutely. No association between postmenopausal hormones and risk of rectal cancer was observed.

Newcomb's finding of a stronger effect with recency of exposure may clarify the null findings of some prior studies. Until recently, clinicians tended to prescribe short-term postmenopausal hormone therapy for the acute effects of menopause. In prior studies conducted among older cohorts of postmenopausal women, few would be recent users. Over time, women have used postmenopausal hormone therapy for longer durations than ever before, increasing the pool of recent users. Thus, studies conducted among more recent generations of postmenopausal women would have the opportunity to observe the protective effect.

Adenocarcinoma of the large bowel is one of the most common cancers in Western populations and is associated with significant morbidity and mortality. If postmenopausal hormones do have a protective effect, their use will have a considerable public health impact.

TAMOXIFEN

Tamoxifen is a nonsteroidal antiestrogenic medication that has been used successfully for 15 years in the treatment of breast cancer. Because tamoxifen acts by binding to estrogen receptor sites, it has been most effective in treating postmenopausal women, who are more likely to have cancers containing estrogen receptors.[56] Currently,

Table 15–5 Relative Risks of Colon and Rectal Cancers According to Use of Hormone Replacement Therapy

		Colon Cancer		*Rectal Cancer*	
*Use of HRT**	*No. of Controls*	*No. of Cases*	*RR† (95% CI)*	*No. of Cases*	*RR† (95% CI)*
Ever	541	113	0.73 (0.56–0.94)	65	1.17 (0.83–1.63)
Former	273	78	0.85 (0.63–1.15)	45	1.32 (0.90–1.92)
Recent‡	268	35	0.54 (0.36–0.81)	20	0.91 (0.54–1.55)
Estrogen only	171	24	0.54 (0.34–0.88)	12	0.90 (0.46–1.76)
Estrogen and progestin	62	11	0.54 (0.28–1.05)	8	1.13 (0.51–2.50)
Never	1044	357	1.00	142	1.00

*The type of HRT (ie, estrogen only or estrogen and progestin) could not be determined for 35 subjects.

†RRs adjusted for age, use of sigmoidoscopy screening, family history of large-bowel cancer, body mass index, and intake of beer or hard liquor.

‡Within year prior to diagnosis or reference date.

Source: Reprinted from P.A. Newcomb and B.E. Storer, Postmenopausal Hormone Use and Risk of Large-Bowel Cancer, *Journal of the National Cancer Institute*, Vol. 87, pp. 1067–1071, 1995, National Cancer Institute.

tamoxifen is being used for treatment of all stages of breast carcinoma among women of any age.[57] A meta-analysis of 61 randomized clinical trials (encompassing 28,986 women with breast cancer) showed that 51% of tamoxifen-treated women were disease-free after 10 years, compared with 45% in the control group.[58]

Of particular importance for the potential primary prevention of breast cancer are data showing that tamoxifen is effective in preventing contralateral (opposite) breast cancers. An overall analysis of breast cancer treatment trials observed a nearly 40% reduction in the odds of contralateral breast cancer among women treated with tamoxifen.[58]

Recently, there has been interest in using tamoxifen to prevent breast cancer. Several studies are currently underway to test prophylactic tamoxifen therapy for healthy women who are at high risk for developing breast cancer.[59–61] Women will take the drug for extended periods to prevent even a first occurrence of cancer. One such recently completed trial is the Breast Cancer Prevention Trial (BCPT), a placebo-controlled clinical investigation involving 16,000 women aged 35 or over who are considered at high risk for breast cancer.[62] All women aged 60 or over are eligible to participate, and women aged 35–59 years are eligible if their 5-year risk of breast cancer, based on the Gail model,[63] is equivalent to or greater than that of a 60-year-old woman. The Gail model uses the age of the woman and the following additional risk factors: number of affected first-degree relatives, age at menarche, age at first live birth, number of previous breast biopsies, and presence of atypical hyperplasia in a biopsy specimen. The BCPT found that tamoxifen can reduce the incidence of breast cancer by nearly half in women at high risk but may increase the risk of endometrial cancer and of thromboembolism.[64] A large breast cancer prevention trial called Study of Tamoxifen and Raloxifene (STAR) has started in the United States. Raloxifene is available for the prevention of osteoporosis. Results should be available in the next 7 years.

In contradiction to its antiestrogenic tumor-suppressive action in the case of breast cancer, tamoxifen has been associated with the development of endometrial carcinoma[65] and several other gynecologic malignancies (Table 15–6).[57] The relative risk of endometrial cancer appears to increase with increasing duration of use and be particularly high in women over 60.[57] Interim results from an ongoing randomized trial found that 15 of 1,419 women randomized to receive tamoxifen developed endometrial cancer.[66] This reflected an annual risk of about 2 per 1,000 women, a risk approximately 3 times greater than that of a similar group of women in the general population.[65]

Whether the observed increased incidence of endometrial adenocarcinoma in tamoxifen-treated breast cancer patients represents a true increase or improved detection of very early lesions is unknown.[67] The action on the endometrium has not yet been clarified. However, the observation that most of the endometrial cancer among tamoxifen users has been diagnosed at an early stage suggests that detection bias may play some role.

Given the current trend toward prolonged tamoxifen treatment and the large-scale trials of tamoxifen for the prevention of breast cancer among high-risk healthy women,[59,68] routine screening for endometrial cancer in tamoxifen users has been recommended.[57,67,69–71] Further studies are required to quantify and assess the long-term benefits and adverse effects of tamoxifen.

Table 15–6 Reports of Endometrial Carcinoma and Other Gynecologic Malignancies in Tamoxifen-treated Breast Cancer Patients

Authors	N	Year	Mean Age (Years)	Menopausal Status	
				Pre	Post
Killackey et al	3	1985	59.3	1	2
Scottish Trial	3	1987			
Hardell*	11	1988	65.4	0	11
Fornander et al	13	1989		0	13
Neven et al†	1	1989			
Atlante et al	4	1989	58.3	1	3
Nuovo et al	2	1989		0	2
Dauplat et al	2	1990	62	0	2
Mathew et al	5	1990	65	0	5
Malfetano	7	1990		0	7
Spinelli et al	3	1991	45.3	3	0
De Muylder et al	2	1991		0	2
Rasmussen and Neilsen	2	1991	76	0	2
Andersson et al	7	1991		0	7
Seoud et al	5	1992	67.4	0	5
Total	70		63.9	5	61

*Hardell L. Tamoxifen as risk factor for carcinoma of corpus uteri. *Lancet.* 1988;2:563. Letter. Hardell L. Pelvic irradiation and tamoxifen as risk factor for carcinoma of corpus uteri. *Lancet.* 1988;2:1432. Letter

†Neven P, De Muylder X, Van Belle Y, Vanderick G, De Mulyder E. Tamoxifen and the uterus and endometrium. *Lancet.* 1989;1:375–376. Letter.

Source: Reprinted with permission from The American College of Obstetricians and Gynecologists (*Obstetrics and Gynecology*, 1993, Vol. 82, pp. 165–169).

DIETHYLSTILBESTROL

Diethylstilbestrol (DES) is a potent synthetic estrogen that was prescribed in the United States between 1940 and 1970 for a wide range of pregnancy-related conditions, in particular, to prevent miscarriage and suppress lactation.[72–75] During this period, anywhere from 500,000 to 2 million women were exposed.[76] By the early 1970s, the carcinogenic properties of DES had become apparent, and in 1971 it was banned for use in pregnant women.[75]

Six cohort studies have examined the future risk of breast cancer in mothers exposed to DES during their reproductive years.[77–85] The majority of these studies suggested the existence of a modest (20% to 50%) increased risk among exposed women, with a latency of about 15 to 20 years. Greenberg et al[84] performed a retrospective cohort study among 3,000 women who had taken DES during pregnancy and a comparable group of unexposed parous women. The authors observed a 50% increased risk of breast cancer 20 or more years after DES exposure. Risk among users and among nonusers continued to diverge over time. Subsequently, the American Cancer Society performed a large prospective cohort study of women exposed to DES during pregnancy in order to determine the risk of subsequent fatal breast cancer.[77] This study had an average follow-up period of more than 30 years and thus included women who had reached an age when breast cancer incidence is high. In contrast to Greenberg's findings, risk of fatal breast cancer did not increase over time.

Several methodologic issues are important to consider in this area. Because women exposed to DES undergo increased surveillance, tumors might be detected that otherwise would have remained occult. If such tumors are detected, those exposed to DES would be expected to have an excess of small early-stage tumors rather than large later-stage tumors. In addition, DES-exposed women might have other characteristics responsible for their exposure to the drug and for their higher incidence of breast cancer as well. The existence of such characteristics could lead to a spurious association between DES and subsequent breast cancer. For example, DES was given to those at risk for miscarriage,[86] and miscarriage has been associated in some studies with a moderate increase in breast cancer risk.[87] In the recent study by Greenberg, however, no difference between cancer stage was observed, and controlling for history of miscarriage did not affect the results.[84] Similarly, in the American Cancer Society study,[77] a history of spontaneous abortion was not associated with fatal breast cancer,[88] and control for this variable did not alter the risk estimates.

Although the risks found are modest and could be due to bias or residual confounding, the similarity of study results, coupled with the known carcinogenic potential of DES,[76] supports the hypothesis that exposure to DES during pregnancy has a weak carcinogenic effect on the breast. Evidence suggests that this effect does not, as was initially feared,[84] increase markedly over time.[77,85]

Although DES is no longer in general use, its impact on breast cancer can be considered in evaluating the risk associated with exogenous hormones taken today. The doses of DES historically administered during pregnancy were massive relative to current doses of estrogen used for replacement therapy or contraception.[77] The relevance of these high doses to the potential effects of current low levels of exogenous estrogens remains somewhat unclear. However, the epidemiological studies provide some reassurance that no large increases in breast cancer risk are observed even with large doses of exogenous estrogens given in pregnancy, a time when breast tissue may be particularly vulnerable to carcinogenic exposure.

SUMMARY

Exogenous hormones and hormone antagonists appear to increase the risk of some cancers and to decrease the risk of others. Oral contraceptives have effects on a wide variety of cancers. The risk of endometrial cancer and ovarian cancer are almost certainly reduced by the use of combined oral contraceptives. For both these cancer sites, the protection provided by oral contraceptives lasts for many years, perhaps even decades, after the use of oral contraceptives has stopped. Protection against cancer of the ovary, in particular, is of great potential importance, since this disease commonly presents at an advanced stage and treatment is often not effective. On the other hand, evidence that early use of oral contraceptives may increase breast cancer risk is of concern.

Findings from recent studies suggest that certain subgroups of oral contraceptive users may be particularly susceptible to risk of breast cancer. The Collaborative Group on Hormonal Factors in Breast Cancer found a small increased risk of breast cancer among current oral contraceptive users that persisted for 10 years after discontinuation. This pattern may be compatible with promotion of tumors that are already initiated, and further research in this area is necessary.

Combined oral contraceptive use is associated with an increased risk of invasive cervical cancer, the risk increasing with increasing duration of use. Studies in this area face complex design and analysis issues, include susceptibility to several important sources of bias.

The association between hormone replacement therapy and breast cancer is an issue of public health importance given the increasing size of the older female population . Although findings rule out a large effect of hormone therapy on breast cancer risk, some risk associated with current or long-term hormone replacement therapy may exist. Additional follow-up in this area is needed to clarify the influence of bias.

Epidemiological evidence consistently indicates that the administration of exogenous estrogen unopposed by progestin increases the risk of endometrial cancer. Current hormone replacement therapies include an opposing hormone, progestin, which inhibits endometrial growth. Although it is not yet certain that the combination therapy completely eliminates the risk of cancer, it unquestionably reduces it to a great extent.

Exogenous hormones are associated with the decreased risk of some diseases. For example, postmenopausal hormones protect against osteoporosis and cardiovascular disease, and oral contraceptives appear to reduce the risk of subsequent endometrial and ovarian cancer by nearly half.[89] The protection lasts for many years, even decades, after the use of oral contraceptives has stopped, and may be related to the duration of use. Note, however, that the current data regarding long-term use are based on the effects of formulations of the pill as it was first available in the 1960s and the following decade. It is not clear that current low-dose formulations will carry the same degree of benefit.

Epidemiological studies of large-bowel cancer suggest that risk of this cancer is reduced by the use of exogenous hormones. Adenocarcinoma of the large bowel is one of the most common cancers in Western populations and is associated with significant morbidity and mortality. If postmenopausal hormones do have a protective effect, it will have a considerable public health impact.

With the current trends of prolonged tamoxifen treatment and the large-scale trials of tamoxifen for the prevention of breast cancer among high risk healthy women,[59,68] routine screening for endometrial cancer in tamoxifen users has been recommended.[57,67,69,71] Further studies are required to quantify and assess the long-term benefits and adverse effects of tamoxifen. Although DES is no longer in general use, its impact on breast cancer can be considered in evaluating the risk associated with exogenous hormones taken today.

With the realization that women's own hormones may affect the risk of cancer, a major research effort has been directed at elucidating the link between medically administered hormones and the incidence of cancer. Two important factors hamper epidemiological studies of the effects of exogenous hormones on cancer risk. First, surveillance bias among those taking exogenous hormones may cause a spurious association between the drug and the cancer risk. Second, hormone use itself may be associated with improved survival after diagnosis.

In summary, the carcinogenic effects of natural and synthetic female hormones, if they exist, are not large, do not pertain to all the drugs that have been used, and are not equally present at all ages.[3] As a result, the epidemiological investigation of the relationship between exogenous hormones and cancer risk faces many challenges. Long-term follow-up of existing drugs and surveillance of the effects of new formulations should be an ongoing focus of cancer epidemiology,[90] but given the low incidence of most cancers, the power to detect relatively weak effects remains limited.

Discussion Questions

1. Discuss the challenges involved in designing a prospective study to examine the effect of exogenous hormones on cancer risk. Compare these to the challenges involved in designing a case-control study.
2. Define detection bias and discuss its threat to studies of exogenous hormones and cancer. How does the presence of detection bias affect observed findings (mention the likelihood, magnitude, and direction of effect)? How can researchers provide evidence that detection bias is not responsible for their findings?
3. Summarize the effects of combined oral contraceptives on breast cancer, endometrial and ovarian cancer, and cancer of the uterine cervix. Given the weight of the evidence, would you recommend oral contraceptives to women of reproductive age today?
4. Explain why future studies are required to quantify and assess the long-term benefits and potential adverse effects of tamoxifen.
5. Although DES is no longer in general use, discuss how its impact on breast cancer sheds light on the risk associated with exogenous hormones taken today.

References

1. Farber E. Possible etiologic mechanisms in chemical carcinogenesis. *Environ Health Perspect.* 1987;75:65–70.
2. Selby JV, Friedman GD, Herrinton LJ. Pharmaceuticals other than hormones. In: Schottenfeld D, Fraumeni JF Jr, eds. *Cancer Epidemiology and Prevention.* 2nd ed. New York: Oxford University Press. 1996:489–501.
3. Harvard Center for Cancer Prevention. Causes of human cancer. Prescription drugs. *Cancer Causes Control.* 1996;7(suppl 1):S45–S47.
4. Ory HW, Rosenfeld A, Landman LL. The pill at 20: an assessment. *Fam Plann Perspect.* 1980;12:278–283.
5. Romeiu I, Berlin JA, Colditz GA Oral contraceptives and breast cancer: review and meta-analysis. *Cancer.* 1990;66:2253–2263.
6. Prentice RL, Thomas DB. On the epidemiology of oral contraceptives and disease. *Adv Cancer Res.* 1987;49:285–401.
7. Bernstein L, Henderson BE. Exogenous hormones. In: Schottenfeld D, Fraumeni JF Jr, eds. *Cancer Epidemiology and Prevention.* 2nd ed. New York: Oxford University Press; 1996:462–489.
8. Collaborative Group on Hormonal Factors in Breast Cancer. Breast cancer and hormonal contraceptives: collaborative reanalysis of individual data on 53,297 women with breast cancer and 100,239 women without breast cancer from 54 epidemiological studies. *Lancet.* 1996;347:1713–1727.
9. Pike MC, Henderson BE, Krailo MD, Duke A, Roy S. Breast cancer in young women and use of oral contraceptives: possible modifying effect of formulation and age at use. *Lancet.* 1983;2:926–930.
10. Rookus MA, Leeuwen FE (for the Netherlands Oral Contraceptives and Breast Cancer Study Group). Oral contraceptives and risk of breast cancer in women aged 20–54 years. *Lancet.* 1994;344:844–851.
11. Collaborative Group on Hormonal Factors in Breast Cancer. Breast cancer and hormonal contraceptives: further results. *Contraception.* In press.
12. Furner SE, Davis FG, Nelson RL, et al. A case-control study of large bowel cancer and hormone exposure in women. *Cancer Res.* 1989;49:4936–4940.

13. Ramcharan S, Pellegrin FA, Ray R, Hsu JP. *The Walnut Creek Contraceptive Drug Study: A Prospective Study of the Side Effects of Oral Contraceptive Use.* Bethesda, MD: US Department of Health, Education, and Welfare; National Institutes of Health; National Institute of Child Health and Human Development; Center for Population Research; 1981. NIH publication Nos. 74-562, 76-563, 81-564.
14. Beral V, Hannaford P, Kay C. Oral contraceptive use and malignancies of the genital tract: results from the Royal College of General Practitioners' Oral Contraception Study. *Lancet.* 1988;2:1331–1335.
15. Schlesselman JJ. Cancer of the breast and reproductive tract in relation to use of oral contraceptives. *Contraception.* 1989;40:1–38.
16. Whittemore AS, Harris R, Itnyre J, Collaborative Ovarian Cancer Group. Characteristics relating to ovarian cancer risk: collaborative analysis of 12 US case-control studies. II. Invasive epithelial ovarian cancers in white women. *Am J Epidemiol.* 1992;136:1184–1203.
17. Bernstein L, Henderson BE. Exogenous hormones. In: Schottenfeld D, Fraumeni JF Jr, eds. *Cancer Epidemiology and Prevention.* Philadelphia: WB Saunders Co; 1982:462–488.
18. Brinton LA, Reeves WC, Brenes MM, et al. Oral contraceptive use and risk of invasive cervical cancer. *Int J Epidemiol.* 1990;19:4–11.
19. World Health Organization Collaborative Study of Neoplasia and Steroid Contraceptives. Invasive squamous-cell cervical carcinoma and combined oral contraceptives: results from a multinational study. *Int J Cancer.* 1993;55:228–236.
20. Thomas DB, Ray RM. Oral contraceptives and invasive adenocarcinomas and adenosquamous carcinomas of the uterine cervix. World Health Organization Collaborative Study of Neoplasia and Steroid Contraceptives. *Am J Epidemiol.* 1996;144:281–289.
21. Ursin G, Peters RK, Henderson BE, et al. Oral contraceptive use and adenocarcinoma of cervix. *Lancet.* 1994;344:1390–1394.
22. Parazzini F, La Vecchia C, Negri E, et al. Risk factors for adenocarcinoma of the cervix: a case-control study. *Br J Cancer.* 1988;57:201–204.
23. Brinton LA, Huggins GR, Lehman HF, et al. Long-term use of oral contraceptives and risk of invasive cervical cancer. *Int J Cancer.* 1986;38:339–344.
24. Brinton LA, Tashima KT, Lehman HF, et al. Epidemiology of cervical cancer by cell type. *Cancer Res.* 1987;47:1706–1711.
25. Schiffman MH, Bauer HM, Hoover RN, et al. Epidemiologic evidence showing that human papillomavirus infection causes most cervical intraepithelial neoplasia. *J Natl Cancer Inst.* 1993;85:958–964.
26. Bosch FX, Munoz N, de Sanjose S, et al. Risk factors for cervical cancer in Colombia and Spain. *Int J Cancer.* 1992;52:750–758.
27. Armstrong BK. Estrogen therapy after the menopause: boon or bane? *Med J Aust.* 1988;148:213–214.
28. Dupont WD, Page DL. Menopausal estrogen replacement therapy and breast cancer. *Arch Intern Med.* 1991;151:67–72.
29. Sillero-Arenas M, Delgado-Rodriguez M, Rodrigues-Canteras R, Bueno-Cavanillas A, Galvez-Vargas R. Menopausal hormone replacement therapy and breast cancer: a meta-analysis. *Obstet Gynecol.* 1992;79:286–294.
30. Colditz GA, Egan KM, Stampfer MJ. Hormone replacement therapy and risk of breast cancer: results from epidemiologic studies. *Am J Obstet Gynecol.* 1993;168:1473–1480.
31. Colditz GA, Stampfer MJ, Willett WC, et al. Type of postmenopausal hormone use and risk of breast cancer: 12-year follow-up from the Nurses' Health Study. *Cancer Causes Control.* 1992;3:433–439.
32. Adami HO, Persson I, Hoover R, Schairer C, Bergkvist L. Risk of cancer in women receiving hormone replacement therapy. *Int J Cancer.* 1989;44:833–839.
33. Colditz GA, Hankinson SE, Hunter DJ, et al. The use of estrogens and progestins and the risk of breast cancer in postmenopausal women. *N Engl J Med.* 1995;332:1589–1593.
34. Adami HO, Persson I, Yuen J, Bergkvist L, Hoover R. Oestrogen replacement therapy and breast cancer: update of an Italian case-control study. In: Mann R, ed. *Hormone Replacement Therapy and Breast Cancer Risk.* Carnforth, England: Parthenon Publishing; 1992:93–98.
35. Hunt K, Vessey M, McPherson K. Mortality in a cohort of long-term users of hormone replacement therapy: an updated analysis. *Br J Obstet Gynaecol.* 1990;97:1080–1086.
36. Grodstein F, Stampfer MJ, Colditz GA, et al. Postmenopausal hormone therapy and mortality. *N Engl J Med.* 1997;336:1769–1775.
37. Paganini-Hill A, Ross RK, Henderson BE. Endometrial cancer and patterns of use of oestrogen replacement therapy: a cohort study. *Br J Cancer.* 1989;59:445–447.

38. Persson I, Adami HO, Bergkvist L, et al. Risk of endometrial cancer after treatment with oestrogens alone or in conjunction with progestogen: results of a prospective study. *BMJ.* 1989;298:147–151.
39. Shapiro S, Kelly JP, Rosenberg L, et al. Risk of localized and widespread endometrial cancer in relation to recent and discontinued use of conjugated estrogens. *New Engl J Med.* 1985;313:969–972.
40. Wynder EL, Hyams L, Shigematsu T. Correlations of international cancer death rates: an epidemiological exercise. *Cancer.* 1967;20:113–126.
41. Jensen OM. Different age and sex relationship for cancer of subsites of the large bowel. *Br J Cancer.* 1984;50:825–829.
42. McMichael AJ, Potter JD. Host factors in carcinogenesis: certain bile-acid metabolic profiles that selectively increase the risk of proximal colon cancer. *J Natl Cancer Inst.* 1985;75:185–191.
43. Weiss NS, Daling JR, Chow WH. Incidence of cancer of the large bowel in women in relation to reproductive and hormonal factors. *J Natl Cancer Inst.* 1981;67:57–60.
44. Wu AH, Paganini-Hill RA, Ross RK, et al. Alcohol, physical activity and other risk factors for colorectal cancer: a prospective study. *Br J Cancer.* 1987;55:687–694.
45. Potter JD, McMichael AJ. Large bowel cancer in relation to reproductive and hormonal factors: a case-control study. *J Natl Cancer Inst.* 1983;71:703–709.
46. Chute CG, Willett WD, Colditz GA, et al. A prospective study of reproductive history and exogenous estrogens on the risk of colorectal cancer in women. *Epidemiology.* 1991;2:201–207.
47. Gerhardsson de Verdier M, London S. Reproductive factors, exogenous female hormone, and colorectal cancer by subsite. *Cancer Causes Control.* 1992;3:355–360.
48. Jacobs EJ, White E, Weiss NS. Exogenous hormones, reproductive history, and colon cancer (Seattle, Washington, USA). *Cancer Causes Control.* 1994;5:359–366.
49. Bostick RM, Potter JD, Kushi LH, et al. Sugar, meat, and fat intake, and non-dietary risk factors for colon cancer incidence in Iowa women (United States). *Cancer Causes Control.* 1994;5:38–52.
50. Calle EE, Moracle-McMahill HL, Thun MJ, et al. Estrogen replacement therapy and risk of fatal colon cancer in a prospective cohort postmenopausal women. *J Natl Cancer Inst.* 1995;87:517–523.
51. Newcomb, PA, Storer BE. Postmenopausal hormone use and risk of large-bowel cancer. *J Natl Cancer Inst.* 1995;87:1067–1071.
52. Davis FG, Furner SE, Persky V, et al. The influence of parity and exogenous female hormones on the risk of colorectal cancer. *Int J Cancer.* 1989;43:587–590.
53. Peters RK, Pike MC, Chang WW, et al. Reproductive factors and colon cancers. *Br J Cancer.* 1990;61:741–748.
54. Wu-Williams AH, Lee M, Whittemore AS, et al. Reproductive factors and colorectal cancer risk among Chinese females. *Cancer Res.* 1991;51:2307–2311.
55. Risch HA, Howe GR. Menopausal hormone use and colorectal cancer in Saskatchewan: a record linkage cohort study. *Cancer Epidemiol Biomarkers Prev.* 1995;4:21–28.
56. Leis HP. The role of tamoxifen in the prevention and treatment of benign and malignant breast lesions: a chemopreventive. *Int Surg.* 1993;78:176–182.
57. Daniel Y, Inbar M, Bar-Am A, Peyser MR, Lessing JB. The effects of tamoxifen treatment on the endometrium. *Fertil Steril.* 1996;65:1083–1089.
58. Early Breast Cancer Trials' Collaborative Group (EBCTCG). Systemic treatment of early breast cancer by hormonal cytotoxic, or immune therapy. *Lancet.* 1992;339:71–85.
59. Powles TJ, Tillyer CR, Jones AJ, et al. Prevention of breast cancer with tamoxifen: an update on the Royal Marsden Hospital pilot programme. *Eur J Cancer.* 1990;26:680–684.
60. Davidson NE. Tamoxifen: panacea or Pandora's box. *N Engl J Med.* 1992;326:885–886.
61. Nayfield SG, Karp JE, Ford LG, Dorr FA, Kramer BS. Potential role of tamoxifen in prevention of breast cancer. *J Natl Cancer Inst.* 1991;83:1450–1459.
62. McKeon VA. The breast cancer prevention trail: evaluating tamoxifen's efficacy in preventing breast cancer. *J Obstet Gynecol Neonatal Nurs.* 1997;26:79–90.
63. Bush TL, Helzlsouer KJ. Tamoxifen for the primary prevention of breast cancer: a review and critique of the concept and trial. *Epidemiol Rev.* 1993;15;233–243.
64. Overmoyer BA. The breast cancer prevention trial (P-1 study): the role of tamoxifen in preventing breast cancer. *Cleve Clin J Med.* 1999;66:33–40.
65. Seoud MA-F, Johnson J, Weed JC. Gynecologic tumors in tamoxifen-treated women with breast cancer. *Obstet Gynecol.* 1993;82:165–169.

66. Fisher B, Costantino JP, Redmond CK, Wickerham DL, Cronin WM. Endometrial cancer in tamoxifen-treated breast cancer patients: findings from the National Surgical Adjuvant Breast and Bowel Project (NSABP) B-14. *J Natl Cancer Inst.* 1994;86:527–537.
67. Wolf DM, Jordan VC. Gynecologic complications associated with long-term adjuvant tamoxifen therapy for breast cancer. *Gynecol Oncol.* 1992;45:118–128.
68. Seoud MAF, Johnson J, Weed JC. Gynecologic tumors in tamoxifen-treated women with breast cancer. *Obstet Gynecol.* 1993;82:165–169.
69. Boccardo F, Guarneri D, Rubagoti A, et al. Endocrine effects of tamoxifen in post-menopausal breast cancer patients. *Tumori.* 1984;70:61–68.
70. Guesberg SB. Tamoxifen for breast cancer: associated with endometrial cancer. *Cancer.* 1990;65:1463–1464.
71. De Muylder X, Neven P, De Somer M, Van Belle Y, Vanderick G, De Muylder E. Endometrial lesions in patients undergoing tamoxifen therapy. *Int J Gynaecol Obstet.* 1991;36:127–130.
72. Marselos M, Tomatis L. Diethylstilboestrol. I. Pharmacology, toxicology, and carcinogenicity in humans. *Eur J Cancer.* 1992;28A:1182–1189.
73. Smith OW. Diethylstilbestrol in the prevention and treatment of complications of pregnancy. *Am J Obstet Gynecol.* 1948;56:821–834.
74. Smith OW, Smith G, Van S. The influence of diethylstilbestrol on the progress and outcome of pregnancy based on a comparison of treated with untreated primigravidas. *Am J Obstet Gynecol.* 1949;58:994–1009.
75. Giusti RM, Iwamoto K, Hatch E. Diethylstilbestrol revisited: a review of the long-term health effects. *Ann Intern Med.* 1995;122:778–788.
76. Noller KL, Fish CR. Diethylstilbestrol usage: its interesting past, important present, and questionable future. *Med Clin North Am.* 1974;58:793–810.
77. Calle EE, Mervis CA, Thun MJ, Rodriguez C, Wingo PA, Heath CW Jr. Diethylstilbestrol and risk of fatal breast cancer in a prospective cohort of US women. *Am J Epidemiol.* 1996;144:645–662.
78. Bibbo M, Haenszel WM, Wied GL, Hubby M, Herbst AL. A twenty-five-year follow-up study of women exposed to diethylstilbestrol during pregnancy. *N Engl J Med.* 1978;298:763–767.
79. Hubby MM, Haenszel WM, Herbst AL. Effects on the mother following exposure to diethylstilbestrol during pregnancy. In: Herbst AL, Bern HA, eds. *Developmental Effects of Diethylstilbestrol (DES) in Pregnancy.* New York: Thieme-Stratton; 1981:120–128.
80. Beral V, Colwell L. Randomised trial of high doses of stilboestrol and ethisterone in pregnancy: long-term follow-up of mothers. *BMJ.* 1980;281:1098–1101.
81. Vessey MP, Fairweather DVI, Norman-Smith B, et al. A randomized double-blind controlled trial of the value of stilboestrol therapy in pregnancy: long-term follow-up of mothers and their offspring. *Br J Obstet Gynaecol.* 1983;90:1007–1017.
82. Meara J, Vessey M, Fairweather DV. A randomized double-blind controlled trial of the value of diethylstilboestrol therapy in pregnancy: 35-year follow-up of mothers and their offspring. *Br J Obstet Gynaecol.* 1989;96:620–622.
83. Hadjimichael OC, Meigs JW, Falcier FW, et al. Cancer risk among women exposed to exogenous estrogens during pregnancy. *J Natl Cancer Inst.* 1984;73:831–834.
84. Greenberg ER, Barnes AB, Resseguie L, et al. Breast cancer in mothers given diethylstilbestrol in pregnancy. *N Engl J Med.* 1984;311:1393–1398.
85. Colton T, Greenberg ER, Noler K, et al. Breast cancer in mothers prescribed diethylstilbestrol in pregnancy. *JAMA.* 1993;269:2096–2100.
86. Noller KL, Fish CR. Diethylstilbestrol usage: its interesting past, important present, and questionable future. *Med Clin North Am* 1974;58:793–810.
87. Kelsey JL, Hildreth NG, eds. *Breast and Gynecologic Cancer Epidemiology.* Boca Raton, FL: CRC Press, 1983.
88. Calle EE, Mervis CA, Wingo PA, et al. Spontaneous abortion and risk of fatal breast cancer in a prospective cohort of United States women. *Cancer Causes Control.* 1995;6:460–468.
89. La Vecchia C, Franceschi S, Bruzzi P, Parazzini F, Boyle P. The relationship between oral contraceptive use, cancer and vascular disease. *Drug Saf.* 1990;5:436–444.
90. Skegg D. Other drugs. In: Vessey MP, Gray M, eds. *Cancer Risks and Prevention.* Oxford: Oxford University Press; 1985:211–230.

Chapter 16

Diet and Cancer

Harris Pastides

People have an obvious interest in determining whether the foods and drinks they consume can increase or decrease their risk of developing cancer. Substantial evidence from epidemiological and laboratory-based research connects cancer to aspects of diet, yet relatively few etiological relationships have been definitively established. Observational studies of migrant populations and international comparisons of dietary habits and cancer incidence rates provide limited information. Cohort studies of diet and cancer are preferable but are often impractical owing to the relatively long induction and latency periods characteristic of cancer development. Case-control studies have been used more commonly but are constrained by the retrospective nature of the study design. Part of the difficulty in achieving high levels of validity in case-control studies is determining individuals' past nutritional intake and related food consumption behaviors with sufficient accuracy. Numerous methods of dietary assessment are used routinely in epidemiological studies, and each has its inherent strengths and weaknesses. Improvements in dietary measurement and commensurate increases in the validity of epidemiological study findings regarding diet and cancer continue to occur. Although changing dietary behavior is difficult, there is reasonable hope that, as we learn more about dietary cancer risk factors as well as the cancer prevention characteristics of certain foods, the epidemiological community will be able to make recommendations leading to a reduction of population cancer rates.

Of all the potential causes of cancer, few attract as much attention from the public and from scientists as diet. This is hardly surprising given the cultural and behavioral determinants and consequences of what we eat and drink. Consider the vast number of habits and social influences that affect our dietary choices. Also, consider a small sampling of the items about diet and health that attract our attention in the news media. For example, a recent study performed in Greece found that increased olive oil consumption was independently associated with a reduced breast cancer risk whereas margarine intake was associated with a higher risk.[1] Another study reported a link between the consumption of charbroiled and well-done meats and the risk of developing breast cancer.[2] Then there was the Dutch prospective study that observed a deficit of lung cancer in individuals who had relatively high intakes of the micronutrient selenium.[3] These three examples represent the tip of the iceberg when it comes to the information provided to the public. And because dietary modification is within our personal control, reports of an association between a food item and cancer risk frequently touch off nutritional fads, many of which fizzle because the initial findings are not supported by subsequent research findings, the recommended dietary modifications are not embraced by the medical community, or the requirements are too difficult to comply with. Of all the areas of cancer epidemiological research, the investigation of dietary factors may hold the most promise for the primary prevention of cancer, but the road to conclusive and complete knowledge will be a difficult one.

The view that food can be responsible for causing a chronic disease or a symptom complex seemed somewhat far-fetched until the causes of the primary nutritional deficiency diseases came to be understood in the 19th and early 20th centuries. The classic discoveries regarding scurvy as a vitamin C deficiency and beriberi as a thiamin deficiency paved the way for the development of research models for the purpose of studying additional nutrient-disease associations.[4] Still, it was difficult to imagine how dietary factors could be related to disorders other than those of the gastrointestinal system, including metabolic and degenerative diseases and malignancies. Now it is much more widely accepted that our food and drink contain some mutagens and carcinogens in addition to a variety of chemicals that may be able to block carcinogenesis, at least as demonstrated in animal tumor bioassay systems.[5]

In their classic review of the causes of cancer, Doll and Peto found it difficult to pinpoint the proportion of cancer deaths in the United States attributable to dietary factors. Ultimately, they suggested the exact percentage fell somewhere in the very wide range of 10% to 70%.[6] A more recent update by Willett concluded that approximately 32% of cancer deaths may be preventable through dietary modification.[7] Any cause of cancer for which primary prevention could mitigate even 10% of a population's total cancer mortality burden offers an impressive opportunity for research and public health action.

This chapter begins with an overview of the terminology related to foods and nutrients as a necessary basis for understanding epidemiological research on nutrition and cancer. Next, the chapter reviews the methods and limitations of epidemiological studies of diet, including modern techniques for assessing an individual's diet. The chapter then summarizes the state of epidemiological knowledge about important associations between dietary factors and cancer causation, although a detailed description of every dietary factor associated with one or more cancers is beyond its scope. The chapter concludes with a presentation of the American Cancer Society Guidelines for nutrition and cancer prevention.

AN OVERVIEW OF FOODS AND NUTRIENTS

Following is the framework provided by Willett[8] for classifying the vast number of constituents of foods consumed by humans. The categories are not necessarily exclusive:

- *Energy sources.* Energy sources, including proteins, carbohydrates, fats, and alcohol, are transformed into energy to sustain life.
- *Nutrients.* Nutrients, including vitamins, minerals, lipids, and amino acids, are required for good health.
- *Other natural compounds.* Countless enzymes and enzyme inhibitors, specialized lipids, genetic material, and other substances are required to sustain animal and plant cell structure and function. Cholesterol, for example, is an important structural component of animal cell membranes.
- *Natural toxins.* Although most people consider pesticides to be chemical food contaminants, some pesticides are produced naturally by plants as a defense

mechanism. The toxins that make some plants poisonous to humans provide an obvious example of natural toxins.

- *Microbial contamination.* Foods are easily contaminated, especially during processing or storage, by fungi. Aflatoxins such as aspergillus have received much attention because of their etiologic link to liver cancer.
- *Food additives.* Substances are added to foods to preserve them or to improve their color, taste, or consistency. These chemicals attract a great deal of public attention and concern, yet they are among the best characterized and most intensively regulated.
- *Agricultural contaminants.* These substances include fungicides, herbicides, pesticides, and growth hormones.
- *Inorganic contaminants.* Inorganic substances, including metals, such as lead and cadmium, and synthetic compounds, such as polychlorinated biphenyls, can contaminate our food supply.
- *Chemicals formed by cooking.* Numerous substances are created by cooking foods. Some specific agents created by cooking or charring meats have been hypothesized to cause cancer of the gastrointestinal system.

It should be clear that this wide array of food constituents presents a great challenge to cancer researchers engaged in the investigation of dietary factors. Even when an association between a food and cancer risk is observed through epidemiological study, disentangling the specific dietary component likely to be the cancer cause usually presents many difficulties.

TYPES OF STUDIES USED TO INVESTIGATE THE RELATIONSHIP BETWEEN DIET AND CANCER

Experimental Studies

Epidemiological studies of diet and cancer are extremely difficult to design and carry out. One reason is that the many behavioral, cultural, and demographic determinants of what and how a person eats and drinks create a large potential for confounding. Experimental researchers use the tool of randomization to prevent confounding, but those conducting an observational epidemiology study have no such option. For example, researchers interested in learning whether persons who consume a relatively large amount of their daily caloric consumption from "fast foods" have an increased risk of cancer would have to contend with the high probability that frequenters of fast-food establishments have different socioeconomic and employment backgrounds, different smoking and alcohol intake patterns, and different weights than nonfrequenters. Randomized, controlled trials remove much of the threat of confounding by these extraneous factors by allocating subjects to "treatment" or "control" groups in a way that distributes these factors fairly evenly. Unfortunately, except for certain randomized trials of vitamins or other micronutrients, experimental studies are incapable of addressing most diet and cancer hypotheses. The numerous potential problems that would typically arise include subject compliance (eg, maintaining the interest of subjects in taking supplements for an extended period of time with no obvious benefit), the required duration of follow-up to determine whether an intervention has caused an effect (eg, following persons to determine the incidence of a solid cancer of the gastrointestinal system following a chemoprevention regimen), and ethical concerns (eg, randomizing women to different alcohol consumption levels to observe the impact of alcohol use on breast cancer risk). Nevertheless, several notable chemoprevention randomized trials have been completed successfully, including the Physician's Health Study.[9]

Population-based Cohort and Case-Control Studies

One problem common to most population-based epidemiological studies of diet and cancer is the lack of significant variability in the diets of persons who live in the same society. If the range of dietary intake is limited by the availability of foods or by the habits or preferences of individuals, a study may not have sufficient power to identify disease outcomes caused or prevented by exposure to a dietary factor. This is likely to be a problem in more fully developed nations, where food consumption patterns tend to be more stable. Greater dietary variability is more likely to occur in nations whose economies are undergoing rapid development or where population shifts are taking place, especially from rural to urban locations. The rapidly evolving economies and social systems of Southeast Asia, for example, present an opportunity to study sizable groups possessing dietary patterns marked by both agrarian and urban lifestyles.

Case-control studies are additionally constrained by measurement error. While this problem is not unique to studies of diet, it may be a more serious problem for them given the generally low variation in dietary patterns referred to above.[10] Other conventional methodological challenges presented by case-control studies also must be dealt with, including identifying controls in institutionally based studies who have conditions etiologically unrelated to the dietary factor being studied; avoiding selective participation by groups of individuals, including those who are more prone to have positive health behaviors than nonparticipants; and mitigating the potential for differential recall of former dietary habits based on the influence of having been diagnosed with what may be perceived to be a diet-related cancer.

Methods for trying to enhance the validity of dietary recall are discussed later. The conduct of prospective cohort studies would certainly prevent some of the biases that plague case-control studies, since the reporting of dietary intake precedes the development of any hypothesized cancer. These studies also may incorporate serial measurements of dietary intake over time, thus allowing the assessment of intraindividual dietary variability. However, there are serious practical barriers to the conduct of prospective studies, including the large number of subjects required to study even the most common cancers and the great organizational effort, expense, and time that prospective studies require.

Migrant Studies

According to the conventional view, if cancer risk is genetically determined, group members who migrate from their place of origin to a new location should maintain cancer rates that are similar to those of the friends and neighbors they left behind. Alternatively, if cancer risk is greatly influenced by environmental, cultural, or lifestyle factors, including dietary constituents, cancer rates in a migrant population should eventually mimic those of the population in the new location. A cancer rate intermediate between those of the new and old locations indicates that the rate results from both genetic and external risk factors or that a gradual adjustment toward the rate in the new location is occurring. In the latter case, migrant studies can be useful in helping estimate the induction and latency periods for cancers caused by specific causal factors. Countries of the Mediterranean region of Europe have seen notable population transitions to urban centers in the past two decades. Researchers who are able to control for the nondietary environmental influences that accompany this pattern of intranational migration have a useful opportunity to examine how shifts in dietary pattern influence cancer rates.

Special Dietary Exposure Groups

Occasionally, researchers are given the chance to conduct epidemiological studies in populations with distinct dietary patterns. For example, groups like the largely vegetarian Seventh-Day Adventists have been reported to have markedly lower rates of colon cancer.[11] This fact seemingly supports the hypothesis that meat or dietary fat is a cause of colon disease. As intuitively plausible as this hypothesis is, the danger of confounding is great, since there are numerous other dietary characteristics (eg, lower alcohol consumption) and nondietary characteristics (eg, geographic location) common to this group but not to the comparison groups that could be selected by epidemiologists.

Occasionally, researchers uncover highly specific dietary customs that are strongly associated with elevated cancer rates. One example is the noted association between betel-nut chewing, a practice common among men and women in India and other Asian countries, and cancer of the esophagus. Indian men and women who chew betel nuts have been reported to have greater than a 15-fold and 6-fold excess risk, respectively, of this aggressive fatal cancer.[12] Ironically, persons who smoke a local type of cigarette (bidi) in addition to chewing the betel had lower risks, perhaps because they spit out the liquid extract, unlike nonsmokers, who do not spit it out.[13] Another example is the association between consumption of highly salted fish, which is a staple of certain southern Chinese populations, and cancer of the nasopharynx. A large, consistent body of epidemiological evidence, mainly from case-control studies, has confirmed the existence of a strong association. According to one estimate, as many as 90% of the new cases of this relatively common cancer in some Cantonese populations may be attributable to consumption of salted fish.[14]

Ecologic Studies

Early studies of possible associations between diet and cancer mostly compared cancer rates in populations with varying intake levels of dietary constituents, such as fat or alcohol. A strong correlation between a nutritional constituent and a cancer was taken as evidence of a possible causal relationship. The findings of these studies then provoked more concerted and detailed studies to ascertain whether the observed trends were reproducible at the individual level. Yet, as described in the preceding section, numerous risk factors for cancer apart from the dietary constituents being investigated are likely to vary between geographic regions. For example, cancer rates for specific organ sites differ significantly in Japan and in the United States, but so do countless lifestyle and environmental factors, not to mention hereditary factors. A positive correlation between a dietary factor and cancer incidence may serve to stimulate a new theory and may provide limited evidence in support of an existing theory, but in and of itself it cannot provide an adequate basis for concluding that a causal association exists.

METHODS FOR DETERMINING DIETARY INTAKE

A detailed review of the tools and methods for discovering individuals' short- and long-term dietary patterns is beyond the scope of this chapter. Those wishing to pursue this topic further are advised to consult other texts.[8] Nevertheless, it is important to understand the complexities involved in studying diet and cancer epidemiologically, and therefore a brief overview is presented here.

Per Capita Food Intake

Cross-sectional studies, including those performed on migrant populations, sometimes make use of population-based "food-basket" estimates of consumption. A per capita estimate may be reached by aggregating data on the quantities of local, domestic, and imported foods produced and purchased; subtracting the amount of food exported, fed to livestock, and used for nonfood purposes; and dividing the remainder by the estimated population. Among other limitations, this method does not account for foods produced at home or for foods purchased but not eaten due to waste and other factors. Food-basket estimates are obviously very imprecise as measures of food actually eaten by any individual and therefore have very limited value in epidemiological studies.

Food Inventories

After researchers define a fixed period, they can acquire data on average per capita food intake by having trained interviewers guide the principal household food preparers through a standardized, structured interview about foods purchased, prepared, and consumed. Usually, this method is not able to elicit exact details on actual food consumption by individual members of a family (except for small children) because it fails to capture information on foods consumed outside the home or not in the presence of the preparer. Nevertheless, food inventories are able to estimate familial dietary patterns with greater sensitivity and specificity than the food-basket technique.

Individual Dietary Intake

Etiologic studies must rely on data collected about an individual's nutritional exposures during the time period relevant to the presumed induction and latency period of the particular cancer under scrutiny. Nearly always, gathering such data requires asking the subject—or possibly a surrogate, such as the parent of a young child or a family member who has survived a deceased subject—about food consumption.

Recent Recall

In this commonly used technique, research participants are asked to report consumption of a limited number of food items or of all foods consumed over a recent defined time, such as 1 day, several days, or an entire week. It is usually assumed that the 24-hour recall will be more "accurate" than longer term recall because memory of recent intake is likely to be greater. On the other hand, 24-hour recall is likely to lead to a poorer estimate of a person's typical diet than if the report included a longer period, such as 3 days (including at least 1 weekend day) or 1 week, because there is a fair amount of variation in a person's dietary pattern (eg, the person may be ill or traveling on a given day). As is evident, there is a tradeoff between the expected loss of accuracy associated with a longer recall period and the higher probability of nonrepresentativeness associated with the 24-hour recall period. If the researcher's goal is to measure group dietary intake, 24-hour recall information collected on a large cross-section of some defined population may lead to a reasonable estimate.

Short-term recall data may be recorded directly by a subject on a form or a computer screen or may be "entered" orally on a tape recorder for future coding and microcomputer entry by a research staff member. Gathering recall data can be facilitated by using trained interviewers operating face to face or over the telephone, although trained interviewers add considerably to the expense of doing a study. In order to increase the reliability of short-term recall data, subjects are sometimes asked to complete a food frequency questionnaire as well.

Food Diaries

Participants in nutritional surveys are sometimes provided with structured forms and asked to record all foods consumed over a defined period of up to one week. They are asked to carefully record the type and amount of food consumed, including relatively precise data on the size and weight of each food item. Accommodation must be made for portions of food served on a plate but not consumed as well as for all foods consumed outside of the home. The pros and cons of this technique are quite evident. The prospective nature of the technique should enhance the accuracy of the reporting and lead to the acquisition of potentially valuable quantitative information about food portions. On the other hand, the relatively high burden placed on the participants often requires that they be compensated or have a special interest in the nutritional issues under investigation, and, if the latter, their interest may render them different from nonparticipants in ways that affect the research findings (ie, selection bias may occur). Also, the fact that participants are being "observed" may influence them to change their consumption patterns during the follow-up period. A participant may, for example, forgo a midday snack consisting of a candybar in favor of a piece of fruit or no snack at all. Depending on how the diary results are to be used, this "Hawthorne effect" may adversely impact the validity of the findings.[15]

All of the above methods for collecting data on dietary patterns have at best limited value for etiologic cancer epidemiology, since they do not address dietary patterns that would be relevant to the possible causation of a cancer. Considering that latency periods are between 5 and 30 years for most cancers, eating habits must be assessed for the relevant induction period, which terminates only when the latent cancer is established.

For this reason, epidemiologists tend to rely on dietary history techniques, recognizing that these have their own limitations.

Dietary Histories

Dietary histories are used to estimate former dietary patterns of relevance to the specific purpose of a study. In a case-control study of esophageal cancer, for example, the dietary history questionnaire would perhaps focus on the consumption of foods containing nitrites (which can be converted in the body to cancer-related nitrosamines). The researchers might use the questionnaire to inquire about a case subject's consumption of a range of nitrite-containing foods during the theorized induction period for the subject's cancer and about a control subject's consumption of such foods during the same period. Data are typically recorded as frequencies of consumption (eg, "When you were between 30 and 40 years of age, how many times per week, on average, did you eat deli meats?"). Food models and/or photographs can help subjects estimate portion sizes and can thus improve the quality of the reporting. Information from individual questionnaires would likely be summed to arrive at a cumulative nitrite amount or other quantitative estimate.

Dietary history data are usually collected through a written questionnaire or a personal interview. Careful training of interviewers and subjects is required if this technique is to provide a reasonable estimate of former food consumption. Additional strategies for increasing the accuracy of dietary history data include interviewer probing (eg, asking questions not only about food consumption but also about food preparation techniques) and asking subjects for related information in two different ways or in different sections of the questionnaire. Dietary histories lack the precision of dietary logs but can be used to assess food intake during a relevant exposure period.

Use of Surrogates

When studying aggressive fatal cancers, it is sometimes impossible to obtain the necessary historical dietary data from case subjects (and even control subjects, of course, can die before being questioned). Depending on the amount of specificity required, the relevant dietary information may be collected from a surviving family member, such as a spouse or an adult child. Studies that compared dietary information collected from case subjects while still alive and from family surrogates show mixed results. For example, Lerchen and Samet asked wives of men who died of lung cancer to report their husbands' typical intake of six foods selected from the original questionnaire (carrots, chili, eggs, liver, and peaches).[16] The reliability of the two reports was judged to be good, but complete information was reported for only about 80% of the case subjects, and owing to the extent of the missing data, an index of vitamin A intake could not be computed for about 10% of the subjects based on the wives' responses.[17]

Using similar methodologies, it has been shown that the level of agreement between subjects and their surrogates in reporting the type and amount of foods consumed seems to depend on the food being assessed. In two studies from Hawaii and New York State, researchers found agreement to be higher for meats than for fruits and vegetables.[18,19] One possibility is that agreement is greater for foods most often consumed inside the home; another is that agreement is better for "unusual foods" (eg, quiche, Brussels sprouts) than for "everyday foods" (eg, milk, fruit).

Biological Markers

Biological markers are discussed at length in Chapter 6. Much of the rationale for using biomarkers rests on an underlying theory of disease causality. They are particularly relevant for the study of cancer because it generally has a long induction period and because mutational events are thought to be common first steps in the progression of cancer. The use of biomarkers may thus allow detection of cellular changes associated with cancer to occur earlier than otherwise possible and may enable treatment to begin earlier. In addition, biomarkers may reduce bias and misclassification and may enhance our understanding of the pathology of cancer. Most importantly, biomarkers may be extremely valuable as adjunct tools in the measurement of dietary intake.

Biological markers serve a dual purpose in studies of dietary intake. They may be used as surrogates for or indicators of nutrient intake and they may be used for validating other methods of quantifying dietary assessment. Examples of specific biochemical indicators for nutrients include retinol and retinyl esters for vitamin A, adipose α-tocopherol for vitamin E, ascorbic acid for vitamin C, lycopene for tomato products, and isoflavonoids for soy products. As measures of dietary intake, biomarkers have the advantage of being relatively objective and quantifiable and not being subject to the inconsistencies of individual recall. In addition, they often work extremely well for foods that exhibit a high degree of variability in nutrient content.

However, the use of biomarkers does have some drawbacks. They may be subject to the individual homeostatic mechanisms that control the concentration of many of the body's nutrients and therefore may not exhibit a linear relationship with nutrient intake. Another factor affecting the measurement of biomarkers is the bioavailability of specific nutrients. In addition, some biomarkers may only be sensitive to recent food intake, making these less desirable for the study of chronic diseases such as cancer. Most importantly, individual lifestyle, genetic, and other environmental factors may play a significant role in the level of nutrients measured in the body, and their relationship with potential biomarkers must be given due attention. Although biomarkers represent an advance in nutritional epidemiology, the above considerations must be taken into account to avoid the misclassification of subjects with respect to dietary intake.

As for specific dietary biomarkers implicated in the development of cancer, many have been hypothesized but few have been established unequivocally through empirical research. Aflatoxin, a mycotoxin produced by fungi on foods such as corn and peanuts, has been strongly implicated in the occurrence of liver cancer. The DNA adduct AFB-N-7-guanine has been established as a reliable biomarker for aflatoxin and has a demonstrated significant association with liver cancer.[20] However, research on other biomarkers has not led to significant results. Perhaps the most studied group of biomarkers are those associated with the nutritional compounds known as antioxidants (eg, carotenoids, ascorbic acid, and α-tocopherol). Because antioxidants are thought to mitigate the oxidative damage to cells from free radical compounds, one hypothesis is that they may be protective for a variety of cancers. This hypothesis is controversial, and evidence from a randomized clinical trial showed no beneficial and perhaps even some harmful effects of α-tocopherol and β-carotene in relation to lung and other cancers.[9] Another class of compounds, heterocyclic amines, that occur when meats are charred or cooked to "well done," are well established as potent mutagens.[21] While etiologic relationships between heterocyclic amines and specific cancers have yet to be strongly established, there is some evidence for an association between heterocyclic amines and gastric cancer.[22] Another group of biochemical markers recently studied consists of isoflavonoids, which are derived mainly from soy intake. Results from a study in Shanghai, where soy intake is high, indicated that the risk of breast cancer was inversely related to the excretion rates of isoflavonoids.[23]

EPIDEMIOLOGICAL EVIDENCE REGARDING DIET AND CANCER

This section summarizes what is known about some specific dietary constituents. For nearly every constituent listed, there are insufficient or inconsistent data, and so scientists and public health officials need to temper the advice they offer the general public about making changes in individual dietary behaviors. Because changing eating behaviors is extraordinarily difficult, a recommendation to reduce or increase a dietary constituent should be made only when the weight of evidence clearly favors the change. Given the established casual association between certain fats and coronary disease, the reduction in colorectal cancer that seems to result from decreasing fat intake can be presented as simply an additional benefit of a low-fat diet. Unfortunately, most of the dietary constituents listed below have only been associated with an increase or decrease in cancer risk in epidemiological studies, and their etiologic effects have received little confirmation from experimental research in the medical and related health sciences.

As summarized by Willett[10] and others (as noted), dietary constituents reported to raise or lower the risk of cancer include the following:

- *Additives.* Thousands of substances are intentionally added during the processing of food, some of which, like sugar, are consumed in huge quantities. Many others unintentionally contaminate food, but these amount to a minute portion of our total food consumption. Except for studies in the 1970s and 1980s on artificial sweeteners, little epidemiological research has been done on the risks and benefits of food additives with respect to cancer.
- *Agricultural chemicals.* Interest in the potential carcinogenicity of fertilizers, pesticides, crop growth regulators, and related chemicals is high, especially because of the nearly universal recommendation that fruits and vegetables be consumed in high quantities by adults and children alike. It is reassuring that official surveys indicate that the pesticide-limit violation rate is only 1% to 2% for domestic produce and 2% to 4% for imported produce. In 1996, the US Environmental Protection Agency signed into law the Food Quality Protection Act, which governs the ways in which pesticides are regulated, and over the years to come the agency will revise the tolerance limits for the approximately 9,000 pesticides used on US crops. Also, the National Cancer Institute, other collaborating agencies, and manufacturers of agricultural chemicals are placing a new emphasis on research designed to determine the health effects of agricultural chemicals. Note, however, that the information gathered on this issue to date fails to support the conclusion that agricultural chemicals pose an important cancer risk to consumers.

- *Antioxidants.* These nutrients, found especially in fruits and vegetables, resist oxygen-induced damage to tissue. Antioxidants that have received a great deal of public attention recently include vitamins C and E, selenium, and β-carotene. Of three clinical trials designed to determine whether β-carotene, at high doses, lowers individual cancer risk, two found that, among smokers of cigarettes, users of the supplements had a higher lung cancer risk than nonusers.[9,24] Vitamin C has been suggested to confer a reduced risk of developing oral and other gastrointestinal system cancers.[25] However, other factors found in fruits and vegetables rich in vitamin C may be responsible for the salubrious effect attributed to the vitamin. Furthermore, the biochemical mechanisms by which antioxidants would actually impede the development or progression of cancer remain theoretical.
- *Calcium.* Very limited evidence has been reported suggesting that high intake of foods rich in calcium is associated with a decreased risk of colorectal cancer.
- *Cholesterol.* Low blood cholesterol has been associated with cancer, but the reduction in level has been explained as a likely result of the cancer itself.
- *Coffee.* Studies have been inconsistent. Overall, there is no conclusive evidence that coffee consumption affects the risk of cancer.
- *Energy intake.* Total energy intake, as estimated by obesity, has been related to colon cancer in men and endometrial cancer in women. The evidence is less consistent for postmenopausal breast cancer, but high body mass is associated with a decreased risk of premenopausal breast cancer.[26] Willett has suggested that the explanation may be that obese women have more anovulatory menstrual cycles.[10] The evidence regarding height as a risk factor for cancer is even less consistent. Further study of this issue is important, because adult height is closely related to dietary experiences in youth, and therefore an association between height and cancer that reflects an underlying causal mechanism could be quite illuminating.
- *Fat.* The possible role of dietary fat in the development of cancer has received more attention than that of any other dietary constituent. The sites most frequently studied and for which an association has been observed are the breast, colon, and prostate. The data are more convincing for meat intake and colon cancer than for the other sites, and it is conceivable that the observed association could be due to factors in meat other than fat.
- *Fiber.* Insoluble fiber (eg, wheat bran) has been reported to reduce the risk of colorectal cancer, but the data do not conclusively establish the amount of the risk reduction or the level of intake required to produce the effect. One theory is that the fiber reduces the effect of potential carcinogens in the intestinal system by decreasing their transit time through the body. In studies that distinguish various sources of fiber, fiber from fruits and vegetables has been shown to be more beneficial than fiber from cereals.[27,28]
- *Fish oils.* Animal research has suggested that fish oils, which are rich in omega-3 fatty acids, help suppress cancer formation.
- *Folic acid.* This B vitamin is hypothesized to reduce the risk of certain cancers, but the mechanism of its purported action is unclear.
- *Irradiated foods.* Radiation is used as a way to kill harmful organisms in food but does not remain in the food. There is no link with cancer.

- *Nitrites.* Nitrates are used as a preservative in meats and can be converted to nitrosamines in the intestinal system. Nitrosamines are carcinogenic and may cause stomach cancer. Vitamin C blocks the conversion of nitrites to nitrosamines.
- *Salt.* Per capita salt intake has declined in industrialized nations this century, as the need to use it as a food preservative has been obviated. The decline correlates with a decline in stomach cancer, suggesting to some that the association is causal.
- *Tea.* It has been proposed that green tea may be able to reduce the risk of cancer of the skin and other sites based mainly on experimental studies of animals.[29]

As for the mechanism through which nutritional factors could be involved in carcinogenesis, a variety of theories exist. These theories, which relate both to tumor initiation and to tumor promotion, were developed mainly on the basis of animal studies, and further research in human populations must precede their acceptance. For example, one study found that a selenium-supplemented diet inhibited mammary cancer in female rats and that a high-fat diet enhanced initiation.[30] There is no direct evidence linking dietary constituents to the process of DNA repair, and the precise mechanism leading to cancer initiation is speculative. Evidence relating diet to tumor promotion is more abundant but also not conclusive. Studies of the rat mammary gland, mouse skin, rat intestine, and rat and mouse liver have indicated that increased intake of calories and fat enhances tumor promotion and that intake of selected nutrients such as vitamin D and selenium retards it.[31] Finally, certain nutrients have been demonstrated to interfere with the later-stage progression of cancers in animals and perhaps in humans. Retinoids (derived from carotenoids), for example, seem to slow down the progression of certain precancerous lesions in the urinary tract and also to reduce the risk of secondary cancers of the aerodigestive tract in individuals already being treated for primary cancers of the larynx, esophagus, and other organs.

DIET AND CANCER: A GLOBAL PERSPECTIVE

The urbanization of countries, especially those undergoing rapid development, is a continuing phenomenon. Referred to as the "demographic transition," the movement of people from rural locations to cities is difficult to stop, even when government incentives or policies stand in opposition. By the year 2005, half the population of the world will live in cities.[32] The evolution of new dietary patterns that follow urban migration has been termed the "nutrition transition."[33] The transition is toward foods relatively low in starch and fiber and relatively high in animal fat and sugar as well as refined foods. Although it is difficult, because of the parallel sociocultural changes, to establish that the changes in cancer incidence in these countries are due to the nutritional transition, the claim that diet is partly responsible for the changes in incidence is reasonable. Ironically, in most economically developed countries, consumer demand has led to the reintroduction of less refined and processed foods into daily diets during the 1990s. Figure 16–1 offers a picture of dietary patterns in 14 regions of the world. A strong correlation be-

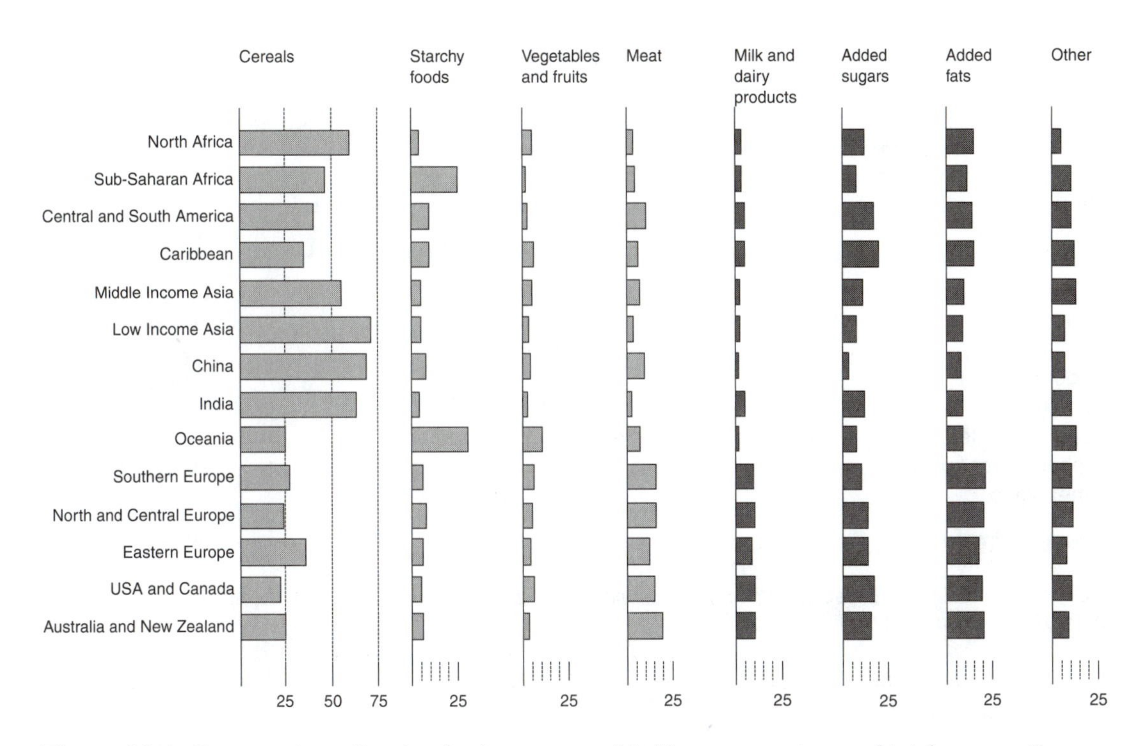

Figure 16–1 Consumption of major food groups worldwide as percentages of total energy. *Source:* From World Cancer Research Fund in Association with American Institute for Cancer Research, *Food Nutrition and the Prevention of Cancer: A Global Perspective*, © 1997. Reprinted by permission of the American Institute for Cancer Research.

---

tween economic development and the consumption of dairy products, meat, and added fats is evident.

Changes in the food supply will continue to be driven by consumer choices as well as governmental policies relating to food health and safety. Recent, highly publicized food-related outbreaks of illnesses such as "mad cow disease" have had a salubrious effect. The public is increasingly considering the health consequences of its eating habits, and if scientists can continue to produce valid findings translatable into practical recommendations regarding cancer prevention, favorable international incidence and mortality trends may start to occur in the next century.

DECREASING THE BURDEN OF CANCER THROUGH DIETARY MODIFICATION

We return now to the question of how to reduce the burden of cancer in a population through individual dietary change. Using available epidemiological evidence on cancer causation, Willett[7] has slightly modified the Doll and Peto[6] estimates and has calculated a point estimate as well as a range for the percentage of avoidable cancer deaths. Admittedly, Willet's estimates are rough, but they can still play a role in supporting persons wishing to make healthy lifestyle changes. As seen in Table 16–1, prostate cancer mor-

Table 16–1 Cancer Deaths Avoidable by Dietary Change, 1994

Type of Cancer	*Current*	*Avoidable Percentage (%) Range*
Lung	20	10–30
Colon/rectum	70	50–80
Breast	50	20–80
Prostate	75	20–80
Pancreas	50	10–50
Stomach	35	30–70
Endometrium	50	50–80
Gall bladder	50	50–80
Larynx, bladder, cervix, mouth, pharynx, esophagus	20	10–30
Other types	10	—
Overall estimate	32	20–42

Source: Reproduced with permission from *Environmental Health Perspectives*, Vol. 103, Supplement 8, W.C. Willett, Diet Nutrition and Avoidable Cancer, pp. 165–170, 1995.

tality and colorectal cancer mortality have the greatest potential for reduction through dietary change given the current state of knowledge.

Research able to discriminate causal relationships between diet and cancer risk from statistical correlations is now needed. If even a small number of causal connections are found and publicized, the incidence of cancer should begin to decline. Schatzkin et al[34] proposed that observational and experimental epidemiological research be combined with metabolic (clinical) studies and animal research to generate the range of results necessary to discover which relationships are causal.

Dietary recommendations can be used to reduce the risk not only of cardiovascular diseases but also of various cancers. *Social marketing* is a term used to describe the application of business marketing techniques to the cause of improving public health or welfare.[35] Much work is currently being done to identify ways to promote healthy dietary practices in the general population. Programs for educating the public about health matters through the mass media need to adhere to a set of rational principles. In late 1996, the American Cancer Society Advisory Committee on Diet, Nutrition and Cancer Prevention published guidelines for advising the public about dietary habits that could help reduce their individual cancer risk.[36] Summarized in Exhibit 16–1, the guidelines advocate a diet high in fruits and vegetables and low in fats and alcohol, and they also advocate a lifestyle that includes regular, moderate activity and maintenance of a healthy weight. The guidelines lack specific recommendations on the consumption of micronutrients, which is perhaps disappointing to some health professionals. However, the reality is that research has not yet been successful in identifying incontrovertible associations, despite a number of promising leads in the investigation of dietary constituents that may result in true primary prevention opportunities.

Another recent programmatic attempt to reduce cancer risk through dietary behavior modification is the National Cancer Institute's Five A Day Program. The program,

Exhibit 16–1 American Cancer Society Guidelines on Diet, Nutrition, and Cancer Prevention

1. Choose most of the food you eat from plant sources.
   - Eat five or more servings of fruits and vegetables each day.
   - Eat other foods from plant sources, such as breads, cereals, grain products, rice, pasta, or beans several times each day.
2. Limit your intake of high-fat foods, particularly from animal sources.
   - Choose foods low in fat.
   - Limit consumption of meats, especially high-fat meats.
3. Be physically active.
   - Achieve and maintain a healthy weight.
   - Be at least moderately active for 30 minutes or more on most days of the week.
   - Stay within your healthy weight range.
4. Limit consumption of alcoholic beverages, if you drink at all.

Source: From *CA: A Cancer Journal for Clinicians*, Vol. 46, pp. 325–341, © 1996 by the American Cancer Society. Reprinted with permission from Lippincott-Raven Publishers.

which encourages individuals to eat five or more servings of fruits and vegetables daily, has forged partnerships with many state health departments and with many industrial partners in the food and agriculture sectors to market its message and to evaluate the message's impact.

Finally, it is notable that several diets, more popular internationally, are now being followed by increasing numbers of Americans. Most evident are the traditional Mediterranean diet and the macrobiotic diet. Ecologic data show that overall cancer rates and several site-specific cancer rates are lower in populations where these diets are prevalent. Also, case studies indicate that some cancer patients, following a macrobiotic diet, appear to have overcome cancer following a grave prognosis.[37] Systematic research is needed to address these claims and it is likely that studies of this topic will be planned.

SUMMARY

In the 21st century, the potential role of nutrients and other dietary factors as primary etiologic agents in human carcinogenesis will continue to be investigated. Although the public seems to have grown somewhat weary of being apprised of epidemiological results of dietary studies that have not stood the test of time, the quest for well-founded dietary recommendations that can reduce individual cancer risk remains a high priority. If specific results are not forthcoming in the near future, it will still be possible for the public health community to continue to recommend adherence to general guidelines aimed at stemming obesity and reducing the proportion of dietary calories derived from fat. There is sufficient evidence that the same guidelines that promote healthy living from a cardiovascular disease point of view also can lower cancer risk. Even if overestimates of the reduction in cancer incidence possible through healthful diets abound, meaningful decreases can be achieved by using the information already in hand.

Discussion Questions

1. For each of the following diet-cancer associations, provide some evidence in support of an etiologic hypothesis, and, if possible, also provide counter-evidence indicating why the association may not be causal: fiber and colon cancer, alcohol and breast cancer, and antioxidants and cancer in general.
2. Compare the methods of the "recent recall" with the "dietary record" in terms of their (1) potential validity and (2) consumer acceptability. Assume that the goal is to assess current dietary behavior rather than former behavior.
3. Identify one or more diets that have been promoted as protective against cancer (eg, macrobiotic diet, Mediterranean diet, etc.). Based on current epidemiological evidence, what characteristics of these diets, if any, would likely reduce cancer risk? In general terms, is there enough information in your opinion to publicize these diets as anticarcinogenic? Why or why not?

References

1. Trichopoulou A, Katsouyanni K, Stuver S, et al. Consumption of olive oil and specific food groups in relation to breast cancer risk in Greece. *J Natl Cancer Inst.* 1995;87:110–116.
2. Ward MH, Sinha R, Heinman EF, et al. Risk of adenocarcinoma of the stomach and esophagus with meat cooking method and doneness preference. *Int J Cancer.* 1997;7:14–19.
3. Van den Brandt PA, Van't Veer P, Goldbohm RR, et al. A prospective cohort study on selenium status and the risk of lung cancer. *Cancer Res.* 1993;53:4860–4865.
4. National Research Council. *Diet, Nutrition, and Cancer.* Washington, DC: National Academy Press; 1982.
5. Prochaska HJ, Sanatamaria AB, Talay P. Rapid detection of inducers of enzymes that protect against carcinogens. *Proc Natl Acad Sci USA.* 1992;89:2394–2399.
6. Doll R, Peto R. The causes of cancer: quantitative estimates of avoidable risks of cancer in the United States today. *J Natl Cancer Inst.* 1981;66:1191–1308.
7. Willett WC. Diet, nutrition and avoidable cancer. *Environ Health Perspect.* 1995;103(suppl 8):165–170.
8. Willett WC. *Nutritional Epidemiology.* New York: Oxford University Press; 1998.
9. Hennekens CH, Buring JE, Manson JE, et al. Lack of effect of long-term supplementation with beta carotene on the incidence of malignant neoplasms and cardiovascular disease. *N Engl J Med.* 1996;334:1145–1149.
10. Willett WC. Diet and nutrition. In: Schottenfeld D, Fraumeni JF Jr, eds. *Cancer Epidemiology and Prevention.* 2nd ed. New York: Oxford University Press; 1996:438–461.
11. Phillips RL, Garfinkel L, Kuzma JW, Beson WL, Lotz T, Brin B. Mortality among California Seventh-Day Adventists for selected cancer sites. *J Natl Cancer Inst.* 1980;65:1097–1107.
12. Jussawalla DJ, Deshpande VA. Evaluation of cancer risk in tobacco chewers and smokers: an epidemiologic assessment. *Cancer.* 1971;28:244–252.
13. Munoz N, Day NE. Esophageal cancer. In: Schottenfeld D, Fraumeni JF Jr, eds. *Cancer Epidemiology and Prevention.* 2nd ed. New York: Oxford University Press; 1996:681–706.
14. Yu MC, Huang T-B, Henderson BE. Diet and nasopharyngeal carcinoma: a case-control study in Guangxi, China. *Int J Cancer.* 1989;43:1077–1082.
15. Block G, Woods M, Potosky A, Clifford C. Validation of a self-administered diet questionnaire using multiple diet records. *J Clin Epidemiol.* 1990; 43:1327–1335.
16. Lerchen ML, Samet JM. An assessment of the validity of questionnaire responses provided by a surrogate spouse. *Am J Epidemiol.* 1986;123:481–489.
17. Samet JM, Alberg AJ. Surrogate sources of dietary information. In: Willett W. *Nutritional Epidemiology.* New York: Oxford University Press; 1998:157–173.
18. Kolonel LN, Hirohata T, Nomura AM. Adequacy of survey data collected from substitute respondents. *Am J Epidemiol.* 1977;106:476–484.

19. Marshall J, Priore R, Haughey B, Rzepka T, Graham S. Spouse-subject interviews and the reliability of diet studies. *Am J Epidemiol.* 1980;112:675–683.
20. Groopman JD, Hall AJ, Whittle H, et al. Molecular dosimetry of aflatoxin-N7-guanine in human urine obtained in The Gambia, West Africa. *Cancer Epidemiol Biomarkers Prev.* 1992;1:221–227.
21. Weisburger JH, Rivenson A, Reinhardt J, et al. Genotoxicity and carcinogenicity in rats and mice of 2-amino-3,6-dihydro-3-methyl-7H-imidazole [4,5-f] quinolin-7-one: an intestinal bacterial metabolite of 2-amino-3-methyl-3H-imidazo [4,5-f] quinoline. *J Natl Cancer Inst.* 1994;86:25–30.
22. Correa P, Fontham E, Pickle LW, et al. Dietary determinants of gastric cancer in south Louisiana inhabitants. *J Natl Cancer Inst.* 1985;75:645–654.
23. Zheng W, Dai Q, Custer LJ, Shu XO, Wen WQ, Jin F, Franke AA. Urinary excretion of isoflavonoids and the risk of breast cancer. *Cancer Epidemiol Biomarkers Prev.* 1999;8:233–239.
24. Omenn G, Goodman GE, Thornquist MD, et al. Effects of a combination of beta carotene and vitamin A on lung cancer and cardiovascular disease. *N Engl J Med.* 1996;334:1150–1155.
25. American Cancer Society, Advisory Committee on Diet, Nutrition, and Cancer Prevention. Guidelines on diet, nutrition, and cancer prevention: reducing the risk of cancer with healthy food choices and physical activity. *CA Cancer J Clin.* 1996;46:325–341.
26. Le Marchand L, Kolonel LN, Earle ME, Mi MP. Body size at different periods of life and breast cancer risk. *Am J Epidemiol.* 1988;128:137–152.
27. Potter JD, McMichael AJ. Diet and cancer of the colon and rectum: a case-control study. *J Natl Cancer Inst.* 1986;76:557–569.
28. Slattery ML, Schumacher MC, Smith KR, West DW, Abdeighany N. Physical activity, diet, and risk of colon cancer in Utah. *Am J Epidemiol.* 1988;128:989–999.
29. Mukhtar H, Katiyar SK, Agarwal R. Cancer chemoprevention by green tea components in diet and cancer. In: Jacobs MM, ed. *Markers, Prevention, and Treatment.* New York: Plenum Press; 1994.
30. Wattenberg LW. Inhibition of carcinogenesis by minor dietary constituents. *Cancer Res.* 1992;52(suppl 7):2085S–2091S.
31. Pariza MW. Fat, calories, and mammary carcinogenesis: net energy effects. *Am J Clin Nutr.* 1987;45 (suppl 1):261–263.
32. *United Nations World Urbanization Prospects: The 1994 Revision.* New York: United Nations; 1995.
33. Popkin BM. The nutrition transition in low-income countries: an emerging crisis. *Nutr Rev.* 1994;52:285–298.
34. Schatzkin A, Dorgan J, Swanson C, Potischman N. Diet and cancer: future etiologic research. *Environ Health Perspect.* 1995;103(suppl 8):171–175.
35. Fox KF, Kotler P. *The Marketing of Social Causes: The First Ten Years, in Cancer, Diet, and Nutrition: A Comprehensive Sourcebook.* Chicago: Marquis; 1985.
36. American Cancer Society. *American Cancer Society Guidelines on Diet, Nutrition, and Cancer Prevention.* Atlanta, GA: American Cancer Society; 1996.
37. Kushi M. *The Macrobiotic Approach to Cancer: Towards Preventing and Controlling Cancer with Diet and Lifestyle.* Garden City Park, NY: Avery Pub. Group; 1991.

Appendix A

Informational Web Sites

Agency for Toxic Substances and Disease Registry
http://www.atsdr.cdc.gov/atsdrhome.html

Cancer Registries Resources
http://www-dep.iarc.fr/resour/software.htm

Centers for Disease Control and Prevention
http://www.cdc.gov/

Centers for Disease Control and Prevention
Morbidity and Mortality Weekly Report
http://www.cdc.gov/epo/mmwr/mmwr.html

Centers for Disease Control and Prevention
National Program of Cancer Registries
http://www.cdc.gov/cancer/npcr/reg97.htm

Epidemiology Sites
http://www.uwo.ca/epidem/other.html

Health Canada, Population and Public Health Branch
Cancer Bureau
http://www.hc-sc.gc.ca/hpb/lcdc/bc/index.html

Health on the Net Medical Search
http://www.hon.ch/

International Agency for Research on Cancer
http://www.iarc.fr

International Agency for Research on Cancer
Cancer Data Bases and Other Resources
http://www.iarc.fr/pageroot/database.html

Medical/Clinical/Occupational Toxicology Resource Home Page
http://www.pitt.edu/~martint/welcome.htm

National Academy of Sciences
http://www.nas.edu/

National Cancer Institute
CancerNet Statistics
http://cancernet.nci.nih.gov/statistics.shtml

National Center for Health Statistics
http://www.cdc.gov/nchswww/default.htm

National Institutes of Health
http://www.nih.gov/

National Toxicology Program
http://ntp-server.niehs.nih.gov/

NCRA (National Cancer Registrars Association)
http://www.ncra-usa.org/history.html

Surveillance, Epidemiology and End Results (SEER)
National Cancer Institute
http://www-seer.ims.nci.nih.gov/AboutSEER.html

US Census Bureau
http://www.census.gov

Welcome to PubMed (Medline Literature Search)
http://www.ncbi.nlm.nih.gov/PubMed/

Welcome to CDC WONDER on the Web
http://wonder.cdc.gov/

World Health Organization
http://www.who.int/

The World Wide Web Virtual Library: Epidemiology
http://www.epibiostat.ucsf.edu/epidem/epidem.html

Glossary

acetylaldehyde Major metabolite of ethanol and a known carcinogen in animals.

acquired immune deficiency syndrome (AIDS) Syndrome caused by a retrovirus, the human immunodeficiency virus (HIV), which infects and destroys $CD4^+$ helper T cells, leading to suppression of the immune system. Individuals infected with HIV become more susceptible to certain types of cancers and infections.

acquired immunodeficiency Immunodeficiency acquired as a result of exposure to agents such as drug therapy or HIV.

acquired mutations Changes in DNA acquired through exposure to external agents such as ultraviolet light or chemical agents.

acute lymphocytic leukemia (ALL) A type of leukemia that progresses rapidly and affects immature lymphocytes.

acute nonlymphocytic leukemia (ANLL) A type of leukemia that does not involve lymphocytes and can be caused by alkylating agents.

acylation A chemical process in which an acyl group is added to a molecule.

adduct The addition product between two molecules

adenocarcinoma A type of cancer that originates from the glandular epithelium.

adenosquamous carcinoma A tumor that affects both glands and squamous cells.

adjuvant chemotherapy Drug therapy given as a secondary treatment after primary treatment by another method such as surgery.

adrenal androgens Steroid hormones secreted by the adrenal glands.

adult T-cell leukemia A form of leukemia associated with the HTLV-I virus and characterized clinically by hypercalcemia.

aerodigestive tract cancer Malignant neoplasm of the oral cavity, pharynx, larynx, and esophagus.

aflatoxin A toxic compound produced by the mold *Aspergillus flavus*. The toxin binds to the DNA, thereby preventing replication and transcription, and it causes acute liver damage and liver cancer.

agammaglobulinemia of Bruton An inherited immune deficiency disease that is characterized by low levels of all classes of gamma globulin.

aldehyde dehydrogenase 2 (ALDH2) Enzyme that is responsible for eliminating acetylaldehyde from the body.

alkaline phosphatase (AFOS) Serum biomarker.

alkylation A chemical process in which an alkyl group is substituted for a hydrogen atom.

allele One of the alternate forms of a gene.

allergy Abnormal immune response to an antigen, such as dust, pollen, food, drugs, or animal dander.

Ames test A type of bioassay used to test agents for mutagenicity in bacterial systems.

amino acids Water soluble organic compounds, 20 of which make up proteins. The sequence of the amino acids determines the shape, properties, and biological roles of proteins.

anaplasia Loss of cell differentiation.

androgen A male hormone that stimulates the development of the testes and male secondary characteristics.

angiogenesis Development of new blood vessels.

angiosarcoma Lethal type of cancer that affects blood vessels of the liver.

ankylosing spondylitis Immobility and consolidation of a vertebral joint due to degenerative disease.

antagonist An agent that interferes with the normal action of a biological agent.

anterior pituitary The anterior lobe of the pituitary gland that is located at the base of the brain; it is responsible for the secretion of hormones that facilitate the proper functioning of the endocrine organs.

antibody A protein that is produced by B lymphocytes in response to an antigen.

antigen Any substance, but usually a protein, that the body regards as foreign and that elicits an immune response.

antineoplastic agent Chemotherapeutic agent used in the treatment of cancer.

antioxidant Synthetic or natural substance that eliminates free radicals from the body.

aplastic anemia A type of anemia in which the blood cells are not fully developed.

apoptosis Programmed cell death; the death of a cell that occurs as a normal process during cell development.

asbestos Fibrous minerals used commercially in the fabrication of insulation products because of their heat resistant properties.

Aspergillus flavus A mold that produces the toxin aflatoxin.

asthma Chronic disease of the respiratory system; the constriction of the alveoli that is characterized by wheezing, coughing, and difficulty in breathing.

astrocyte A type of cell that forms the structural support for the central nervous system.

ataxia-telangiectasia A type of hereditary disease (genetic instability) in which individuals are more susceptible to leukemias and lymphomas.

attributable risk The percentage of disease in a population that can be attributed to a causal factor.

atypia The condition of being irregular.

autoimmunity Disorder of the immune system in which the body's immune system begins to attack its own tissues.

avian leukosis virus A virus that causes leukemias in chickens.

Azathioprine A drug that causes immune suppression.

B lymphocyte (B cell) A type of blood cell that matures in the bone marrow and is involved in the production of antibodies.

basal cell carcinoma Tumor of the epithelial tissues.
basement membrane The extracellular material that separates the epithelium from the underlying support tissue.
BCG (Calmette-Guerin) tuberculosis vaccine A live attenuated vaccine that stimulates the immune system.
benign neoplasm Tumor that is well differentiated and remains confined to the point of origin.
benzo[*a*]pyrene An established carcinogen in animals.
beriberi A disease caused by a deficiency of vitamin B_1.
beta carotene Yellow or red pigment that is found in carrots or sweet potatoes and converted by the body into vitamin A.
bioassay A biological test that occurs outside of the body (eg, estrogen receptor assay).
biomarker Biochemical measure used to detect genetic, cellular, or molecular alterations.
biopsy The removal of tissues or cells from a living body for the purposes of microscopic examination. It is used to determine if cells are cancerous.
blastoma A neoplasm that originates from embryonic tissues.
Bloom syndrome A hereditary disease that causes genetic instability and increases the susceptibility of individuals to leukemias and lymphomas.
BRCA-1 A tumor suppressor gene that is associated with familial breast cancer.
Burkitt's lymphoma Non-Hodgkin's B-cell lymphoma. It is commonly found in Central Africa and is caused by the Epstein-Barr virus.
carcinogen Any agent that causes cancer.
carcinoma A neoplasm that originates from epithelial tissue.
causal association Relationship between an illness and an exposure that has been shown to be responsible for its development.
$CD4^+$T helper lymphocyte CD4 is a cell surface glycoprotein found on T helper cells; a $CD4^+$T helper lymphocyte is the cell that controls both humoral and cell-mediated immunity.
cell cycle Cell division occurring in four steps: G_1, S, G_2, and M; the result is the formation of two daughter cells each containing the same number of chromosomes as the parent cell.
cell-mediated response A branch of the immune response system that is mediated by T lymphocytes.
cervical intraepithelial neoplasia (CIN) A preinvasive lesion of the cervix.
cervical lymphadenopathy Regional lymph node enlargement associated with various diseases.
chemotherapy Treatment of cancer with antineoplastic drugs.
Chlamydia trachomatis A sexually transmitted bacterium that can lead to pelvic inflammatory disease (PID).
chlorambucil An antineoplastic agent used in the treatment of cancer; an immunosuppressive agent.
chloramphenicol A commonly used antibiotic that has been associated with an increased risk of leukemia.
cholesterol Fatty acid hydrocarbon found in all tissues of animals. It serves as a precursor for the production of steroid hormones.

chromosome Condensed DNA; the basic genetic material.

chromosome translocation The exchange of segments of DNA between nonhomologous chromosomes.

chronic lymphocytic leukemia (CLL) A type of leukemia that progresses slowly and affects immature lymphocytes.

chronic myelocytic leukemia (CML) A type of leukemia that progresses slowly and originates from the pluripotent stem cell.

cirrhosis Liver degeneration.

cofactor An additional factor that may act in conjunction with the main causal factor in the development of cancer.

collagenase An enzyme that cleaves collagen, which is the supportive protein structure of the skin, tendon, bone, cartilage, and connective tissue.

combined oral contraceptives An oral contraceptive that contains estrogen and progestin.

connective tissue Tissue comprising bone, muscle, and cartilage; it serves as the support structure for the organs.

corticosteroid A hormone commonly given to recipients of organ transplants to prevent organ rejection.

cotinine A metabolite of nicotine that can be measured in urine and saliva in smokers.

cytogenic The origin and the development of cells.

cyclins Proteins that aid in the control of the cell cycle.

cyclin D A protein that has negative effects on the cell cycle.

cyclin-dependent kinases (CDKs) Enzymes that aid in the regulation and control of the cell cycle (the progression of a cell from G_0 to G_1).

cyclophosphamide An immunosuppressive drug.

cyclosporine A An immunosuppressive drug.

cytochrome P-450 A protein that is found in liver cells and other tissues.

cytokines Proteins that regulate the intensity and duration of the immune response (eg, interleukin 2).

cytokinesis Cell division of cytoplasm during mitosis.

cytomegalovirus (CMV) A common viral infection that usually causes no disease but can cause serious disease among infants and immunodeficient and immunosuppressed individuals.

cytoplasm Fluidlike substance surrounding the nucleus of a cell.

cytotoxic drugs Drugs that have the ability to kill cells.

cytotoxic T cells A type of T lymphocyte that is capable of killing foreign cells.

deletion The loss of nucleotide sequences.

dephosphorylation The removal of phosphates from a protein.

diethylstilbestrol (DES) A synthetic estrogen used in the United States between 1940 and 1970 to prevent miscarriages.

differentiation The structural changes that a cell undergoes as it become specialized in particular functions.

Diphenylhydantoin (phenytoin) An anticonvulsant drug.

diuretic An agent that promotes the excretion of urine.

DNA Deoxyribonucleic acid; the genetic material of all living organisms.

DNA adduct A covalent chemical addition to the DNA, such as a mutagen or carcinogen, that creates a bulge in the DNA, leading to problems during replication and protein synthesis.

DNA-dependent RNA polymerase II An enzyme that is required during the transcription process. It is involved in the initiation of transcription at the start site so that DNA will be copied to a precursor RNA.

DNA polymerase II The enzyme that replicates DNA.

DNA repair The correction of mistakes made during DNA replication.

dose-response Exposure and disease relationship in which the risk of disease varies with the dose or duration of the exposure.

doubling time The time needed for a tumor to double in mass.

Down's syndrome (trisomy 21) A congenital form of mental retardation resulting from an individual's having three copies instead of the normal two copies of chromosome 21.

dysplasia Abnormal tissue development that may represent an early preneoplastic stage of a cancer.

E2F Transcription factor that works with pRB protein. If pRB protein is bound to E2F, this complex cannot enter the nucleus, and initiation of DNA replication does not occur. If pRB protein is not bound to E2F, then initiation of DNA replication can occur.

E6 and E7 Oncogenes of the human papillomavirus (HPV).

early G_1 Step in the cell cycle where a cell decides to undergo DNA replication.

eczema (Wiskott-Aldrich syndrome) A type of inflammatory response that involves the epidermis, causing redness and itching.

electromagnetic fields Non-ionizing radiation made up of electric and magnetic fields.

electrophil A molecule that is electron deficient.

endogenous hormones Hormones that originate within the body.

enhancer regions Transcriptional regulatory elements on DNA located upstream or downstream from the start site of a gene.

endometrium The cells that line the uterus.

environmental tobacco smoke (ETS) Sidestream smoke and mainstream smoke exhaled by active smokers. ETS of both types may be inhaled by nonsmokers.

enzyme A protein that functions as a catalyst in biochemical reactions.

ependymal The membrane lining of the ventricles of the brain and the spinal cord.

epidermal growth factor (EGF) An external growth factor that binds to epidermal growth factor receptors to initiate the cell cycle.

epidermal growth factor receptor (EGFr) A receptor that binds epidermal growth factor.

epidermoid Derived from epidermal cells.

epithelial tissue Tissue that forms the covering surface of the body and the lines of the internal organs.

Epstein-Barr virus (EBV) A DNA virus that causes Burkitt's lymphoma and nasopharyngeal carcinoma.

***erb* A** An oncogene product with homology to a steroid receptor.

***erb* B** An oncogene product of the epidermal growth factor receptor that causes unregulated cell division.

estrogen A steroid hormone that is produced mainly by the ovaries and is responsible for the development of female secondary characteristics and regulation of the menstrual cycle.

estrogen and progesterone receptor assay A type of assay used to determine if a patient's breast cancer responds to estrogen or progesterone and also to determine the clinical treatment of the breast cancer.

ethanol Major ingredient in alcoholic beverages.

etiology The study of the factors that lead to the development of disease.

eukaryotic cell Cells that have genetic material contained within a distinct nucleus.

exogenous hormones Hormones that originate outside of the organism or cell.

exons Nucleotide sequences that will code for a protein.

exposure matrix Tools used in developing exposure ratings for individuals who work in specific industries or occupations.

Fanconi's anemia A hereditary disease (recessive) that is characterized by genetic instability and results in higher incidences of leukemias and lymphomas.

fatty acid An organic compound made up of a hydrocarbon chain and a terminal carboxyl group. It is found in fats and oils.

ferritin An iron complex that stores iron in the body in places such as liver, spleen, bone marrow, and reticuloendothelial cells.

flavivirus The family name of a group of viruses that cause yellow fever or Dengue fever; its molecular structure is similar to that of the Hepatitis C virus.

folate Salt of folic acid.

folic acid A vitamin of the vitamin B complex; deficiency results in poor growth and nutritional anemia.

follicular phase First half of the menstrual cycle (days 1–14). During this phase plasma estrogen levels in the woman's body begin to increase and the levels of progesterone remain low. The endometrium becomes thickened and at day 14 ovulation occurs.

fos Immediate early gene product, a short-lived transcription factor that becomes activated within one hour after the growth factor binds to its receptor.

free radical A molecule that has unpaired electrons, is highly reactive, and can induce mutations in DNA.

G_0 Resting state of the cell cycle.

G_1 (gap 1) Point in the cell cycle at which the cell prepares to duplicate its DNA.

G_2 (gap 2) Point in the cell cycle at which duplicated DNA is condensed into chromosomes in preparation for separating into two daughter cells.

gamma rays Type of ionizing radiation.

gastric cardia Part of the stomach surrounding the junction where the esophagus and stomach meet.

gene Region of DNA that codes for precursor messenger RNA.

genome Complete DNA or RNA sequence of an organism. Some viruses such as oncornavirus, polio virus, and influenza virus use RNA as their genome.

genotoxicity Gene damage caused by mutagens.

genotype The genetic makeup of an organism.

germ cells Cells that produce the reproductive cells; in humans, the germ cells are found in the ovaries and testes.

glioma A type of brain cancer.
glomerulonephritis Inflammation of the kidneys.
glutathione S-transferase (GTS) Enzyme system that plays an important role in determining an individual's ability to metabolize various carcinogens, including benzo[*a*]pyrene, styrene, ethylene oxide, halomethanes, and methyl bromide.
glycoproteins Proteins that are covalently associated with carbohydrates.
glycosylation The addition of carbohydrates (sugars) to proteins.
gray (Gy) Unit of measure for ionizing radiation (1 gray = 100 rad).
hematopoietic system Cells of the circulatory system.
hemoglobin Oxygen-carrying red blood cells.
hepadnavirus A virus that infects liver cells in several mammalian and avian species.
hepatitis B virus (HBV) A DNA virus that causes hepatocellular carcinoma.
hepatitis C virus (HCV) A RNA virus that causes hepatocellular carcinoma.
hepatocellular carcinoma Liver cancer.
hepatocytes Liver cells.
herpes virus type 1 A virus causing an infection that occurs in early childhood and can recur as cold sores throughout adolescence and adulthood.
herpes virus type 2 A virus that mainly infects adults as a sexually transmitted disease and can recur as genital lesions.
heterocyclic amines Well-established animal carcinogens produced during high-temperature cooking of animal foods.
heteropeptide Molecule containing two or more different peptides.
heterozygous Having different alleles at a given locus
high-density lipoprotein (HDL) Lipoprotein that transports endogenous cholesterol from the tissues to the liver.
high-grade lymphomas Histological subtypes of non-Hodgkin's lymphoma; small, noncleaved, large-cell, immunoblastic B lymphocytes.
histadine One of the 20 amino acids.
histone A protein that DNA wraps into chromosomal structures.
HIV-1 The primary virus responsible for AIDS.
HIV-2 A variant form of HIV-1 that spreads more slowly than HIV-1.
Hodgkin's disease A tumor of the lymphatic system.
homeostasis Maintaining the stability of the organism by the coordinated responses of the organ system to environmental changes.
homopeptide A molecule containing two or more identical peptides.
homozygous Having the same allele at a given locus
horizontal transmission The transmission of a viral agent from person to person through blood products and sexual contact.
hormone A chemical produced by granular structures that affects the activity of cells in a distant organ.
hormone replacement therapy Exogenous hormones given to postmenopausal women.
human herpes virus 8 Also called Kaposi's sarcoma herpes virus (KSHV); associated with Kaposi's sarcoma among HIV-infected and non-HIV-infected individuals.
human immunodeficiency virus (HIV) Retrovirus responsible for causing AIDS.

human papillomavirus (HPV) DNA virus responsible for cancer of the uterine cervix, anal cancer, and cancer of the aerodigestive tract.

human T-cell leukemia virus type I (HTLV-I) Retrovirus that causes adult T cell leukemia.

humoral response A branch of the immune system involving B lymphocytes and antibodies.

hydrophilic The property of a substance preferentially found in water extracts as opposed to lipids.

hypercalcemia An excess of calcium in the blood.

hyperplastic polyps Precursor of colon cancer.

IL-2 receptor (IL-2r) A receptor that binds interleukin 2.

immunodeficiency A deficiency in either the humoral or the cell-mediated immunological response.

immunofluorescent antibody An antibody conjugated with a fluorescent probe.

immunosuppressive agent Any agent that suppresses the immune system.

in situ In the natural or normal place. In situ cancer is limited to the first layer of epithelial cells.

in vitro In glass; in an artificial environment. In vitro experiments use living cells grown in a culture medium.

inborn immunodeficiency Immunodeficiency that is present at the time of birth.

incubation period The time period between contact with an infectious agent and the first clinical evidence of the disease.

induction period The time period between first exposure and initiation of a tumor.

inherited immune deficiency diseases Germ line mutations that lead to defects in the immune system.

inherited mutagenic disorders Germ line mutations that affect the genes involved in DNA repair.

initiating agent A carcinogen that causes the development of a tumor by causing mutations.

initiation A permanent mutation in the DNA caused by biological, chemical, or physical agents; such a change can be due to radiation, chemicals, retroviruses, random mutations during replication, DNA amplification, or a random loss of a DNA segment.

interferon A family of glycoproteins produced by a variety of cells to help regulate the immune system.

interferon a A protein derived from leukocytes. It is secreted from virus-infected cells.

interferon-stimulated response element (ISRE) Found in the promoter region on a number of genes whose transcription protects a cell from virus infection.

interleukin 2 (IL-2) T-cell growth factor; it stimulates the growth of T cells.

intermediate early genes Genes that code for proteins involved in the initiation of the G_1 phase of the cell cycle.

intermediate grade lymphomas Histological subtypes of non-Hodgkin's lymphoma: diffuse or large B-cell lymphocytes.

International Agency for Research on Cancer (IARC) Unit of the World Health Organization that evaluates the potential carcinogenicity of specific chemicals and physical agents.

International Classification of Diseases (ICD-9) Detailed coding system based on the primary anatomic site of the tumor.

International Classification of Diseases for Oncology (ICD-O) Developed by the International Agency for Research on Cancer (IARC), ICD-O is a coding system based on the primary anatomic site and histological classification of the tumor.

introns Intervening sequences of nucleotides that do not code for a protein; these sequences are removed after transcription and before translation of the processed messenger RNA.

invasive Said of a primary tumor that has spread beyond it original site.

ionizing radiation Removal of electrons when atoms or cellular molecules absorb this type of energy. It can induce damage to cells. The two types consist of gamma rays and X-rays.

jun Immediate early gene products; a short-lived transcription factor that becomes activated within one hour after the growth factor binds to its receptor.

Kaposi's sarcoma A type of vascular neoplasm common among AIDS patients.

Kaposi's sarcoma herpes virus (KSHV) Also known as human herpes virus 8, it is associated with Kaposi's sarcoma among HIV-infected and non-HIV-infected individuals.

karyotype The number and structure of chromosomes in the nucleus.

late G_1 A step in the cell cycle in which the cell has made its decision to begin DNA replication.

latency period The time between first exposure to a carcinogen and the development of a tumor.

latent cancer Subclinical cancer (a cancer that has not yet manifested); early stages of a cancer before any clinical manifestation.

latent period The time period between exposure to a carcinogen and the development of a tumor.

latent virus A virus that has inserted its DNA or RNA into the host genome and is not currently causing clinical disease.

leader sequence Sequence of DNA that comes before the gene.

leukemias Tumors that arise from the bone marrow, which is the blood-forming organ. It is clinically defined by duration and characteristic (acute or chronic), cell type (myeloid, lymphoid, or monocytic), and increase or no increase in the number of abnormal cells (leukemic or aleukemic [subleukemic]).

Li-Fraumeni syndrome A rare, hereditary cancer susceptibility that leads to the development of multiple kinds of tumors; it results from inherited mutations of the p53 tumor suppressor gene.

ligand The portion of the receptor that a protein molecule recognizes and binds to.

ligation The connecting of neighboring nucleotide sequences.

lipids A diverse group of organic compounds that are insoluble in water and are classified into two categories: (1) complex lipids, such long-chain fatty acids, and (2) simple lipids, such as steroids not containing long-chain fatty acids.

locally invasive Said of cancer that has spread to adjacent organs.

locus Position of a gene on a chromosome.

luteal phase Second half of the menstrual cycle (days 15–28). This phase is characterized by high levels of both estrogen and progesterone.
lymph node Lymphoid organ that contains dendritic cells, lymphocytes, macrophages; this organ serves as the site for filtration of antigen and the activation of lymphocytes.
lymphatic leukemia Leukemia associated with the lymphatic tissue.
lymphatic system System encompassing lymphatic vessels and tissues involved in the immune system (lymph nodes, spleen, tonsils, and thymus).
lymphoma A neoplasm of the lymphoid tissue, such as Hodgkin's disease.
lymphoreticular tumor Neoplasm of the reticuloendothelial cells of the lymph nodes.
macromolecules Large molecular weight molecules.
macrophage Phagocytic cell of the immune system; myeloid cell.
mainstream smoke (MS) Smoke drawn directly into the mouth of an active smoker.
malignancy Another term for cancer.
mammography An X-ray screening tool for detecting breast cancer in an early, potentially treatable clinical stage.
maximum tolerated dose The dose of a chemical that may be administered without shortening the longevity of the animals as a result of noncarcinogenic toxic effects.
melanoma Skin cancer of the melanocytes.
melatonin A protein that pigments cells.
mesothelioma Cancer of the mesothelial tissue, a rare lung cancer associated with exposure to asbestos.
messenger RNA (mRNA) RNA molecule copied from DNA; after processing, mRNA serves as a template for protein synthesis
metalloproteinases Proteins that contain metal ions.
metastasis The spread of a primary cancer to distant sites of the body via blood and lymphatic vessels and the formation of distant tumors.
methoxsalen (8-MOP) Photosensitizing agent (psoralens) that is used to treat psoriasis or vitiligo.
mitosis (M) Cell division in which the daughter cells each contain the same number of chromosomes as the parent cell.
monocytic leukemia Leukemia of the monocytes.
mucopolysaccharides Group of polysaccharides that contain a hexosamine.
multifocal lesions Two or more tumors at the same site.
multiple myeloma Cancer of the mature B-lymphocytes.
multiple primary cancers Two separate and distinct primary tumors in the same individual.
mutagenic The ability to induce mutations.
mutation An alteration in the base sequence of DNA
myasthenia gravis Autoimmune disease affecting the muscular system, marked by fatigue and exhaustion and progressive paralysis of the muscle.
myc Immediate early gene product; a short-lived transcription factor that becomes activated within one hour after the growth factor binds to its receptor.
mycotoxins Fungal toxins.
myelofibrosis Replacement of the bone marrow by fibrous tissue.

myelogenous leukemia Leukemia of the myeloid tissue.

myeloid leukemia A type of leukemia that originates from the myeloid tissue.

***N*-acetyltransferase** An enzyme that helps purge the body of various environmental carcinogens.

nasopharyngeal carcinoma (NPC) Carcinoma in the part of the pharynx that lies above the soft palate.

necrosis The death of a tissue or organ.

neoplasm Abnormal and uncontrolled growth of a cell; also called a *tumor.*

nervous system The system that makes up the brain and spinal cord (central nervous system) and the peripheral nervous system.

nested case-control study A case control study in which the cases and controls are selected from a cohort study.

neuroblastoma A type of childhood cancer involving embryonic neural cells and caused by a deletion in chromosome 1.

Nf-kB A transcriptional factor that binds to TATA box–binding protein (TBP) and other sites.

nicotine An addictive chemical present in tobacco products.

nitrites Chemicals used as preservatives in meats and converted to nitrosamines by the digestive system.

nitrosamines A carcinogen that may lead to the development of stomach cancer.

NK cells (natural killer cells) Lymphocytes having the ability to recognize and kill some tumor cells.

***N*-methyl-*N*-nitrosourea (MNU)** A potent carcinogen. Animal studies have shown that it acts synergistically with alcohol in the formation of tumors.

non-Hodgkin's lymphoma Any type of lymphoma that is not Hodgkin's lymphoma.

non-ionizing radiation Energy that does not remove electrons from molecules. It is less likely to cause damage to cells. Two types are radio waves and microwaves.

nonmelanotic skin cancer Skin cancer of the basal or squamous cell type.

nucleotide Sequence of DNA that is held together by covalent bonds.

nucleosome Composed of four histone proteins to which DNA wraps to form the chromosome.

nucleus A macromolecule that contains protein, DNA, and ribosomal RNA.

O^6-alkyldeoxyguanine-DNA alkyltransferase DNA repair enzyme system that repairs DNA damage caused by *N*-nitroso compounds in cigarette smoke and various pollutants.

oncogene A cancer-causing gene.

oncogenesis The process whereby oncogenes lead to the development of cancer.

open reading frame (ORF) A section of the DNA that contains no stop codons (stop codons are three nucleotide sequence that signal the halt of protein synthesis).

osteogenic sarcoma A connective tissue tumor originating in the bone.

osteoporosis A decrease in bone density that occurs among menopausal women due to a decrease in estrogen.

osteosarcoma A tumor of the bone.

p15 A cyclin-dependent kinase inhibitor that has a negative effect on the cell cycle in which the differentiated cells stop dividing; it works in conjunction with Rb and p21.

p16 A cyclin-dependent kinase inhibitor that has a negative effect on the cell cycle in which the differentiated cells stop dividing; it works in conjunction with Rb and p21.

p21 A cyclin-dependent kinase inhibitor that is regulated by p15, p16, and p27.

p27 A cyclin-dependent kinase inhibitor that has a negative effect on the cell cycle in which the differentiated cells stop dividing; it prevents a cell from entering the early G_1 stage; it works in conjunction with Rb and p21.

p53 A tumor suppressor protein that inhibits the cell cycle.

Pap test A cytological cancer screening test used for the early detection of carcinoma of the uterine cervix.

papillary carcinoma An epithelial tumor that has fingerlike projections.

passive smoking Inhalation of environmental tobacco smoke, which includes sidestream smoke from another person's burning cigarette and mainstream smoke exhaled by the active smoker.

penetrance The probability of displaying a phenotype given a specific genotype.

peptides Two or more amino acids that are linked together by a peptide bond.

peritoneal cavity The body cavity located between the thigh and pelvis.

person-years A measure of the amount of time a person is at risk for a disease.

pesticides Chemicals used to kill insects and weeds.

pestivirus A virus that causes various animal diseases; its molecular structure is similar to that of the hepatitis C virus.

phenacetin An analgesic.

phenotype The observable characteristics of an organism that are determined by genes.

Philadelphia chromosome Translocation of chromosome 22 and the *abl* oncogene from chromosome 9, causing chronic myelogenous leukemias.

phosphorylation The addition of a phosphate to a protein.

photosensitizing agent Any agent that becomes active when exposed to light, such as ultraviolet light.

plasma membrane The lipid bilayer that surrounds the cell.

platelet-derived growth factor (PDGF) An external growth factor that binds to the PDGF receptor to initiate the cell cycle.

platelet-derived growth factor receptor (PDGFr) A receptor that binds PDGF.

pleomorphism The assumption of various distinct forms by an organism; common among neoplastic cells.

point mutation A change in a single nucleotide of DNA.

poly A signal A stretch of adenine nucleotides that varies in length from 30 to more than 200 nucleotides on the 3′ end of messenger RNA (mRNA); it is thought to provide stability for mRNA.

polycyclic hydrocarbons A class of organic chemicals consisting of carbon and hydrogen molecules formed into linked ring structures.

polycythemia vera A disease characterized by an increase in the total mass of red cells and an increase in total blood volume; often caused by leukocytosis.

polymerase chain reaction (PCR) A molecular biology technique that allows small amounts of DNA to be made into multiple copies.

polymorphic An occurrence of two or more alleles for a given locus in a population where at least two alleles appear with frequencies of more than 1%.

polyvinyl chloride Chemical widely used in the plastics industry; causes angiosarcoma of the liver.
poorly differentiated Said of neoplastic cells that have a primitive appearance and loss of normal functioning.
postmenopausal hormones Exogenous hormones given to postmenopausal women.
pRB Tumor suppressor protein that prevents the cell from entering the S phase of the cell cycle.
precursor RNA A complementary sequence of nucleotides of genes; the sequence is processed and then translated into proteins.
premalignant A neoplastic cell that has not developed the ability to invade surrounding tissue.
prevalence The total number of cases of a disease at a certain point in time.
primary cancer A new cancer; not a metastatic cancer.
primary prevention Activities designed to reduce the incidence of a disease.
progestogen A type of steroid hormone that is secreted by the corpus luteum and prepares the endometrium for the implantation of the egg.
progression The process by which initiated, replicating cells grow into a tumor.
prolactin Steroid hormone that is produced by the pituitary gland and stimulates milk production in the breast tissue.
proliferation Multiplication of cells through cell division.
promoter sequences Cis-acting regulatory elements located between the 5′ enhancer region and the 5′ start site of the gene.
promotion The process of cellular proliferation of an initiated cancer cell.
protease An enzyme that cleaves proteins.
protein A string of amino acids coded for by a gene.
protein kinase An enzyme that phosphorylates a protein.
proto-oncogenes Genes that produce normal proteins involved in cell growth, replication, differentiation, and death.
psoriasis Chronic, recurrent, hereditary dermatosis.
radiogenic cancers Cancers caused by radiation.
radionuclides Radioactive disintegration products of ionizing radiation.
radon An inert gas formed by the decay of radioactive radium and uranium; exposure to radon increases the risk of lung cancer in humans.
rads Units in which ionizing radiation is measured; amount of radiation that is absorbed by the tissue.
ras An oncogene.
receptors Protein structures that are found on the surface of the plasma membrane and that have a high affinity for particular ligands.
Reed-Sternberg cell A cell that shows characteristics of Hodgkin's disease.
reliability A measure of how well multiple measurements agree with each other.
replication The process by which a cell makes a duplicate copy of its DNA.
reserpine An antihypertensive drug.
reticuloendothelial system A system that is made up of red and white blood cells and that provides nutrients to other tissues.
retinoblastoma A type of childhood cancer of the eye.
retrovirus An RNA virus that contains an enzyme called reverse transcriptase.

reverse transcriptase (RNA-dependent DNA polymerase) The enzyme that a retrovirus uses to make an RNA genome into a DNA copy and to integrate this copy into the host chromosome.

rheumatoid arthritis An autoimmune disease characterized by chronic inflammation of the joints.

ribonucleoprotein A complex consisting of RNA and a protein; the existence of these complexes allow mRNA to be transported from the nucleus to the cytoplasm, where translation can take place.

ribosome An organelle responsible for the translation of mRNA into the sequence of amino acids that forms a protein.

Rous sarcoma virus A virus that causes solid tumors in chickens; the first oncogene (SRC) was identified in this virus.

S (synthesis) The stage of the cell cycle in which DNA replication occurs.

sarcoma A neoplasm of the connective tissue.

screening A program design to detect cancer at an early stage among asymptomatic individuals.

scurvy A disease caused by a deficiency in vitamin C in the diet; the symptoms include weakness, anemia, and spongy gums.

secondary cancer Metastatic spread of cancer from the primary site of origin to another organ in the body.

secondary prevention Activities aimed at reducing the progression of a disease; an example is a cancer screening program to detect cancer at an early stage.

selenium A micronutrient that is known to have antioxidant effects.

sensitivity A measure of the ability of a test to identify an individual with a disease.

sentinel event Observational link that is made between an exposure and a disease.

serine/threonine kinases A protein kinase that phosphorylates serine or threonine in a protein.

seroconversion The development of antibodies to an antigen; the process of going from seronegative to seropositive.

seronegative The absence of antibodies to a particular antigen.

seropositive The presence of antibodies to a particular antigen.

serum gamma-glutamyl transferase (GGT) A serum marker used to monitor alcohol consumption.

serum marker A biomarker, such as high-density lipoprotein or alkaline phosphatase, that can be detected in a blood sample.

7,12-dimethylbenz[*a*]anthracene (DMBA) Potent carcinogen; animal studies have shown that it acts synergistically with alcohol in the formation of tumors.

7-methyl guanosine cap Posttranscriptional processing in which 7 methyl guanosine cap is added to the 5′ end of the precursor RNA.

severe combined immunodeficiency syndrome (SCIDS) A disease that affects both the humoral and cell-mediated response; individuals with SCIDS are susceptible to viral, bacterial, fungal, and protozoan diseases.

sex hormone–binding globulin (SHBG) A globulin that binds to testosterone, reducing the amount of testosterone in the body.

sidestream smoke (SS) Smoke produced at the burning end of the cigarette when a smoker is not actively drawing in smoke.

sis Oncogene product that binds to the PDGFr, resulting in cell division at an inappropriate time and in an unregulated manner.

sister chromatid exchange (SCE) The chromosomal exchange of sister chromatids (sister chromatids are the two duplicate halves of the condensed chromosome).

Sjogren's syndrome An autoimmune disease affecting the salivary glands, liver, kidney, and thyroid.

small nuclear RNAs Short nucleoproteins that bind precursor RNAs and are involved in posttranscriptional processing events.

solid tumors Tumors that are classified as carcinomas and sarcomas.

somatic mutations Mutations that arise from nonreproductive cells and are not inheritable.

SOS repair DNA repair that does not correct the DNA sequence, allowing the mutated cell to undergo cell division and pass the mutation onto the daughter cells.

Southern blot A laboratory technique that uses nucleic acid sequence probes to identify various alterations in DNA, such as gene amplification, deletions, or rearrangements.

Sp1 A transcriptional factor that binds to TATA box–binding protein (TBP).

specificity The probability that an individual who has a negative test result does not have the disease.

spontaneous mutations Permanent changes in the DNA sequence that are not caused by external factors.

squamous cell A flat epithelial cell.

squamous-cell carcinoma A type of cancer that occurs in the flat epithelial cells.

start site Site on the DNA where transcription begins.

steroid hormones Group of hormones that include estrogen, androgen, progesterone, and glucocorticoids; these hormones are lipid soluble and therefore can directly pass through the cell membrane.

Surveillance, Epidemiology, and End Results (SEER) Population-based cancer registries located in various parts of the United States.

synergistic Said of the combination of two agents (eg, a drug and a hormone) that produces a greater effect than either agent produces alone.

synthetic hormone A hormone that is not naturally occurring, such as diethylstilbestrol (DES).

syphilis A sexually transmitted disease; syphilis is divided into primary, secondary, and tertiary stages.

T lymphocyte A type of white blood cell (lymphocyte) that is involved in the cell-mediated immune response.

tamoxifen An estrogen antagonist used in the treatment of breast cancer.

TATA box The region of DNA that is located near the 5′ start site of the gene; a nucleotide region that is AT rich.

TATA box–binding protein (TBP) A type of transcriptional factor that binds to the TATA box, leading to the binding of other transcriptional factors and to the activation of a gene.

TATA box binding protein associated protein (TAP) A transcriptional factor that binds to TATA box–binding protein.

tax A gene found in HTLV-I that codes for a protein that is a transactivator.

testosterone A steroid hormone that is produced by the testes and stimulates the development of male sexual characteristics.

thiamin deficiency A deficiency of vitamin B; it is characterized by edema (accumulation of excess fluid) and polyneuritis (inflammation of the nerves).

thrombocytopenia A decrease in the number of blood platelets.

thymic hypoplasia of DiGeorge Underdevelopment of the thymus leading to immunodeficiency.

thymine-thymine dimers Linkage of adjacent thymines due to ultraviolet light; leads to problems with DNA replication.

thymoma Tumor of the thymus; either epithelial or lymphoid in origin.

tinea capitis Fungal infection of the scalp.

TNM system Tumor staging system that is based on tumor size (T), the extent of regional lymph node involvement (N), and metastases (M).

transactivator Binds to the 5′ end of precursor RNA; allows for transcription of full-length RNA.

transcription The synthesis of messenger RNA (mRNA) from a DNA template; first step in protein synthesis; it takes place inside the nucleus.

transcription factors Proteins that bind to specific regions on the DNA to initiate transcription.

transforming growth factor beta A protein that prevents the cell from entering into the early G_1 stage of the cell cycle.

translation A process of protein synthesis in which mRNA is translated into a sequence of amino acids; this process takes place in ribosomes in the cytoplasm of the cell.

tumor A mass resulting from abnormal and uncontrolled growth of cells; also called a *neoplasm.*

tumor grading Assessment of degree of cell differentiation based on histological examination of a tumor cell; based on morphology and rate of cell division.

tumor progression The increasing malignancy of a tumor; the continued growth of a tumor.

tumor promoters Any factor that leads to tumor development.

tumor suppressor factor Any factor that suppresses the development of a tumor; most tumor suppressor factors are protein molecules.

tumor suppressor gene A gene that inhibits the development of a tumor.

tyrosine kinase (TK) An enzyme that phosphorylates tyrosine.

ubiquitin Protein/peptide that is found in cells and gets attached to a protein as a "tag" signaling the degradation of that protein.

ultraviolet radiation (UV) A type of solar radiation.

urethane An animal carcinogen.

vertical transmission Transmission of genetic material from parents to child through the egg or sperm.

vinyl chloride monomer (VCM) A chemical that serves as a building block to make vinyl chloride.

virus Infectious particles that can only replicate within living cells.

vitamin B_{12} A vitamin required in the production of red blood cells.

vitamin B_6 A vitamin important in amino acid metabolism; commonly found in cereal grains, yeast, liver, and milk.

vitamin C Ascorbic acid, a water-soluble vitamin found in citrus fruits; deficiency in vitamin C leads to scurvy; vitamin C blocks the conversion of nitrites to nitrosamines.

vitamin E A fat-soluble vitamin; acts as a scavenger of free radicals; commonly found in cereal grains and green vegetables.

vitiligo An autoimmune disease of the melanocytes that results in patches of depigmentation in the skin.

well differentiated Said of neoplastic cells that are morphologically similar to normal cells found in the tissue where the tumor originated.

Wilms' tumor A childhood cancer of the kidney.

Wiskott-Aldrich syndrome An inherited syndrome associated with chronic eczema and immunodeficiency.

X chromosome A chromosome that partially determines the gender of the organism; two X chromosomes give rise to a female.

X-rays A type of ionizing radiation.

xeroderma pigmentosum An inherited (recessive) skin disease in which individuals are sensitive to ultraviolet light. Individuals with the disease are unable to repair DNA from exposure to ultraviolet light and have a high incidence of skin cancer.

Y chromosomes A chromosome that partially determines the sex of an organism; one X and one Y give rise to a male.

years of potential life lost (YPLL) A measure of the impact of a particular disease; this measure can be calculated by subtracting the age at which each individual dies of a disease from age 65 or from average life expectancy.

Index

B

C

D

E

J

K

N

O

P

Q

R

S

T

U

V

W

X

Z